HIV and Aging

# Interdisciplinary Topics in Gerontology and Geriatrics

## Vol. 42

Series Editor

Tamas Fulop Sherbrooke, Que.

# HIV and Aging

Volume Editors

Mark Brennan-Ing New York, N.Y.
Rosanna F. DeMarco Boston, Mass.

12 figures, and 12 tables, 2017

KARGER Basel · Freiburg · Paris · London · New York · Chennai · New Delhi · Bangkok · Beijing · Shanghai · Tokyo · Kuala Lumpur · Singapore · Sydney

**Mark Brennan-Ing, PhD**
Director for Research and Evaluation
ACRIA Center for HIV and Ageing
575 8th Avenue, Suite 502
New York, NY 10018 (USA)

**Rosanna F. DeMarco, PhD**
Chair and Professor, College of Nursing and Health Science
University of Massachusetts Boston
100 Morrissey Boulevard
301-66 Science Center
Boston, MA 02125-3393 (USA)

Library of Congress Cataloging-in-Publication Data

Names: Brennan-Ing, Mark, editor. | DeMarco, Rosanna F., editor.
Title: HIV and aging / volume editors, Mark Brennan-Ing, Rosanna F. DeMarco.
Other titles: HIV and aging (Brennan-Ing) | Interdisciplinary topics in gerontology and geriatrics ; v. 42. 2297-3508
Description: Basel ; New York : Karger, 2017. | Series: Interdisciplinary topics in gerontology and geriatrics, ISSN 2297-3508 ; vol. 42 | Includes bibliographical references and indexes.
Identifiers: LCCN 2016039580| ISBN 9783318059458 (hard cover : alk. paper) | ISBN 9783318059465 (electronic version)
Subjects: | MESH: HIV Infections--complications | Aging--physiology
Classification: LCC RA643.8 | NLM WC 503.5 | DDC 618.97/69792--dc23
LC record available at https://lccn.loc.gov/2016039580

Bibliographic Indices. This publication is listed in bibliographic services, including Current Contents® and PubMed/MEDLINE.


www.karger.com
Printed in Germany on acid-free and non-aging paper (ISO 9706) by Kraft Druck GmbH, Ettlingen
ISSN 2297–3508
e-ISSN 2297–3486
ISBN 978–3–318–05945–8
e-ISBN 978–3–318–05946–5

# Contents

VII **Preface**
Sprague, C. (Boston, Mass.)

Introduction

1 **Local and Global HIV Aging Demographics and Research**
Sprague, C. (Boston, Mass./Johannesburg); Brown, S.M. (Boston, Mass.)

Part I: Physiological Changes and Clinical Biomarkers in HIV and Aging

11 **Are HIV-Infected Older Adults Aging Differently?**
Karpiak, S.E.; Havlik, R. (New York, N.Y.)

28 **Cellular Senescence, Immunosenescence and HIV**
Fülöp, T. (Sherbrooke, Que.); Herbein, G. (Besançon); Cossarizza, A. (Modena); Witkowski, J.M. (Gdansk); Frost, E.; Dupuis, G. (Sherbrooke, Que.); Pawelec, G. (Tübingen); Larbi, A. (Singapore)

47 **Biomarkers and Clinical Indices of Aging with HIV**
Fitch, K.V.; Feldpausch, M.N.; Looby, S.E.D. (Boston, Mass.)

Part II: Multimorbidity and Geriatric Care of HIV Patient

59 **Multimorbidity and Burden of Disease**
Brown, T.T. (Baltimore, Md.); Guaraldi, G. (Modena)

74 **Polypharmacy, Using New Treatments to Customize Care for Aging Patients and Adherence Present and Future**
Alberts, L.H. (Boston, Mass.)

85 **Behavioral Health**
Pantalone, D.W.; Czajkowski, S.E.; Taylor, S.W. (Boston, Mass.)

101 **Disability among Persons Aging with HIV/AIDS**
Leveille, S.G.; Thapa, S. (Boston, Mass.)

119 **Application of Geriatric Principles and Care Models in HIV and Aging**
Sangarlangkarn, A. (New York, N.Y./Bangkok); Avihingsanon, A. (Bangkok); Appelbaum, J.S. (Tallahassee, Fla.)

Part III: Psychosocial Issues in Aging with HIV

134 **Sexual Health, Risk and Prevention**
Aronowitz, T. (Boston, Mass.)

144 **Stigma in an Aging Context**
Emlet, C.A. (Tacoma, Wash.)

159 **Social Support Systems and Social Network Characteristics of Older Adults with HIV**
Brennan-Ing, M.; Seidel, L.; Karpiak, S.E. (New York, N.Y.)

173 **Remediating HIV-Associated Neurocognitive Disorders via Cognitive Training: A Perspective on Neurocognitive Aging**
Vance, D.E.; Cody, S.L.; Moneyham, L. (Birmingham, Ala.)

187 **Mental Health, Psychosocial Challenges and Resilience in Older Adults Living with HIV**
Halkitis, P.N.; Krause, K.D.; Vieira, D.L. (New York, N.Y.)

204 **Medical, Social and Supportive Services for Older Adults with HIV**
Cox, L.E. (Galloway, N.J.); Brennan-Ing, M. (New York, N.Y.)

222 **The Relevance of Palliative Care in HIV and Aging**
Shorthill, J. (Tigard, Oreg.); DeMarco, R.F. (Boston, Mass.)

Part IV: Concluding Remarks

234 **Ageism, Aging and HIV: Community Responses to Prevention, Treatment, Care and Support**
DeMarco, R.F. (Boston, Mass.); Brennan-Ing, M. (New York, N.Y.); Brown, S.M.; Sprague, C. (Boston, Mass.)

240 **Author Index**

241 **Subject Index**

# Preface

### Overview of National and Global Data

An estimated 3.6 million people aged 50 years or older were living with HIV in 2013, of a total population of 35.3 million with HIV worldwide. The majority – numbering 3 million – reside in low- and middle-income countries (LMICs), primarily in sub-Saharan Africa, with the remaining 600,000 in high-income countries (HICs), encompassing the regions of Western and Central Europe and North America. In HICs today, an estimated 30% of people with HIV are aged 50 years or older [1]. In countries in North and South America, including the United States and Brazil, this figure is an estimated 50% [2, 3]. These figures are underpinned by 2 simultaneous shifts: an increasing proportion of individuals with HIV are living longer and aging with HIV globally; and older individuals are newly acquiring HIV [4].

Despite decades of attention on building a global HIV research and programming agenda, HIV in older populations has generally been neglected until recently [1, 2]. Indeed, Demographic Health System and HIV prevalence data captured by UNAIDS, as well as other national and global prevalence surveys, largely report data for age groups up to age 49 only [4, 5]. In spite of data limitations, the overall trend is clear: the increasing proportion of those with HIV over 50 years of age, who are living longer across countries, comprises a significant aspect of the changing global HIV epidemic today [1, 4].

This phenomenon – aging with HIV – is attributed primarily to 3 factors: (a) greater access to combination antiretroviral therapy (cART) and increasing effectiveness of cART in prolonging life and reducing mortality; (b) declining HIV incidence in younger populations, shifting the burden of HIV to older populations; and (c) HIV risk behaviors evident among older individuals [4]. Age at HIV infection appears to be increasing significantly. At the same time, age at HIV diagnosis has increased; and HIV incidence (new HIV infections) is increasing in older adults as a consistent pattern worldwide [6].

Generally, trends vis-à-vis HIV and aging are informed by 2 larger transitions. The first is an unprecedented demographic shift, or change in birth and death rates across regions of the world, whereby mortality rates have declined in an unprecedented manner and life expectancy at birth has increased over the last 50 years [7, 8]. The effect is that people are living longer in each country, with a few exceptions. With a global population that is aging, the health and medical needs of the world's population are also changing, including those with HIV [2, 10]. The second marked shift is a global health transition, particularly in the LMICs. In the developing world, infectious diseases like tuberculosis and HIV have historically been significant causes of death. While HIV is the sixth leading global cause of deaths among adults, HIV and other communicable diseases combine with maternal, perinatal, and nutritional conditions to comprise over 60% of mortality in the Africa region. In recent years, however, non-communicable diseases (NCDs), led by ischemic heart disease and stroke, have become significant causes of death and are expected to increase further [7]. Economic growth in LMICs and increasing urbanization have been associated with poor nutrition; lack of exercise and obesity are other factors associated with increases in NCD prevalence [9]. Other causes of injury and premature death in LMIC settings, such as road accidents, maternal mortality, and malnutrition, are likely to remain significant causes of injury and death in particular regions. This suggests that NCDs are likely to supplement infectious diseases like HIV as leading causes of morbidity and mortality in those aging with HIV. In addition, there is increasing evidence that mental illness has been under-documented in the developing countries to date and may contribute greatly to mortality and morbidity than previously thought, leading to a triple or quadruple burden of disease in LMIC. Evidence indicates that depressive symptoms in older populations are likely to increase; those living with or at risk of HIV have particular mental health and social support needs that must be addressed through health and social services [2, 7, 9].

Taken together, the demographic and health transitions have significance, not only for HIV diagnosis and treatment but also for HIV risk factors and health determinants including social determinants, which affect global and national burdens of disease. These transitions influence planning, including health workforce preparation, health service delivery, clinical care, and health systems [8–10]. Equally, there is some indication that, with health financing and health care reform underway in many regions, HIV will need to maintain its position as a priority global health concern amid a changing landscape of other health conditions and diseases [10, 11].

The chapters presented in this book represent what we have learnt thus far as well as the emerging knowledge related to 'aging' of the HIV experience. More than 30 years into the global HIV epidemic, 10% of the world's HIV positive population is now aged 50 or older, with this number projected to increase [4]. One of the most important conclusions drawn by the international community vis-à-vis HIV responses, now a key assumption embedded in national strategic plans on HIV and AIDS, is to understand the unique features of this epidemic, the populations affected, and tailor responses, giving rise to the 'know your epidemic, know your response' approach led by UNAIDS [4]. Developing priority agendas on existing research and evidence must be in accordance with national health priorities. This renders a research or programming agenda across many regions emergent and exploratory. At the same time, the need for health promotion and protection in older populations who have acquired HIV or are at risk of transmission – once obscured – is becoming much more visible, requiring multiple points of research and intervention. It is our intention to bring visibility to aging and HIV, in order to inform research, policy and clinical practice.

*Courtenay Sprague*, Boston, Mass.

## References


1 Joint United Nations Programme on HIV and AIDS (UNAIDS): AIDS by the Numbers. Geneva, UNAIDS, 2013.

2 High KP, Brennan-Ing M, Clifford DB, Cohen MH, Currier J, Deeks SG, Deren S, Effros RB, Gebo K, Goronzy JJ, Justice AC, Landay A, Levin J, Miotti PG, Munk RJ, Nass H, Rinaldo CR Jr, Shlipak MG, Tracy R, Valcour V, Vance DE, Walston JD, Volberding P; OAR Working Group on HIV and Aging: HIV and aging: state of knowledge and areas of critical need for research. A report to the NIH office of AIDS research by the HIV and aging working group. J Acquir Immune Defic Syndr 2012;60(suppl 1):S1–S18.

3 Cardoso SW, Torres TS, Santini-Oliveira M, Marins LM, Veloso VG, Grinsztejn B: Aging with HIV: a practical review. Braz J Infect Dis 2013;17:464–479.

4 UNAIDS: HIV and Aging: Special Supplement to the UNAIDS Report on the Global AIDS Epidemic 2013. Geneva, UNAIDS, 2013. http://www.unaids.org/sites/default/files/media_asset/20131101_JC2563_hiv-and-aging_en_0.pdf.

5 Negin J, Cumming RG: HIV infection in older adults in sub-Saharan Africa: extrapolating prevalence from existing data. Bull World Health Organ 2010;88:847–853.

6 Costagliola D: Demographics of HIV and aging. Curr Opin HIV AIDS 2014;9:294–301.

7 World Health Organization: World Health Statistics. Geneva, WHO, 2014.

8 Bloom D, Canning D: Global Demographic Change: Dimensions and Economic Significance. National Bureau of Economic Research (NBER) Working Paper No. 10817 (September) JEL No. J11, O40 Cambridge (MA): NBER 2004.

9 Chatterji S, Kowal P, Mathers C, Naidoo N, Verdes E, Smith JP, Suzman R: The health of aging populations in China and India. Health Aff (Millwood) 2008;27:1052–1063.

10 UNAIDS: Access to Antiretroviral Therapy in Africa: Status Report on Progress Towards 2015 Targets. Geneva, UNAIDS, 2013. http://www.unaids.org/sites/default/files/media_asset/20131219_AccessARTAfricaStatusReportProgresstowards2015Targets_en_0.pdf.

11 UNAIDS: The Gap Report. Geneva, UNAIDS, 2014. http://www.unaids.org/sites/default/files/media_asset/UNAIDS_Gap_report_en.pdf.

Brennan-Ing M, DeMarco RF (eds): HIV and Aging. Interdiscipl Top Gerontol Geriatr.
Basel, Karger, 2017, vol 42, pp 1–10 (DOI: 10.1159/000448532)

# Local and Global HIV Aging Demographics and Research

Courtenay Sprague[a–c] • Shelley M. Brown[a, d]

[a]University of Massachusetts Boston, Department of Conflict Resolution, Human Security, and Global Governance, John W. McCormack Graduate School of Policy and Global Studies, [b]University of Massachusetts Boston, Department of Nursing, College of Nursing and Health Sciences, Boston, Mass., USA; [c]University of the Witwatersrand, Wits Reproductive Health and HIV Institute, Johannesburg, South Africa; [d]Boston University, Department of Health Sciences, College of Health and Rehabilitation Sciences: Sargent College, Boston, Mass., USA

## Abstract

This introduction serves to foreground current patterns associated with HIV and aging, globally. We highlight key trends by World Health Organization sub-region, and identify gaps in existing knowledge. HIV and aging is insufficiently documented, as prevalence data for those over age 49 have not generally been captured by many countries, or by UNAIDS. Despite limited data and data systems, several dominant trends among adults aged 50 and older are discernible, including: growing HIV risk and prevalence is increasingly evident among maturing adults, worldwide; older individuals at risk of or living with HIV, and their health providers, fail to recognize risk and symptoms, leading to disease progression and delayed treatment. Cross-sectoral strategies will be needed to mount responses; public health campaigns will be essential in educating and informing individuals about HIV risk, prevention and care; and special efforts to tailor interventions to key populations most vulnerable or stigmatized in countries will be critical. 

Over the last 30 years, unprecedented high-level efforts have been made to arrest the global HIV epidemic, including securing access to affordable combination antiretroviral therapy (cART) for global populations, as part of Millennium Development Goal 6, agreed by 189-member United Nations countries in 2000. Global commitments, financed through the Global Fund to Fight AIDS, Tuberculosis and Malaria and other mechanisms, gave rise to multi-sectoral national strategic plans that govern the country responses to HIV and AIDS in their populations [1]. This introduction offers a brief overview of HIV and aging among WHO sub-regions, globally, while offering a preliminary set of themes that emerge from the literature.

## Demographics by Global Region

In different sub-regions, people are aging at different rates, and the total number of people with HIV aged 50 and over varies, as does their risk of contracting HIV [2]. With respect to patterns of HIV infection among older adults, several trends are discernible. A summary snapshot of what is known for each WHO sub-region follows.

## Africa

Sub-Saharan Africa (SSA) is home to the majority of people with HIV or 74% of the global total. HIV prevalence ranges by country, from 0.1% in the North African countries of Morocco and Egypt to 26.5% in Swaziland [3][1]. A number of Southern African countries including Lesotho, Botswana, and South Africa exceed 10% HIV prevalence, with some subgroups in these countries, including women of reproductive age and female sex workers, exceeding 30% HIV prevalence [1, 4]. In 2012, there were 1.6 million new HIV infections in SSA [5]. This is about one million fewer infections than were reported in 2001, indicating great strides in stemming the epidemic, reflected in the expanded coverage of cART, as well as reductions in mortality [3, 6]. For decades, while most of the rest of the world gained life expectancy, SSA experienced a reversal [7, 8].

Understanding of the demographics of aging in SSA is limited because demographic data in older African populations are scarce: only 10 countries in SSA have vital registration systems that are useable and just 2 cover 80% of their national population (Mauritius and Seychelles) [8]. It is clear that fertility has declined and life expectancy at birth in SSA is improving. The size and age distribution of the population in most SSA countries has changed significantly due to HIV-related mortality. For example, Velkoff and Kowal [8] estimated that in 2006 Botswana and Tanzania had 251,000 and 134,000 fewer people, respectively, than without the HIV epidemic. Tanzania had an estimated 134,000 fewer people than without the HIV epidemic. For a number of countries in East and Southern Africa, this means that their overall population today is smaller, and the percent of the population that is aging is also smaller, though the size and effects vary by country. Despite these figures, with the rollout of cART, mortality in SSA has declined and is expected to decline further. The SSA population aged over 60 is expected to reach 67 million by 2030 [6]. Today, the life expectancy in SSA countries is increasing, with greater numbers of individuals initiating cART and higher threshold CD4 cell counts. In South Africa, for example, life expectancy had declined to 56.5 years, but increased to 60 years in recent years, attributed primarily to the rollout of treatment [9].

[1] Data are not reported for Libya and Sudan.

While data systems related to HIV have improved in some of these countries, with annual reporting on national HIV and AIDS strategic plans and improved health and surveillance data, HIV in individuals aged over 50 is insufficiently captured in data sources and reporting. Few quantitative studies of HIV incidence, national HIV prevalence surveys and Demographic and Health Survey (DHS) of older African adults have been conducted, including data collection on sexual, health, and HIV risk behaviors to identify trends or establish baselines [10]. Nonetheless, available studies from Kenya, South Africa, and Swaziland indicate that the HIV prevalence in older African populations is high [2].

In Kenya, for instance, HIV prevalence in those aged 50–64 years in a 2006/2007 survey by the Ministry of Health was 5%, compared with 7.4% in those aged 15–49 years. In Swaziland, 13% of men and 7% of women aged 60–64 years were HIV-positive, compared with 27% HIV prevalence in those aged 15–49 years [4]. HIV prevalence in South Africa's 2012 national HIV prevalence survey was 13% in individuals aged 50–54 years, compared to 18% in the age group 15–49 years [4]. In a study conducted in a more rural province of South Africa, Mpumalanga, Bendavid et al. [11] found that HIV prevalence in those aged 55–59 years was high, an estimated 35% in men and 27% in women; 20% in men aged 60–64 years, compared with 13% in women; and 17% in men aged 65–69 years, compared with 10% in women.

In terms of patterns of HIV risk and sexual behavior, existing literature indicates that sexual behavior in older African populations is consistent, but knowledge of HIV is low [12]. A national household survey conducted in South Africa in 2005 found that 50% of people aged over 50 indicated having sex 1–4 times within the previous 30 days, and more than 25% had sex more than 5 times during the same time period. Surveys conducted in East, West, and Southern Africa indicated that older individuals may have less knowledge about risk factors for HIV, compared to younger cohorts [12]. Research by Negin et al. [12] found that they may be less likely to take an HIV test, leading to late HIV diagnosis and entry into care. Trends reported from UNAIDS indicated that older individuals were less likely to use condoms than younger people [6]. Additional research on HIV attitudes, awareness, and testing among older adults is needed. Some African studies assumed a less frequent sexual activity among older populations, without attempts to confirm those assumptions [6]. Other less recent studies have drawn attention to such 'ageist' ideas as limiting understanding of HIV acquisition in more mature adults [13]. This problem is not limited to SSA, given that Brazilian, European, and American studies have documented that older individuals are diagnosed later by health providers, after AIDS-defining conditions are present – indicating that health providers do not connect risk factors with symptom monitoring and detection [14]. Lastly, as with other regions, mortality in those aged over 50 was higher, compared with younger people living with HIV (PLHIV). At the same time, comorbidities have been demonstrated, including the progression of noncommunicable diseases (NCDs) in older Africans with HIV [15].

### Europe and the Americas

Data from the CASCADE collaboration (Concerted Action on SeroConversion to AIDS and Death in Europe) indicate that the median age at HIV infection has increased, from 26.2 years before 1986, to 33.2 years between 2006 and 2010. CASCADE includes data from 29 cohorts, representing 14 European countries, along with data from Australia, Canada, and Africa. An EU collaboration (EUROCOORD) that includes 23 cohorts in 35 countries indicated that older age was associated with a higher risk of delayed presentation and cART initiation, with mature individuals more likely to present with AIDS-related symptoms, and with lower CD4 cell counts at initiation [16]. Data for individuals newly enrolled in cART indicates an increase for those aged over 50 years, from 8.5 to 19.1% in men, between 1993 and 2012, and from 6.6 to 19.5% in women in the North American AIDS Cohort Collaboration on Research and Design (NA-ACCORD) representing 25 cohorts in the US and Canada. From 1997 to 2007, the proportion of individuals presenting for HIV care who were at least 50 years old increased from 17 to 27% based on the NA-ACCORD data. This is attributed to older age at onset of infection, but also to late entry into HIV care for individuals over 50 years of age [16]. Research also indicates that these factors affect optimal health and survival times for older cohorts of PLHIV. Mature individuals, though initiated rapidly on cART, showed evidence of poorer immunologic response than their younger counterparts, which underscores the need for further research to understand immunological changes and effects. In Europe and North America, Costagliola notes, older patients presented with lower CD4 cell count and remained longer with low CD4 cell counts following initiation on cART, which puts them at risk for disease progression and death when compared with younger patients [16].

Stall and Catania found that high-risk individuals over 50 years were much less likely to adopt AIDS prevention strategies than younger individuals engaging in the same behavioral risks [17]. This suggests that behavioral and health systems' research is needed to ensure health providers recognize HIV risk behaviors and symptoms and initiate cART promptly [18].

### Eastern Mediterranean[2]

Historically, the Eastern Mediterranean (EM) region had one of the lowest HIV prevalence rates, attributed to cultural and social norms that discouraged sex before and outside of marriage. HIV prevalence was an estimated 0.2% in 2012, but new HIV infections have been increasing in some countries. As of 2010, 560,000 individuals

[2] Afghanistan, Bahrain, Djibouti, Egypt, Iran (Islamic Republic of Iran), Iraq, Jordan, Kuwait, Lebanon, Libya, Morocco, Oman, Pakistan, Qatar, Saudi Arabia, Somalia, Sudan, Syrian Arab Republic, Tunisia, United Arab Emirates, Yemen.

were living with HIV, and the HIV epidemic is concentrated primarily in three key affected groups: sex workers, men who have sex with men, and people who inject drugs [19]. Little is known about older individuals aging with HIV or those at risk of being infected. This region has one of the two fastest growing rates of new infections, compared to other regions, thus HIV prevalence and incidence data must be improved to identify those at risk [19]. In addition, only 1 in 5 people with HIV were able to access cART [20, 21]. EM has one of the lowest cART coverage rates globally, with particularly poor coverage in Sudan, South Sudan, Iran, Somalia, and Pakistan, estimated at 10% coverage [22].

There are widespread regional differences in the mode of transmission and access to treatment. HIV prevalence among injecting drug users is high in Pakistan, Islamic Republic of Iran, Libya, Afghanistan, and Egypt [19]. There are rising epidemics in MSM in Egypt and Tunisia, and in female sex workers in Dijibouti, Morocco, and Somalia. HIV services are often free in EM countries but are hampered by stigma, discrimination, lack of HIV information, few locations where HIV services are provided, lack of HIV drugs, stockouts, and a shortage of health staff and poor health and medical infrastructure in some countries [19]. Compounding these issues is the challenge of understanding the effects of HIV on the large number of migrants, poor, and mobile populations in many countries of the EM. This has been identified as a key vulnerable population for this region [21].

There is still a lack of adequate information on local trends in the HIV epidemic, including little to no data on aging populations. Most data and program planning for the region reflect trends in the 15–49 year-old population. There is significant stigma associated with HIV risk in this region, which results in insufficient methods of prevention and treatment. A 2013 joint WHO and UNAIDS advocacy report focused on reducing stigma, normalizing HIV testing, and increasing cART access in the EM [22]. However, the report neglected to address these challenges within those over 50 . This is troubling because almost 70% of the countries in the EM have life expectancies over 70 years of age. People are living longer, and if initiatives to increase access and reduce stigma are successful, routine surveillance in the population over 50 living with or at risk for HIV is essential to adequately prevent, treat, and manage HIV/AIDS in this region.

## South-East Asia

The South-East Asia Region (SEAR) has 3.4 million people living with HIV/AIDS, 32% cART coverage, and 230,000 new infections in 2013 [23]. This region has the second highest burden of HIV, in terms of absolute numbers, with widely disparate epidemics in each country. India has 1.2 billion people, so despite the low overall adult HIV prevalence of 0.26% on average, there are over 2,000,000 individuals with HIV, the third largest epidemic in the world [24]. Thailand has the highest HIV prevalence in the region, at 1.1%. It has seen an increase in HIV-associated premature deaths in recent years, while India has witnessed a decline in new HIV infections and deaths as people are living longer on cART, which has implications for aging populations with HIV [25]. In this region, stigma and discrimination are still key barriers to testing, counseling, diagnosis, and treatment of HIV. Data on HIV in populations over 50 in the SEAR is poor.

WHO's SEAR office released a Regional Health Sector Strategy for 2011–2015 outlining the key challenges and future priorities, which included scaling up cART; building infrastructure; reducing HIV transmission in at-risk populations; and increasing epidemiologic capabilities for countries and research for key populations [24]. Notably, this strategy did not include a specific focus on transmission risk, or treatment and management of HIV in older populations. Country-level surveillance on HIV and AIDS in those aged over 50 is insufficient in this region, and this report demonstrates the lack of attention paid to this population on a regional level. A review of existing literature resulted in very little information on the implications of aging people living with HIV in the region. Though many countries in SEAR are still working to increase cART access and reduce premature HIV-related deaths, it is imperative that future health sector strategies focus on increased surveillance and research for this neglected population.

### Western Pacific

The overall HIV prevalence in the Western Pacific Region (WPR) is below 1% in most countries, with the 2012 prevalence among adults at 1% [26]. In 2013, an estimated 1.3 million people were living with HIV in the region [27]. WHO estimates that 110,000 people were newly infected with HIV in 2012. The region has strengthened HIV surveillance systems, but still lacks comprehensive data on high-risk groups, with poor information on aging populations living with HIV and AIDS [28]. The highest HIV prevalence centers around only five countries: Cambodia, China, Malaysia, Papua New Guinea, and Vietnam, with prevalence above 5%, constituting 90% of the burden of HIV disease in this region [27]. Estimates for Vietnam are 4% of the population, or 250,000–300,000 people with HIV [29]. The countries of Melanesia (Vanuatu, Solomon Islands, Fiji, Papua New Guinea) continue to experience a high burden of HIV while facing emerging NCD challenges [30].

China is the most populous country in the WPR, and primary modes of HIV transmission among adults are intravenous drug use and heterosexual contact, female sex workers, and men who have sex with men. The latter 2 groups are particularly vulnerable to infection due to infrequent condom use [30, 31]. Characteristic of other upper middle income countries (MICs), people with HIV in China are living longer due to increased access to cART. HIV has transitioned from an acute to chronic illness, and both China and Australia are experiencing a documented surge in people living longer with HIV [31]. A 2011 study found an emerging epidemic among older adults in

China, indicating that the number of individuals with HIV increased to 42.7% in 2011, up from 16.5% in 2007 in the capital city of Guangxi Province, in Nanning, home to the second largest number of people with HIV in China [31]. Though the Chinese Ministry of Health reported an 11-fold increase in PLHIV from 2000 to 2011, an increase from 1.9 to 21.1%, very little epidemiological data exists to track trends and regional data [32]. This study noted that unlike other HIV populations in China, heterosexual contact is the major mode of transmission and the primary reason for the increased number of cases in this older population.

The prevalence of older adults, aged 50–64 years, living with HIV in Australia has increased from 6.1% in 2006 to 10.6% in 2009. And the population aged over 50 represents 20% of new HIV diagnoses in 2013 [33]. The average age of those living with HIV is 45 years and the number over age 55 years is 25.7%, with this expected to increase to 44.3% by 2020 [34].

Though the incidence and prevalence of older individuals with HIV has witnessed increases in this region, little research, outside of Australia and China, has focused on those over 50 living with or at risk of HIV transmission. Rural areas of China are where most of the older adults reside, and where blood and plasma donations in the 1990s were a main mode of transmission [31]. A study by Zhang et al. [30] found that more women over 50 in affected rural areas were living with HIV than men, with significant differences in educational attainment between those living with HIV and those who were not. A quantitative analysis of HIV and aging in the Asia Pacific, with reliance on data from people with HIV in Australia, concluded that patients over 50 on cART demonstrated better virological control, but experienced somewhat poorer CD4 cell response, and with an all-cause mortality risk two times higher than in younger patients [34]. Older adults were more likely to need personal care assistance and relied heavily on social support systems [34, 35]. These differences are important reasons why more comprehensive surveillance and research efforts are needed to better understand the behaviors of people with HIV.

Higher income countries (HICs) and upper MICs within this region, including Australia and China, are beginning to examine the impacts of aging and HIV within their population. However, this remains an underappreciated at-risk group in the region. There is a lack of routine surveillance data in the Western Pacific specific to this aging population, few studies on risks and protective factors for living with HIV, and a lack of information on the impacts this will have as the population shifts to managing more chronic disease than acute illness as it relates to HIV.

## Evolving Research Themes

Failure to collect routine HIV data in older populations is a resounding theme across countries. While some data exist, for particular regions such as the EM and North African countries, data are scant. Gains made in SSA countries, which reduced HIV-associated deaths 30% in the six years from 2006 to 2012, indicate that concerted efforts can produce dramatic results when data are marshalled to inform action [1, 3, 36]. To do so, interventions need to be underpinned by accurate data on prevalence, incidence, risk, and health behaviors. National and global surveys must begin to include older ages in existing routine sources and reporting, particularly DHS, UNAIDS, and national prevalence surveys [2, 6, 10]. As the UNAIDS/Lancet Commission stated, 'It is imperative that all countries affected by the HIV epidemic gather detailed epidemiological data, including behavioral and response data… as part of standard practice' [1, p. 3].

A second dominant theme, across regions, whether HICs or lower MICs (LMICs), is that little is known about sexual risk practices and beliefs about HIV in older populations, including social and behavioral factors, attitudes, behaviors, frequency of sex, number of partners, perceptions and beliefs about risk of HIV infection, knowledge about modes of HIV transmission, prevention, and willingness to be tested and take HIV treatment. Evidence to date indicates that regardless of region, older people are practicing unsafe sex, which pushes them into a category of risk-prone behaviors that individuals and their health providers appear not to connect to HIV risk. Disturbing findings indicating ageist and other assumptions about older individuals not having sex need to be debunked and reinforced in the research literature and in health settings. At the same time, age-disparate partnerships, long-established in SSA and elsewhere (e.g., between older men and younger women), may influence HIV infection patterns in younger age groups as well, indicating that isolating aging populations as a separate group, without considering interactions, may not be appropriate in research or programming, and that attention to social context and other social and structural factors remains essential in HIV research [2, 6, 11, 12, 17].

A third theme emerging from the research literature is that those living and aging with HIV experience greater co-morbidities, side effects, and drug interactions, posing challenges to effective adherence and management for older patients with HIV and providers alike, with research needed in these areas. In addition, HIV and/or accompanying cART influences the aging process and the onset of illness associated with advanced age. As a result, experts have called for cellular and immunological research to understand disease progression and the preservation of function, particularly immune function [1, 2, 5, 10, 18, 37, 38].

The fourth theme points to the absence of and need for prevention in older individuals. Particular prevention interventions have been effective in target populations and warrant consideration for people with HIV aged over 50. Examples include pre-exposure or post-exposure prophylaxis for those HIV-exposed, as well as provision of services such as testing and treatment for tuberculosis, hepatitis or other infections and diseases in particular settings, which pose risk factors for HIV. Research is needed on effective prevention methods and strategies and their acceptability and uptake by older individuals to avert new HIV infections.

A fifth theme for an emerging research agenda is that the vast majority of research on HIV and aging is being generated in the HICs or in better-resourced upper MICs with substantial HIV responses, such as Brazil and South Africa. Research is needed within LMIC countries, particularly, to add to the global evidence base of knowledge across and within settings where there may be differences in factors shaping national epidemics. Mentoring and funding support for researchers to publish in international journals and participate in international policy and research conferences should be made available by international funding agencies, such as those that have traditionally supported researchers in LMICs, including European, British, and Canadian funding bodies.

As we progress with this book, we hope that the demographic and research data summarized here will serve as an entry point to engage challenges and opportunities associated with HIV and aging across regional contexts. Constellating an inclusive approach to this problem calls us, as researchers and practitioners, to integrate and apply existing knowledge, while responding to an increasingly pressing need for a new phase of research, policy development, clinical and social services delivery, that responds to the needs and lived experiences of those living with or at risk of acquiring HIV around the world.

## References


1 Piot P, Karim SA, Hecht R, Legido-Quigley H, Buse K, Stover J, Resch S: UNAIDS Lancet commission: defeating AIDS-advancing global health. Lancet 2015;386:171–218.

2 UNAIDS: HIV and Aging: Special Supplement to the UNAIDS Report on the Global AIDS Epidemic 2013. Geneva, UNAIDS, 2013. http://www.unaids.org/sites/default/files/media_asset/20131101_JC2563_hiv-and-aging_en_0.pdf.

3 UNAIDS: Access to Antiretroviral Therapy in Africa: Status Report on Progress Towards 2015 Targets. Geneva, UNAIDS. 2013. http://www.unaids.org/sites/default/files/media_asset/20131219_AccessARTAfricaStatusReportProgresstowards2015Targets_en_0.pdf (accessed April 23, 2015).

4 Shisana O, Rehle T, Simbayi LC, Zuma K, Jooste S, Zungu N, Labadarios D, Onoya D: South African National HIV Prevalence, Incidence and Behaviour Survey, 2012. Cape Town, Human Sciences Research Council Press, 2014.

5 Joint United Nations Programme on HIV and AIDS (UNAIDS): AIDS by the Numbers. Geneva, UNAIDS, 2013.

6 UNAIDS: The Gap Report. Geneva, UNAIDS, 2014. http://www.unaids.org/sites/default/files/media_asset/UNAIDS_Gap_report_en.pdf.

7 World Health Organization: World Health Statistics 2014. Geneva, WHO, 2014.

8 Velkoff V, Kowal P: US Department of Health and Human Services. Population Aging in Sub-Saharan Africa: Demographic Dimensions 2006. Washington, US Government Printing Office, US Census Bureau, 2007.

9 Bradshaw B, Dorrington R, Laubscher R: Rapid Mortality Surveillance Report 2011. Cape Town, Medical Research Council (South Africa), 2012. http://www.mrc.ac.za/bod/RapidMortality2011.pdf.

10 Negin J, Cumming RG: HIV infection in older adults in sub-Saharan Africa: extrapolating prevalence from existing data. Bull World Health Organ 2010; 88:847–853.

11 Bendavid E, Ford N, Mills EJ: HIV and Africa's elderly: the problems and possibilities. AIDS 2012; 26(suppl 1):S85–S91.

12 Negin J, Nemser B, Cumming R, Lelerai E, Ben Amor Y, Pronyk P: HIV attitudes, awareness and testing among older adults in Africa. AIDS Behav 2012;16:63–68.

13 Ory MG, Zablotsky DL, Crystal S: HIV/AIDS and aging: identifying a prevention research and care agenda. Res Aging 1998;20:637–652.

14 el-Sadr W, Gettler J: Unrecognized human immunodeficiency virus infection in the elderly. Arch Intern Med 1995;155:184–186.

15 Greig J, Casas EC, O'Brien DP, Mills EJ, Ford N: Association between older age and adverse outcomes on antiretroviral therapy: a cohort analysis of programme data from nine countries. AIDS 2012; 26(suppl 1):S31–S37.
16 Costagliola D: Demographics of HIV and aging. Curr Opin HIV AIDS 2014;9:294–301.
17 Stall R, Catania J: AIDS risk behaviors among late middle-aged and elderly Americans. The national AIDS behavioral surveys. Arch Intern Med 1994; 154:57–63.
18 High KP, Brennan-Ing M, Clifford DB, Cohen MH, et al: HIV and aging: state of knowledge and areas of critical need for research. A report to the NIH office of AIDS research by the HIV and aging working group. J Acquir Immune Defic Syndr 2012;60(suppl 1):S1–S18.
19 World Health Organization Eastern Mediterranean Region: AIDS and Sexually Transmitted Diseases. Geneva, World Health Organization, 2010.
20 UNAIDS: Global AIDS Response Progress Reporting 2014. Geneva, UNAIDS, 2014. http://www.unaids.org/sites/default/files/media_asset/GARPR_2014_guidelines_en_0.pdf.
21 Population Reference Bureau: HIV and AIDS in the Middle East and North Africa. June 2014. http://www.prb.org/Publications/Reports/2014/middle-east-hiv-aids.aspx (retrieved September 22, 2015).
22 World Health Organization and United Nations Programme on HIV and AIDS: Accelerating HIV Treatment in the WHO Eastern Mediterranean and UNAIDS Middle East and North Africa Regions. Geneva, WHO/UNAIDS, 2013.
23 World Health Organization Regional Office for South-East Asia: HIV Early Diagnosis/Treatment. Geneva, WHO, 2013. http://www.searo.who.int/entity/hiv/en/.
24 National AIDS Control Organisation: Department of AIDS Control, Ministry of Health & Family Welfare, Government of India: Annual Report 2012–2013. http://www.naco.gov.in/upload/Publication/Annual%20Report/Annual%20report%202012-13_English.pdf.
25 World Health Organization South-East Asia Regional Office: Regional Health Sector Strategy on HIV, 2011–2015. Geneva, WHO, 2012.
26 World Health Organization Western Pacific Region (WPRO): HIV in the Western Pacific Region. Geneva, WHO, 2012.
27 World Health Organization Western Pacific Region: WPRO Data and Statistics, 2013. http://www.wpro.who.int/hiv/data/en/.
28 Yu D, Wi T, Calleja JG: How are countries in the Western Pacific Region tracking the HIV epidemic? Results from a 2011 survey of ministries of health. Western Pac Surveill Response J 2013;3:3–8.
29 Messersmith LJ, Semrau K, Hammett TM, Phong NT, Tung ND, Nguyen H, Glandon D, Huong NM, Anh HT: 'Many people know the law, but also many people violate it': discrimination experienced by people living with HIV/AIDS in Vietnam – results of a national study. Glob Public Health 2013;8(supp 1): S30–S45.
30 World Health Organization WPRO: The health of older people in selected countries of the Western Pacific Region. Geneva, WHO, 2014. http://hesp-news.org/2014/08/25/the-health-of-older-people-in-selected-countries-of-the-western-pacific-region/.
31 Zhang Y, Fuller-Thomson E, Anne Mitchell C, Zhang X: Older adults with HIV/AIDS in rural China. Open AIDS J 2013;7:51–57.
32 Liu H, Lin X, Xu Y, Chen S, Shi J, Morisky D: Emerging HIV epidemic among older adults in Nanning, China. AIDS Patient Care STDS 2012;26:565–567.
33 Kirby Institute for Infection and Immunity in Society: HIV in Australia. Annual Surveillance Report. Sydney, Centre for Social Research in Health, 2015. http://kirby.unsw.edu.au/surveillance/2015-annual-surveillance-report-hiv-viral-hepatitis-stis.
34 McDonald K, Elliott J, Saugeres L: Ageing with HIV in Victoria: findings from a qualitative study. HIV Aust 2013;11:13.
35 Han N, Wright ST, O'Connor CC, Hoy J, Ponnampalavanar S, Grotowski M, Zhao HX, Kamarulzaman A: HIV and aging: insights from the Asia Pacific HIV observational database (APHOD). HIV Med 2015;16:152–160.
36 United Nations Programme on HIV and AIDS: World AIDS Day Report. Geneva, UNAIDS, 2012.
37 Costagliola D: Demographics of HIV and aging. Curr Opin HIV AIDS 2014;9:294–301.
38 Cardoso SW, Torres TS, Santini-Oliveira M, Marins LM, Veloso VG, Grinsztejn B: Aging with HIV: a practical review. Braz J Infect Dis 2013;17:464–479.

Courtenay Sprague, MD
University of Massachussetts, Department of Conflict Resolution
Human Security and Global Covernance
100 Morrissey Blvd, Boston MA, 02125-339 (USA)
E-Mail Courtenay.Sprague@umb.edu

Brennan-Ing M, DeMarco RF (eds): HIV and Aging. Interdiscipl Top Gerontol Geriatr.
Basel, Karger, 2017, vol 42, pp 11–27 (DOI: 10.1159/000448539)

# Are HIV-Infected Older Adults Aging Differently?

Stephen E. Karpiak · Richard Havlik

ACRIA, ACRIA Center on HIV and Aging, New York University College of Nursing, New York, N.Y., USA

**Abstract**

With increasing success in treating HIV, infected persons are living longer, and a new challenge has emerged – the need to understand how HIV-infected adults are aging. What are the similarities with typical aging and what are the unique aspects that may have resulted from HIV infection, interacting with characteristic life style factors and other comorbid conditions? Are specific diseases and conditions (comorbidities), typically seen as part of the aging process, occurring at accelerated rates or with higher frequency (accentuated) in HIV-infected adults? At this juncture, conclusions should be tentative. Certainly, biological processes that correlate with aging occur earlier in the older adult HIV population. Clinical manifestations of these biological processes are age-associated illnesses occurring in greater numbers (multimorbidity), but they are not accelerated. Specifically cardiovascular disease, certain cancers, and renal disease are more common with other comorbidities less certain. Management of this elevated risk for developing multimorbidity is a major concern for patients and their health care teams. The medical system must respond to the evolving needs of this aging and growing older adult population who will dominate the epidemic. Adopting a more holistic approach to their health care management is needed to achieve optimal health and well-being in the HIV-infected older adult. Geriatric care principles best embody this approach. 

Those with an HIV/AIDS diagnosis prior to the mid-1990s faced a rapid and often miserable death due to the total collapse of the immune system, exhibiting rarely seen AIDS-related diseases such as pneumocystis pneumonia, Kaposi's sarcoma, dementia, lymphoma, and toxoplasmosis. Death was due to one or more of these comorbidities that could not be effectively managed due to decreasing immune system function. When these infections spread to different organ systems, the course was most often fatal, with death occurring often in isolation fueled by AIDS-based stigma [2].

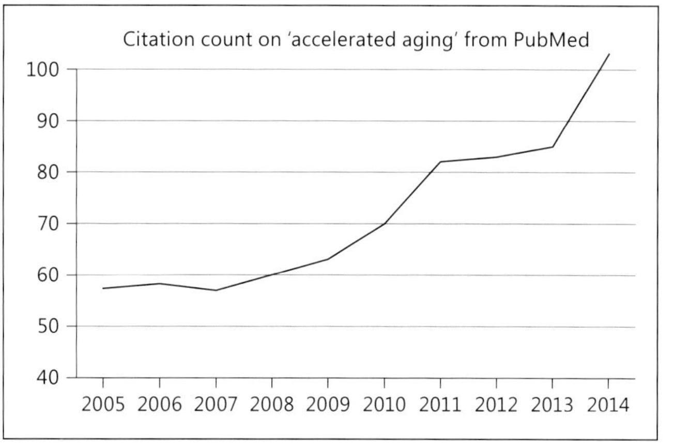


**Fig. 1.** Increase in published articles on HIV and 'accelerated aging'.

In 2015, almost 35 years since the HIV epidemic was recognized, it is estimated that half of all people living with HIV (PLWH) in the US are aged over 50. This is the result of effective combinations of antiretroviral treatments (ARTs), first available in the mid-1990s. In 2013, it was estimated that a 20-year-old diagnosed with HIV who takes ART can expect to live into his/her 7th decade [3].

There is a complication to this extraordinary success of ART [2]. As this population ages, it exhibits increased frequency of age-associated illnesses. The words 'accelerated aging' are often used to describe this aging arc of the older adult with HIV. This descriptor is in part premised on certain data that show these older adults developing illnesses, typically associated with aging at an earlier age than would be expected [4]. This chapter will assess if these older adults are aging differently if infected with HIV. Embracing the high impact conclusion that accelerated aging is occurring in the growing aging HIV-infected population requires scientific evidence including replication.

## Origin of the Accelerated Aging Hypothesis

Increasingly, providers of clinical care for PLWH are spending less time managing HIV drug resistance and associated short-term ART toxicities and are spending more time managing age-associated illnesses [6]. This shift in care has caused many to ask – are people infected with HIV aging faster? Are they experiencing more comorbid age-associated illnesses? (fig. 1).

HIV-treating physicians and researchers observed that there was an increase in the deaths of PLWH , most often from non-AIDS related illnesses. In one representative study sample of 9,858 patients, 55.7% died from non-AIDS-defining causes (cardiovascular disease, end-stage liver disease, and non-AIDS malignancies) [1] (fig. 2).

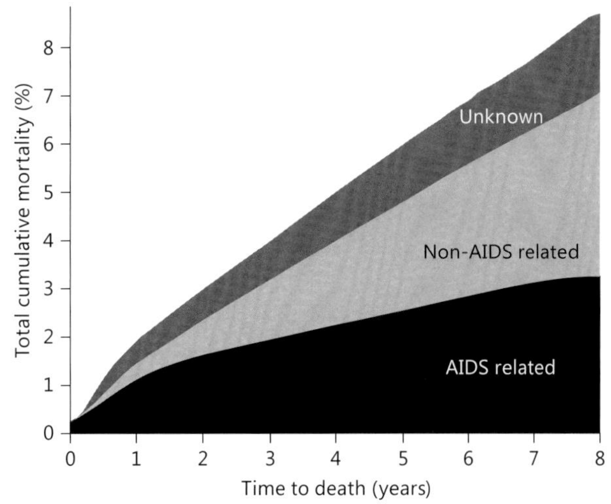


**Fig. 2.** People infected with HIV are dying more often of non-AIDS related disorders (adapted from Marin et al. [1]).

ART has been shown to reduce total mortality, including AIDS deaths, as indicated by the increase in life expectancy. However, an important question is whether ART has the same effect on non-AIDS deaths. In addition, will early ART treatment, when CD4 counts are above 350, be particularly beneficial. Two long-standing NIH cohorts provide insight into these questions, especially since they include access to that always elusive and critical well-matched comparator control group (see below) – Multicenter AIDS Cohort Study (MACS) begun in 1983 which enrolls men who have sex with men (MSM) only, and the Women's Interagency HIV Study (WIHS) began in 1993. A high proportion of both cohorts – 60% or 6,699 individuals – were included in the 2014 study [7] where comparisons were made among 3 subgroups, early initiators of ART (CD4 greater than 350), intermediate initiators (CD4 201–350), and low initiators (CD4 200 or less). The median age at death in the control group was 75 years, and in the early initiators the age was 72 years, while in the other subgroups the age was lower (69 and 66 years, respectively). When further mortality analyses were completed, including statistical adjustment for other known risk factors, mortality rates from non-AIDS causes in those HIV-infected persons who had begun ART early were almost identical to controls. These data reinforce the now overwhelming conclusion that starting ART early is recommended because it reduces both AIDS and non-AIDS mortality.

Other observations that contribute to discussions of whether the aging process is different in the older adult HIV populations are reports from the US and globally that older PLWH exhibit a significantly higher frequency of multimorbidity [4]. Multimorbidity is defined as having 2 or more chronic diseases, but, it is not synonymous with aging The need to manage multimorbidity in the older adult HIV-infected population is causing inexorable tectonic shifts in how care delivery is provided [8].

**Table 1.** Comparisons of typical aging and aging with HIV – appearance

| Factor | Typical aging | HIV | Comment |
|---|---|---|---|
| Loss of hair | Often | Similar | |
| Skin wrinkles | Often | Similar | |
| Loss of subcutaneous fat | Often | Especially in face | Result of older HIV ART drugs |
| Increase in abdominal fat | Often | More frequent | Result of older HIV ART drugs |
| Loss of muscle mass | Common [43] | Especially arms and legs | |

## A Field Still in Its Infancy: Testing the Hypothesis of Accelerated Aging

According to Martin and Volberding [9], accelerated aging in older adults with HIV is an 'intriguing' hypothesis, and, that we should not allow it to become ingrained in the culture of HIV before it has been supported. Most would agree that by 2015 the perception that accelerated aging was occurring is common. What factors must be addressed in the research literature that can allow the accelerated aging hypothesis to be embraced?

To understand what constitutes accelerated aging, researchers need to comprehend 2 intertwined scientific issues: accelerated (premature, faster) aging and accentuated (more) aging. Although untangling these 2 issues completely may not be necessary to address the health care management needs of older persons living with HIV.

What is aging? The first problem, which is more than a semantic issue, is the fundamental understanding of what aging in humans represents and how to measure it. Rare progeria syndromes, such as Hutchinson–Guilford, show manifestations of accelerated aging reflected in early mortality [10]. The major challenge is to describe and quantify 'normal' aging or better the term 'typical' aging in the general population. Yet the complexity of findings has prevented a simple definition that can be used to address questions arising from the need to compare HIV-infected and HIV-uninfected individuals when testing for aging differences. Adding to this challenge is the need to separate physiological changes/processes that occur with aging from diseases and conditions that are common as one ages. Although the dictum 'aging is not a disease' is often cited, the truth of the matter is that physiology and pathology are difficult or impossible to separate when used to define/describe aging. A summary of these differences is found in tables 1–4.

Without valid measures of aging, we are left to operationally define both accelerated and accentuated aging. Accelerated aging occurs when a certain pathology occurs earlier than would be expected in a study population, and accentuated aging occurs when there is an increase in the frequency of any given age-associated pathology (fig. 3).

**Table 2.** Comparisons of typical aging and aging with HIV – organ systems

| Factor | Typical aging | HIV | Comment |
|---|---|---|---|
| Hearing | Diminished | Low and high tone loss [45] | Possible acoustic trauma |
| Vision | Near sightedness | Macular degeneration [43] | |
| Kidney function | Decrease in GFR | Decreased function, especially in African Americans | |
| Menopause | Usual time window | Earlier? | |
| Osteoporosis | Women greater than men | Common in 15% [51] | In HIV, may be from other factors [21] |
| Impaired energy balance | Decreased endurance | More fatigue [57] | |
| Vascular stiffness | Loss of elasticity and increased fibrosis | Increased atherosclerosis and calcium in coronaries and carotids | |
| Neurocognition | Slowing of processing speed | Decreased processing and executive function | |
| Telomeres | Shortening with age | Shorter length and shortening with age [58] | Decrease with age similar in 2 groups [59] |
| T cells | Less due to thymus shrinkage | Cannot replenish naïve or functional CD4 cells | |
| T cells | CD28 negative markers of immune senescence | Similar and produce cytokines | Occurs in HIV even with ART |
| Inflammation | Loss of homeostatic function [43] | Persistent low levels | Occurs in HIV even with ART |
| Testosterone | Low [12] | Low | |
| Other organisms | Not affected | Cytomegalovirus, hepatitis C, bacteria from gut | |

### Comparator Group Challenge: Isolating the HIV Effect

How does HIV affect the aging of older adults? A significant challenge remains in finding comparison groups that are adequate to yield valid results. To effectively answer this question, researchers must control as many variables as possible to isolate the HIV effect. But, many HIV-infected adults bring with them a constellation of characteristics and life experiences that are unique, exerting significant impact on a person's health status. This spectrum of variables must be controlled in analyses that focus on testing the accelerated aging hypothesis. These variables include:

**Table 3.** Comparisons of typical aging and aging with HIV – diseases and conditions

| Factor | Typical aging | HIV | Comment |
|---|---|---|---|
| Vascular diseases | CVD, stroke hypertension type 2 diabetes | MI and CVD 50% higher [48, 49] | |
| Cancer (common) | Increased colon, prostate and breast | Less breast and prostate | |
| Cancer (environmental) | Increased lung | Increased lung | Both due to smoking |
| Cancer (AIDS) | Kaposi sarcoma rare | Kaposi sarcoma associated with AIDS | |
| Cancer (HIV) | Anal, oral, Hodgkin's increased with age | Anal, oral, Hodgkin's at least 2–3 times higher [50] | |
| Renal | End stage due to diabetes and hypertension | Immune activation is the cause [55] | |
| Frailty | Loss of reserve frequent | More frequent in MSM (12 vs. 9% in uninfected) [24]. In women associated with low CD4 nadir [21] | |
| Dementia | Vascular/Alzheimer's at old ages | Mild cognitive problems increased [56] | |
| Geriatric syndromes | Falls/fractures common | Increased fracture risk with overall of 2.9 vs. 1.8 patients with fractures per 100 persons [53] | |
| Depression | Less common with age (may be related to decreased telomere length [46]) | 3–5 times rate of uninfected [54] | |
| Hepatitis C | Usual frequency | Increased due to IV drug use | |

**Table 4.** Comparisons of typical aging and aging with HIV – treatment

| Factor | Typical aging | HIV | Comment |
|---|---|---|---|
| Multimorbidity | Common with elevated inflammation markers [47] | High frequency requiring targeted treatment | In HIV, long-term survivors who took toxic ART and life style factors are contributory |
| Polypharmacy | Common and multimorbidity requires use of many medications | Even more common due to ART and other drugs for depression and other comorbidities | |
| Use of geriatrician | Some consultation to improve functional status and quality of life | Infrequent consultation and the need to increased referral frequency | |

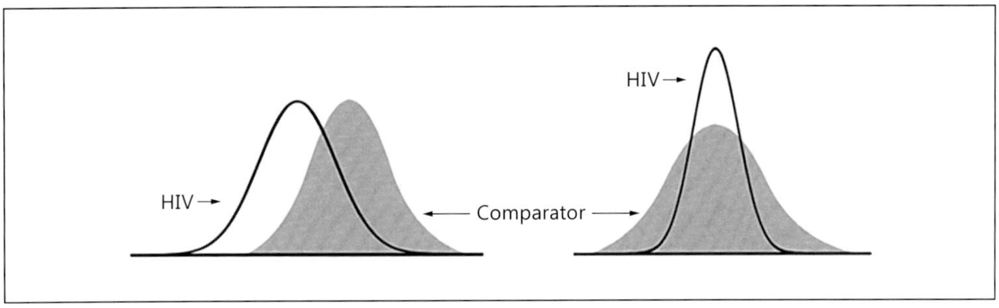


**Fig. 3.** Graphic curves representing the hypothetical occurrence of accelerated or premature aging (left graphic) versus accentuated aging (right graphic). In the accelerated model, a condition/illness/comorbidity occurs at a younger age among those with HIV than among HIV-uninfected comparators. In the accentuated model, the illness occurs at the same age but more often in those infected with HIV when compared to the HIV-uninfected population (adapted from Shiels et al. [5]).

history of drug addiction/use, smoking and alcohol use, hepatitis C, sexually transmitted infections, isolation/depression, post-traumatic stress disorder, financial, housing and food insecurity, as well as gender, race/ethnicity, and sexual identity. Effectively controlling these variables, whose resolution is more often elusive, is a challenge. In the US, large cohorts of HIV-infected people who also have embedded valid comparator groups include the Veteran's Aging Cohort Study (VACS), WIHS, and MACS. In Europe, the Danish HIV Cohort Study contains a comparator group.

Yet even as studies based on these 'ideal' cohorts have added important information, they have not unequivocally resolved whether accelerated or accentuated aging or both are occurring [11]. The complexity and intrinsic nuances of the variables which must be controlled to effectively test the accelerated aging hypothesis are daunting. In addition, variables that control the elevated health risks that characterize this older adult population need to be included. The older adult population living with HIV presents with a common core of risks that are independent of HIV infection/pathology. These include:

- Rates of smoking that are 3–4 times greater (>50%) than the larger US population [12].
- Over 25% are also infected with hepatitis C virus (HCV), and 70–90% have a history of co-infection with hepatitis B virus. HCV is the primary cause of chronic liver disease in the US. In HIV-infected persons, HCV co-infection progresses more rapidly causing liver damage.
- Older adults with HIV, who were infected prior to 1995 when highly effective ART became available, are described as long-term survivors. Many of these took the early ART medications (didanosine, stavudine, zalcitabine, zidovudine (AZT)) that are likely more toxic, given their higher rates of serious side effects and less than optimal efficacy in preventing the collapse of the immune system.

- The duration of long-term survivors living with HIV/AIDS is often greater than 20 years. It is unlikely that these survivors were continuously adherent to ART. During the non-adherent periods, the HIV-associated inflammatory response would have increased/spiked.
- HIV infection is largely occurring within economically underprivileged minority communities wherein good nutrition and emphasis on regular exercise is absent. Economics, ethnicity, and geographic location are examples of primary predictors of health disparities and poor health outcomes.
- Long-term histories of substance use characterize the older adult HIV-infected populations – substances of choice are opiates, cocaine, crack, and alcohol [60].
- Since the beginning of the epidemic to the present, high rates of unmanaged depression contribute to HIV stigma-induced social isolation and concomitant stress.

Holding constant what are almost 2 dozen variables that have been identified as being characteristic of the aging HIV adult population is a significant methodological challenge [12].

## How Does HIV Infection Cause a Different Aging Process: Inflammation?

To monitor the optimal efficacy of ART, viral load and CD4 count are used to monitor the immune system status and HIV replication levels. Biomarkers, which indicate the levels of the HIV-induced inflammatory cascade, such as IL-6 and D-dimer, predict morbidity and mortality [13]. These and other biomarkers of inflammation levels remain elevated in patients who have achieved viral suppression [13]. HIV-induced immune activation leads to inflammatory cascade [14] that is blunted by ART but not eliminated. Inflammation has been shown to be a primary cause of many illnesses evidenced in the older adult HIV population, namely, cardiovascular disease, lymphoma, venous thromboembolism, type 2 diabetes, cognitive dysfunction, and frailty. Inflammation can be induced or exacerbated by co-occurring illnesses or conditions in the HIV-infected population – substance use, depression, smoking, and lack of exercise, poor diet, HCV, and tuberculosis [15].

## Typical Aging versus Aging with HIV

To provide perspective to address the question of whether aging with HIV is different, a detailed listing of both similarities and differences between the characteristics of typical aging and frequent observations and findings regarding older persons with HIV/AIDS are given in tables 1–4. Tables 1–4 summarize the effect of HIV relative to typical aging variables based on appearance, organ systems, diseases and other conditions, and treatment categories. There are both similarities and differences in each of the categories, but the differences do not support accepting the accelerated aging hypothesis.

## Geriatric Syndromes: Frailty and HIV

Several reports chronicle the frailty syndrome to be elevated in older adults with HIV [16–18]. However, various definitions of frailty are used, making comparisons a challenge. These elevations provide impetus to the perception that accelerated aging is occurring in the said population. While chronological age and functional 'age' are correlated, the relationship is markedly reduced when older adults exhibit the frailty syndrome. Frailty is a significant variable since its presence indicates that the person is at greater risk for negative health outcomes including falls, reduced mobility, and independence, accompanied by increased hospitalizations and death. Frailty indicates that a person has markedly reduced reserves needed to recover from even small injuries, illnesses, as well as catastrophic events. Frailty identifies those individual who are in need of increased medical care. As a proxy for advanced aging, the frailty syndrome is usually characterized by associated weakness, decreased energy, lower activity, weight loss, and muscle mass loss. Frailty is a predictor of the older adult's elevated vulnerability to life stressors. It is most often observed in older adults in their 7th and later decades of life. For the US community-dwelling population over 65 years of age, the estimated prevalence of frailty is 10.7% [19]. The prevalence for those aged 80–84 years is 16%, and it increases to 25% and greater in those aged over 85. It is 5–8% for those aged 65–74 years. The prevalence estimates are highest for those in long-term care facilities.

In a literature review, Onen and Overton [20] focused on the presence of premature frailty in HIV-infected persons. The authors contend that the frailty frequency and characteristics were similar to much older adults not infected with HIV, and therefore, represented accelerated aging. Gustafson et al. [21] proposed a similar rationale based on data from middle-aged women with HIV. They studied frailty, as defined by the Fried criteria, in the WIHS cohort and compared 1,449 HIV-positive women, average age 39 years, with 579 HIV-uninfected WIHS controls. The frailty prevalence was 17% in HIV-positive women and 10% in HIV-negative women. A multivariable model showed that HIV infection with a CD4 count less than 200 was a significant correlate of frailty. Other significant predictors were age greater than 40 years, history of smoking, income equal or less than USD 12,000, and other physiological measures. They concluded that the prevalence of frailty in this younger group of women with HIV exceeded the frequency (10%) seen in the uninfected WIHS controls. Why the controls had an elevated rate complicated data interpretation and underlines how difficult and elusive achieving valid frailty data can be. Consistent or replicated study data on frailty is uncommon. In 5 studies that used one of the large HIV cohorts (MACS, WIHS, VACS, ALIVE) with an internal comparator, 2 found increases in frailty [22, 23] and 3 did not find any increase [24–26]. A recent paper [27] assessed the occurrence of a spectrum of geriatric syndromes in a sample of MSM (n = 155; mean age 57). Frailty was found in 9% of the study group and higher percentages of pre-frailty (56%), difficulty with instrumental activities of daily living

(IADLs; 46%), and cognitive impairment (47%) were observed. Non-white race and an increasing number of comorbidities were associated with increased risk of having more geriatric syndromes of frailty, difficulty with IADLs, and cognitive impairment. There was no comparator group.

### Does Function Follow Biology in the Older Adult Aging with HIV?

Biological changes associated with aging in the normal population include immunosenescence, telomere shortening, T cells becoming less available as the thymus shrinks, and increased activation of immune mechanisms leading to increased inflammation. Do these changes, which occur 'early' as a result of HIV infection, translate into clinical manifestations, and particularly the premature onset of associated clinical sequelae in the HIV-infected adult? Wallet et al. [28] in a small study attempted to relate inflammation to physical impairment. The design compared 21 HIV-infected adults, aged 54–69 years and 10 uninfected matched controls on a number of inflammatory biomarkers, physical performance as measured by the speed of a 400-meter walk, a short performance battery, and lower leg muscle strength. Although the HIV-infected group exhibited increased inflammation, even after correcting for comorbidities, the elevated inflammatory markers were unrelated to physical impairment.

Elevated levels of cytomegalovirus-specific immunoglobulin G were found to be associated with impaired physical function in HIV-infected persons [29]. But the authors conclude that given the reductions in the strength of this association in bivariable models, the data suggests only an indirect relationship mediated by systemic inflammation and immune suppression. Functional impairment in HIV-infected persons who are virally suppressed is associated with low muscle mass, low bone mineral density, and low insulin-like growth factor and its binding protein. These factors may be an indication of metabolic aging or early 'somatopause' in middle-aged HIV-infected adults [30].

There are multiple reports of telomere degradation in those infected with HIV [31]. Often telomere shortening is not age dependent, but rather is dependent on HIV infection and independent of ART treatment and viral suppression [32]. In a study of telomere length in 73 HIV-infected patients and 27 controls [31], analysis showed a clear inverse relationship between telomere length and immune suppression. It was estimated that there was a 5-fold acceleration of aging, which translated into HIV patients with an average age of 37 years having telomere length of a 75-year-old. Telomere length is seen as a biomarker of cellular senescence, but there is no clear relationship to the physical function as reflected in the frailty phenotype. In a large study, Woo et al. [33] obtained a sample of about 1,000 men and 1,000 women, and found that there was no relationship between telomere length and the frailty index when physical, psychological, and functional domains were assessed.

## Clinical Reports: Accentuated Aging in HIV-Infected Older Adults Is Common

There is a compendium of research studies that have studied the frequency of comorbid illnesses in older adults with HIV. They share common methods and findings. A close inspection of a few studies reveals interpretation limitations. This recent clinic-based study in Italy [34] yields typical findings. HIV-infected patients were evaluated for specific non-HIV comorbidities as well as 'polypathology', or the presence of 2 or more comorbidities (multimorbidity) and compared to matched controls from the same university center. Polypathology in patients aged 41–50 years were similar to the control group aged 51–60 years. Diabetes, cardiovascular disease, bone fractures, and renal failure were more frequent in the HIV group. These findings were interpreted to support a prematurity of comorbidities (accelerated aging) in HIV-infected persons. In a review of the Italy-based study [35], potential methodological flaws were identified – namely, that the examination of HIV patients may have been more thorough because of their having more frequent medical visits, some of which are driven by the inherent need to follow-up on any medical complaints. In another study [36], researchers compared the immune function in virally suppressed and viremic patients with uninfected individuals on a number of indicators of monocyte activation. They found that elevations of these markers in the HIV-infected individuals were similar to what were found in individuals 4–12 years older. This differential was believed to be consistent with the relationship of inflammation with more frequent and early onset of comorbidities. Yet the study does not take into account the duration of how long the patients were infected with HIV, how long they were on ART therapy, how long they were virally suppressed, and the course of HIV infection. In addition, the variables of increased burden of disease (multimorbidity) resulting in the need for multiple medications, as well as socioeconomic variables and the occurrence of HCV were not addressed.

Data from a large HIV sample from Denmark were compared with population controls [37]. The HIV sample had an increased number of age-related diseases. The relative risks for cardiovascular diseases, most cancers, and severe neurocognitive disease did not increase with age, after HIV diagnosis or ART. There was some variation in the results for chronic kidney disease, hepatitis, and osteoporotic fractures. Overall the results suggest that accelerated aging is not evident in the HIV-infected adults studied. Petoumenos and Law [11] commented on the Denmark study, pointing out that the interpretation of comorbidities and the lack of any acceleration in the HIV group is complicated by the inability to sort out the possible effects of ART, co-infections, and behavioral/life style factors. Interestingly, the study found a general pattern of declining relative risk for comorbidities with advancing age, possibly from selective mortality, although absolute risks continue to rise. This observation supports the current recommendation of early ART and maintenance of undetectable viral load along with reduction of risk factors for comorbidities, especially smoking cessation.

Schouten et al. [38] presented the results from the AGEhIV Amsterdam-based study where patients aged 45 and older with and without HIV infection were studied. The comparison group was matched by age, gender, and ethnic origin. All participants had frequent measures of various non-communicable comorbidities, such as heart attack and kidney disease, and received a comprehensive questionnaire. The groups were reasonably similar on a number of characteristics, and there were greater than 500 participants in each group. The HIV-positive participants had an average of 1.3 age-related illnesses versus 1.0 for the comparison group. This excess held true for every 5-year subgroup measured, and there was a progressive increase by age. In only one 5-year age subgroup (60–64) in the HIV-infected group did the average number of 1.52 equal the 1.51 in the 65+ of HIV negatives, suggesting faster aging. However, overall it did not appear that there was an acceleration of aging due to HIV. Higher frequencies of elevated blood pressure, heart attacks, peripheral vascular disease, and kidney disease were found in the HIV-infected older adults. In analyses, smoking, a treatable risk factor, was a predictor of these outcomes. Also, a CD4 count less than 200 (CD4 nadir) predicted more non-AIDS comorbidities, supporting the now almost universal conclusion that early ART is the standard of care.

Reports show that there are clear increases in the frequency of certain cancers in the older HIV populations. Some reports conclude that cancers occur earlier in HIV patients. To compensate for probable biases in such reports, finding earlier cancer onset because of age differences between AIDS patients and controls, Shiels et al. [5] used data from the large US HIV/AIDS Cancer Match Study, and corrected for age. Then, comparisons were made between medians of the age-adjusted age-at-diagnosis distributions. For most cancers, there was no difference in the age of diagnosis. Although for lung cancer and anal cancer there were earlier diagnoses, which could be a reflection of earlier exposure to risk factors, such as smoking and human papilloma virus.

## HIV Accelerates Aging Is a Hypothesis

In their 2010 editorial titled, HIV and Premature Aging: A Field Still in Its Infancy, Martin and Volberding [9] enumerate the criteria used when considering whether accelerated aging occurs in older adults living with HIV. The authors of the editorial used the Shiels et al. [5] study to illustrate one of the challenges which assessed cancer in the HIV US population (supra), which concludes that certain cancers did not occur earlier and did not support the accelerated aging hypothesis. Martin and Volberding [9] comment that since initial HIV infections predominantly affects a younger population, any analysis will for that reason give the 'appearance' of an early onset of cancer. The editorial ends with 'until scientists have more meaningful and comprehensive methods for measuring subclinical aging, proving that HIV is a true accelerant of the aging process is impossible'.

The VACS utilized a unique resource of a large number (n = 98,687) of HIV-infected (31%) and demographically similar uninfected adults (69%) to address the issue of whether comorbidities occur more frequently and sooner in HIV-infected adults. Validated diagnoses for myocardial infarction (MI), end-stage renal disease (ESRD), and non-AIDS defining cancers (NADC) were used as end points by Althoff et al. [39]. Analyses indicated that the occurrence of MI, ESRD, and NADC was elevated in HIV-infected patients compared to the control group. Also, the mean ages for incidence of MI and NADC were similar between the 2 subgroups. But, ESRD did occur approximately 6 months earlier in the HIV-infected subgroup. However, after correcting for important risk factors, there was no significant difference regarding the age of incidence between the 2 subgroups. These and similar reports support the contention that unless the comparator group is rigorous, it is unlikely that data supporting the accelerated aging hypothesis can be accepted. The authors conclude that the results of this study should reassure HIV patients that it is unlikely that comorbidities will be occurring many years earlier than expected as they age.

### Faster Aging, More Aging, or Both: Our Current Understanding and What Questions Persist?

A thorough review of the literature on issues surrounding accelerated-accentuated aging question and HIV concluded that, 'the answer is probably organ and disease/condition specific' [40]. Specifically, the review recognized that ongoing immune activation is the key mechanism that produces an increase in cytokine and coagulation factors. For specific end organ diseases, the authors reviewed the clinical findings of Guaraldi et al. [4] and found that diabetes, cardiovascular disease, and bone fracture showed accentuated aging and renal failure showed both. Their review provides a mixed answer to the question of faster or more aging, and underlines the need for better biomarkers for studies of aging in older adults with HIV infection. The HIV-infected older adults' immune system status and elevated markers for inflammation occur earlier than in comparator groups. This is not surprising since most HIV infections occur early in life and the virus directly attacks the immune system resulting in immune system changes that mirror the decline seen in non-HIV infected adults over 65. These measures appear to be similar, but are they? These changes occur in patients who are on ART and have achieved sustained viral load suppression. But the biomarkers of reduced immune function and elevated inflammation persist. Can this complicated disconnect between HIV, its treatment and persistent changes in the underlying biology, allow one to conclude that accelerated aging is occurring given that clinical data do not support the biology of accelerated aging?

An important question is whether consistent evidence would be derived from different durations of HIV exposure. A comparison would need to be done between the immune function of individuals infected early and surviving versus those who were infected more recently. Guaraldi et al. [41] divided the study population into those who were seropositive for greater than 20 years and those who had been seropositive for about 10 years or more recently infected and compared to a group in the metabolic clinic for the frequency of multimorbidity. If the population was limited to those 45 years and older, there was a significant increase in the frequency of comorbidities in those who had been seropositive for longer period. This suggested that the subgroup with a longer period of exposure to the HIV virus, even if well treated, may have characteristics leading to more multimorbidity. The variable duration of HIV infection and treatment duration cause researchers to consider whether the long-term survivors in this epidemic are at increased risks. One of the arguments made to support the hypothesis is the fact that these long-term survivors in the late 1980s and early 1990s were exposed to the more toxic ARTs and likely began ART treatment with CD4 levels below 200. They are also most likely to have developed resistance to some of the ARTs, indicating that their adherence behaviors were not always greater than optimal 90% adherence rates needed to sustain viral suppression. Reduced adherence, missing ART doses contribute to increases in immune activation and inflammatory cascade response. A 2015 [27] study of older adults with HIV (mean age 57 years) found that increased risk for developing geriatric syndromes was associated with age and CD4 nadirs. Yet the one factor that significantly reduced risk was whether the patient had taken the early more 'toxic' ART treatments (didanosine, stavudine, zalcitabine, zidovudine (AZT)). This conflicting finding likely represents the ongoing dynamics in the epidemic wherein those least fit succumb before reaching older age.

When comparisons are done with patients very similar to the HIV patients and many times actually imbedded in the same study, such as the VACS [40], the differences in the time of onset of selected diseases is minimal or non-existent, consistent with no acceleration. However, almost universally, whether with excellent or fair comparison groups, the presence of multimorbidity is a prevailing characteristic of reported studies [34]. Whether this is the result of the effect of HIV on multiple systems and organs, such as postulated with chronic inflammation or the interaction with certain disease risk factors, needs further study. Also, depending on the study, there is variability in the conclusions about which diseases and conditions are found to be more prevalent, namely, accentuated aging. These include hypertension, arthritis, diabetes, frailty, and cognitive disorders. In an October 2015 Letter to the Editor in the Journal AIDS [42], Harper concluded that '…current data are not consistent with an accelerated ageing hypothesis', and cumulatively that data does support the view that an increased risk of age-related comorbidities occurs.

We are left considering what interventions would be appropriate to optimize the health of the growing aging HIV populations. Deeks et al. [6] suggest that HIV-infected adults have a high burden of diseases, and there is a health system gap in treatment. This situation needs to change.

## Conclusions

Current data support that HIV infection causes immunosenescence and inflammation at a younger age than seen with typical aging. However, in studies of HIV-infected adults using appropriate comparison groups, HIV-infected older adults have increased number of comorbidities, but they do not occur at a significantly earlier age. Also, it appears that the actual comorbidities occurring in HIV-infected adults may be more limited than previously believed. These include cardiovascular disease, certain cancers, and renal disease, with osteoporosis and related falls being less certain. Data on frailty and other geriatric syndromes is only beginning to emerge. More research with available cohorts with comparable comparison groups embedded is needed to clarify any lingering questions and perceptions that age-related comorbidities are occurring earlier and/or in greater numbers. With the present state of knowledge, there is no doubt that early ART should be initiated in all HIV-positive patients to reduce chronic inflammation. This aggressive action should be paired with cardiovascular risk factor reduction and appropriate screening for cancers, renal disease, and osteoporosis. Finally, improvement in the current health care system is necessary to provide better treatment, prevention and comprehensive care to HIV-infected older adults. Part of the improvement requires embracing geriatric care principles.

## References


1 Marin B, et al: Non-AIDS-defining deaths and immunodeficiency in the era of combination antiretroviral therapy. AIDS 2009;23:1743–1753.

2 Kirk JB, Goetz MB: Human immunodeficiency virus in an aging population, a complication of success. J Am Geriatr Soc 2009;57:2129–2138.

3 Samji H, et al; North American AIDS Cohort Collaboration on Research and Design (NA-ACCORD) of IeDEA: Closing the gap: increases in life expectancy among treated HIV-positive individuals in the United States and Canada. PLoS One 2013.

4 Guaraldi G, et al: Premature age-related comorbidities among HIV-infected persons compared with the general population. Clin Infect Dis 2011;53:1120–1126.

5 Shiels MS, Pfeiffer RM, Engels EA: Age at cancer diagnosis among persons with AIDS in the United States. Ann Intern Med 2010;153:452–460.

6 Deeks SG, Lewin SR, Havlir DV: The end of AIDS: HIV infection as a chronic disease. Lancet 2013;382: 1525–1533.

7 Wada N, et al: Cause-specific mortality among HIV-infected individuals, by CD4(+) cell count at HAART initiation, compared with HIV-uninfected individuals. AIDS 2014;28:257–265.

8 Work Group for HIV and Aging Consensus Project: Summary report from the human immunodeficiency virus and aging consensus project: treatment strategies for clinicians managing older individuals with the human immunodeficiency virus. J Am Geriatr Soc 2012;60:974–979.

9 Martin J, Volberding P: HIV and premature aging: a field still in its infancy. Ann Intern Med 2010;153: 477–479.

10 Dreesen O, Stewart CL: Accelerated aging syndromes, are they relevant to normal human aging? Aging (Albany NY) 2011;3:889–895.

11 Petoumenos K, Law M: HIV-infection and comorbidities: a complex mix. Lancet HIV 2015.

12 Brennan M, et al: Older Adults with HIV: An In-Depth Examination of an Emerging Population. Nova Science Publishers, 2009.

13 Borges AH, et al; INSIGHT SMART and ESPRIT Study Groups and the SILCAAT Scientific Committee: Factors associated with plasma IL-6 levels during HIV infection. J Infect Dis 2015;212:585–595.

14 Desai S, Landay A: Early immune senescence in HIV disease. Curr HIV/AIDS Rep 2010;7:4–10.

15 Deeks SG: HIV infection, inflammation, immunosenescence, and aging. Annu Rev Med 2011;62:141–155.
16 Brothers TD, Rockwood K: Biologic aging, frailty, and age-related disease in chronic HIV infection. Curr Opin HIV AIDS 2014;9:412–418.
17 Womack JA, et al; Veterans Aging Cohort Study Project Team: Physiologic frailty and fragility fracture in HIV-infected male veterans. Clin Infect Dis 2013;56:1498–1504.
18 Pathai S, et al: Frailty in HIV-infected adults in South Africa. J Acquir Immune Defic Syndr 2013;62:43–51.
19 Collard RM, et al: Prevalence of frailty in community-dwelling older persons: a systematic review. J Am Geriatr Soc 2012;60:1487–1492.
20 Onen NF, Overton ET: A review of premature frailty in HIV-infected persons; another manifestation of HIV-related accelerated aging. Curr Aging Sci 2011; 4:33–41.
21 Gustafson DR, et al: Frailty and constellations of factors in aging HIV-infected and uninfected women – the women's interagency HIV study. J Frailty Aging 2016;5:43–48.
22 Desquilbet L, et al; Multicenter AIDS Cohort Study: Relationship between a frailty-related phenotype and progressive deterioration of the immune system in HIV-infected men. J Acquir Immune Defic Syndr 2009;50:299–306.
23 Piggott DA, et al: Frailty, HIV infection, and mortality in an aging cohort of injection drug users. PLoS One 2013;8:e54910.
24 Althoff KN, et al; Multicenter AIDS Cohort Study (MACS): Age, comorbidities, and AIDS predict a frailty phenotype in men who have sex with men. J Gerontol A Biol Sci Med Sci 2014;69:189–198.
25 Terzian AS, et al; Women's Interagency HIV Study: Factors associated with preclinical disability and frailty among HIV-infected and HIV-uninfected women in the era of cART. J Womens Health (Larchmt) 2009;18:1965–1974.
26 Akgun KM, et al: An adapted frailty-related phenotype and the VACS index as predictors of hospitalization and mortality in HIV-infected and uninfected individuals. J Acquir Immune Defic Syndr 2014; 67:397–404.
27 Greene M, et al: Geriatric syndromes in older HIV-infected adults. J Acquir Immune Defic Syndr 2015; 69:161–167.
28 Wallet MA, et al: Increased inflammation but similar physical composition and function in older-aged, HIV-1 infected subjects. BMC Immunol 2015;16:43.
29 Erlandson KM, et al: Physical function impairment of older, HIV-infected adults is associated with cytomegalovirus immunoglobulin response. AIDS Res Hum Retroviruses 2015;31:905–912.
30 Erlandson KM, et al: Functional impairment is associated with low bone and muscle mass among persons aging with HIV infection. J Acquir Immune Defic Syndr 2013;63:209–215.
31 Blanco JR, et al; CoRIS-Biobanco: Shorter telomere length predicts poorer immunological recovery in virologically suppressed HIV-1-infected patients treated with combined antiretroviral therapy. J Acquir Immune Defic Syndr 2015;68:21–29.
32 Monickaraj F, et al: Accelerated aging as evidenced by increased telomere shortening and mitochondrial DNA depletion in patients with type 2 diabetes. Mol Cell Biochem 2012;365:343–350.
33 Woo J, et al: Telomeres and frailty. Mech Ageing Dev 2008;129:642–648.
34 Guaraldi G, et al: A frailty index predicts survival and incident multimorbidity independent of markers of HIV disease severity. AIDS 2015;29:1633–1641.
35 Capeau J: Premature aging and premature age-related comorbidities in HIV-infected patients: acts and hypotheses. Clin Infect Dis 2011;53:1127–1129.
36 Angelovich TA, et al: Viremic and virologically suppressed HIV infection increases age-related changes to monocyte activation equivalent to 12 and 4 years of aging, respectively. J Acquir Immune Defic Syndr 2015;69:11–17.
37 Rasmussen LD, et al: Time trends for risk of severe age-related diseases in individuals with and without HIV infection in Denmark: a nationwide population-based cohort study. Lancet HIV 2015.
38 Schouten J, et al; AGEhIV Cohort Study Group: Cross-sectional comparison of the prevalence of age-associated comorbidities and their risk factors between HIV-infected and uninfected individuals: the AGEhIV cohort study. Clin Infect Dis 2014;59: 1787–1797.
39 Althoff KN, et al; Veterans Aging Cohort Study (VACS): Comparison of risk and age at diagnosis of myocardial infarction, end-stage renal disease, and non-AIDS-defining cancer in HIV-infected versus uninfected adults. Clin Infect Dis 2015;60:627–638.
40 Pathai S, et al: Is HIV a model of accelerated or accentuated aging? J Gerontol A Biol Sci Med Sci 2014; 69:833–842.
41 Guaraldi G, et al: Aging with HIV vs. HIV seroconversion at older age: a diverse population with distinct comorbidity profiles. PLoS One 2015;10.
42 Harper KN: HIV-infected adults experience accentuated but not accelerated ageing. AIDS 2015;29:N3.
43 Margolick JB, Ferrucci L: Accelerating aging research: how can we measure the rate of biologic aging? Exp Gerontol 2015;64:78–80.
44 Jabs DA, et al; Studies of the Ocular Complications of AIDS Research Group: Prevalence of intermediate-stage age-related macular degeneration in patients with acquired immunodeficiency syndrome. Am J Ophthalmol 2015;159:1115–1122.

45 Torre P 3rd, et al: Hearing loss among HIV-seropositive and HIV-seronegative men and women. JAMA Otolaryngol Head Neck Surg 2015;141:202–210.
46 Verhoeven JE, et al: Major depressive disorder and accelerated cellular aging: results from a large psychiatric cohort study. Mol Psychiatry 2014;19:895–901.
47 Stepanova M, et al: Age-independent rise of inflammatory scores may contribute to accelerated aging in multi-morbidity. Oncotarget 2015;6:1414–1421.
48 Islam FM, et al: Relative risk of cardiovascular disease among people living with HIV: a systematic review and meta-analysis. HIV Med 2012;13:453–468.
49 Freiberg MS, et al: HIV infection and the risk of acute myocardial infarction. JAMA Intern Med 2013;173: 614–622.
50 Deeken JF, et al: The rising challenge of non-AIDS-defining cancers in HIV-infected patients. Clin Infect Dis 2012;55:1228–1235.
51 Brown TT, Qaqish RB: Antiretroviral therapy and the prevalence of osteopenia and osteoporosis: a meta-analytic review. AIDS 2006;20:2165–2174.
52 Womack JA, et al; Veterans Aging Cohort Study Project Team: Increased risk of fragility fractures among HIV infected compared to uninfected male veterans. PLoS One 2011.
53 Triant VA, et al: Fracture prevalence among human immunodeficiency virus (HIV)-infected versus non-HIV-infected patients in a large U.S. healthcare system. J Clin Endocrinol Metab 2008;93:3499–3504.
54 Applebaum AB, Brennan M: Mental health and depression; in Brennan M, Karpiak SE, Cantor MH, Shippy RA (eds): Research on Older Adults with HIV: An In-depth Examination of an Emerging Population. New York, Nova Science, 2009.
55 Abraham AG, et al: Kidney dysfunction and markers of inflammation in the multicenter AIDS cohort study. J Infect Dis 2015;212:1100–1110.
56 Heaton RK, et al; CHARTER Group: Neurocognitive change in the era of HIV combination antiretroviral therapy: the longitudinal CHARTER study. Clin Infect Dis 2015;60:473–480.
57 Barroso J, et al: Physiological and psychosocial factors that predict HIV-related fatigue. AIDS Behav 2010;14:1415–1427.
58 Pathai S, et al: Accelerated biological ageing in HIV-infected individuals in South Africa: a case-control study. AIDS 2013;27:2375–2384.
59 Liu JC, et al: Absolute leukocyte telomere length in HIV-infected and uninfected individuals: evidence of accelerated cell senescence in HIV-associated chronic obstructive pulmonary disease. PLoS One 2015;10.
60 Justice AC, et al: Risk of mortality and physiologic injury evident with lower alcohol exposure among HIV infected compared with uninfected men. Drug Alcohol Depend 2016;161:95–103.

Stephen E. Karpiak, PhD
ACRIA, ACRIA Center on HIV and Aging
575 Eighth Avenue, Suite 502
New York, NY 10018 (USA)
E-Mail skarpiak@acria.org

Brennan-Ing M, DeMarco RF (eds): HIV and Aging. Interdiscipl Top Gerontol Geriatr.
Basel, Karger, 2017, vol 42, pp 28–46 (DOI: 10.1159/000448542)

# Cellular Senescence, Immunosenescence and HIV

Tamàs Fülöp[d] • Georges Herbein[a] • Andrea Cossarizza[b] • Jacek M. Witkowski[c] • Eric Frost[e] • Gilles Dupuis[f] • Graham Pawelec[g] • Anis Larbi[h]

[a]Department of Virology, Pathogens and Inflammation Laboratory, University of Franche-Comté, COMUE Bourgogne Franche-Comté University, CHRU Besançon, Besançon, France; [b]Department of Surgery, Medicine, Dentistry and Morphological Science, University of Modena and Reggio Emilia, Modena, Italy; [c]Department of Pathophysiology, Medical University of Gdansk, Gdansk, Poland; [d]Research Center on Aging, Graduate Program in Immunology, [e]Department of Microbiology and Infectious Diseases, and [f]Department of Biochemistry, Graduate Program in Immunology, Faculty of Medicine and Health Sciences, University of Sherbrooke, Sherbrooke, Que., Canada; [g]Second Department of Internal Medicine, Center for Medical Research, University of Tübingen Medical School, Tübingen, Germany; [h]Singapore Immunology Network (SIgN), Biopolis, Agency for Science Technology and Research (A*STAR), Singapore, Singapore

## Abstract

Aging is a complex biological process that leads to several physiological changes. Among these changes, the most striking are those involving the innate and adaptive parts of the immune system. Furthermore, these changes are associated with a low-grade inflammation called inflamm-aging, which is the result of several lifelong antigenic stimulations, including chronic viral infections such as cytomegalovirus. Immunosenescence, concomitantly with inflamm-aging, is considered as the leading cause of age-related diseases including cardiovascular, neurodegenerative and metabolic diseases, and cancer. HIV infection, once considered a unique deadly infectious disease, has now become a chronic disease with efficacious highly active antiretroviral therapy. This signifies that the treatment transforms HIV infection from a chronic infection to a chronic inflammatory disease. Most people with HIV infection become aged, and older adults have been contracting HIV infection. Thus, there is a great interest to study HIV infection in relation to immunosenescence and inflamm-aging to determine whether immunosenescence contributes to HIV infection, or if HIV is causing immunosenescence and, as such, represents a premature immunosenescence and accelerated aging. Although there are many similarities in the immune and inflammatory changes and the occurrence of age-related chronic diseases between normal aging and HIV infection, the interaction between these processes is not well understood, and consequently the concept that HIV infection is an accelerated aging model is questioned. Future studies are needed to effectively answer this question for the better care of HIV-infected elderly patients.

## Introduction

The number of elderly people continues to increase [1]. Aging is a natural process that culminates in physiologic decline and an increased risk of morbidity and mortality [2–4]. This increase is accompanied by an enhanced frequency of age-related diseases, including infectious, neurodegenerative and cardiovascular diseases, and cancer. Many of these diseases have been associated with changes of the immune system, designated 'immunosenescence' [5, 6]. Moreover, one essential characteristic of immunosenescence, which is especially important for the increased incidence of these age-related diseases, is the presence of a chronic low-grade inflammation, dubbed 'inflamm-aging' [7–11]. The overall significance of these immune changes is still controversial in terms of their impact on biological aging process, the biological significance of changes, and the role of chronic antigenic stimulations occurring during the chronological aging. The most important sources of chronic antigen exposure, contributing to immunosenescence, are likely lifelong persistent viral infections such as cytomegalovirus (CMV) and Epstein Barr virus and, probably to less extent, cancer antigens [9, 12, 13].

Among chronic viral infections, HIV occupies a very special place. HIV infection was once a deadly disease of the young in specific populations. In recent times, because of the success of the highly active antiretroviral therapy (HAART), HIV is often seen in older people or those surviving with HIV and are now becoming elderly [14–17]. It is possible to consider HIV infection as a potential model of premature immunosenescence [18–23].

In this chapter, we will discuss the immune changes with aging and the effect of HIV, and explore the relationship between immunosenescence and HIV.

## Effect of Aging on the Immune System

Aging is a complicated biological process involving numerous intricately linked intrinsic and extrinsic factors and alterations affecting all systems of the human body including the immune system, at different levels [2, 24]. The most prevalent concept is that immunosenescence is a general decrease in the functions of the innate and adaptive immune response [5, 6, 11]. It is evident that most of the experimental evidence, obtained mainly in mice and also in humans, tends to support this paradigm. However, it is not established whether the changes that are considered detrimental are adaptations or remodeling of a system which should adapt constantly to the internal and external milieu [25–27]. How did this idea of immunosenescence being detrimental emerge? The reason is that experimental evidence supports the notion that the changes attributed to immunosenescence directly result in age-associated chronic neurodegenerative and cardiovascular diseases and cancer, and in infections and a decreased response to vaccines [9–11, 28]. Even though these diseases are developing over the entire lifespan, it is difficult to conceive that immunosenescence, as we understand it today, could be the only underlying mechanism per se.

We are still unable to accurately assess the most important changes which could be characterized and accepted as biomarkers of immunosenescence. Only a few studies consider the longitudinal changes of the immune response with aging. One of the most important were the Swedish OCTO and NONA studies, which clustered simple immune parameters, including inversion of CD4/CD8 ratio, the expansion of late differentiated $CD8^+$ T cells, CMV seropositivity, poor T cell proliferation, and low B cell number to generate the so-called immune risk phenotype (IRP) [29, 30]. The IRP was associated with increased mortality at 2-, 4- and 6-year follow-ups. Thus far, this study has not been replicated in other aging populations under similar conditions, and it is therefore not possible to generalize these findings [31].

All parts of the immune system are affected by aging, although not to the same extent. The most important function of the innate immune system composed of neutrophils, monocytes/macrophages, dendritic cells, and natural killer cells is to be the first line of protection for an organism against various invaders [6, 32–34]. Most often, this line of defense is enough to eradicate the danger. Because microorganisms are usually phylogenetically conserved, their pathogen-associated molecular patterns are highly conserved and are not shared by mammals; thus, they can be recognized as invaders by non-polymorphic activating receptors expressed on the surfaces of innate immune cells. Innate immune responses strongly influence subsequent adaptive immune responses via antigen processing and presentation, and cytokine and chemokine production. It is now well accepted that the effector functions of cells of the innate immune response decrease with aging [6, 32, 33]. Phagocytosis, chemotaxis, free radical production, and antigen presentation are all altered, but to different extent. Therefore, the first line of immune defense against aggressors is compromised with aging.

The first cells to arrive at the site of a potential infection are neutrophils. There are many changes described in the neutrophil functions with aging [35–42]. Most of the neutrophil functions are decreased, including free radical production, chemotaxis, apoptosis, and intracellular killing. However, some functions remain unchanged, such as phagocytosis and adhesion. In contrast, the production of proinflammatory cytokines is increased, mainly at the resting state, which may contribute to inflamm-aging.

Regarding other innate immune cells, there are few experimental data on the age-related changes of monocytes/macrophages and dendritic cells [43–45]. Phenotypic differences have been described for various monocyte subpopulations, which may have an effect on their functionality. Studies have demonstrated a large increase in the minor population of $CD14^+CD16^+$ monocytes in older subjects [46], which has also been shown to be increased in HIV-infected patients and may play a role in the transport of HIV in the brain. Macrophages in older adults have decreased levels of activation as demonstrated by a decrease in the expression of MHC class II HLA-DR molecules leading to altered functioning.

The microbicidal activity of macrophages also decreases with aging. This is reflected in a weakened respiratory burst, decreases in the production of reactive nitrogen and oxygen intermediate products, and decreased capacity to complete phagocytosis [6, 43]. Similar changes in HIV infections have also been demonstrated [21, 47–51]. These functional changes were shown to be mediated by negative regulatory factor. At the same time, older subjects have elevated basal levels of IL-6 – a proinflammatory cytokine that is secreted by both monocytes and macrophages, and by many other cells types, such as muscle cells, fibroblasts, and hepatocytes. Elevated IL-6 is considered a risk factor for chronic inflammatory diseases of the elderly, especially atherosclerosis [52]. Higher IL-6 levels have already been detected in HIV-infected younger subjects compared to healthy controls, similar to decrease of TH1 cytokines and increased TH2 cytokines that lead to the TH1 to TH2 shift paradigm during the progression of the disease [21, 53]. The dendritic cells appear to be constitutively activated in the elderly, possibly rendering them less reactive to challenges that activate them via the innate Toll-like receptors (TLRs) [50, 54].

NK cells recently have been the subject of increased research interest, as these cells are crucial in defense against virus-infected and cancerous cells [11, 34]. Aging impacts the phenotype of NK cells as their absolute number is increasing, the proportion of CD56$^{bright}$ NK cells are decreasing, and the CD56$^{-}$ NK cells are increasing. This subpopulation has also been shown to expand in certain chronic viral infections, including HIV. There are also changes in surface receptors with decreasing expression of cytotoxicity-activating receptors. This can manifest as functional changes in their main activity, with decreased cytotoxic activity on the single-cell level potentially compensated for by increased NK cell numbers. Interestingly, some parameters such as the expression of CD16 and the antibody-dependent cellular cytotoxicity capacity are not dependent on age. The reasons for these changes or lack of them in aging are not well understood, but some have been related to chronic CMV infection which reshapes the immune system quite similar to aging itself as a result of the requirement for keeping chronic CMV infection in a latent state.

These studies suggest once again that the phenotype of innate immune functioning observed in older subjects matches the phenotype detected in response to HIV infection and may play a role in the hypothesized accelerated aging effects reported in younger HIV-1 infected patients [18–23].

The adaptive immune response is currently considered to be more severely affected by aging than the innate functions, as reflected by changes in the phenotypes and functions of both B and T cells [5, 11, 55]. Lifelong exposure to pathogens activating naïve T cells and thymic involution results in decreasing numbers of naive T cells over the lifespan, especially in the CD8$^{+}$ T cell compartment compared to the CD4$^{+}$ T cell compartment. Concomitantly, differentiation into effector T cells and development of T cell memory is more pronounced in older individuals as a result of these exposures.

This may result in memory 'inflation' (i.e., the accumulation of large numbers of late-stage differentiated memory T cells) by several mechanisms including various antigenic stimulation and insufficient renewal of naïve cells [56–58]. Therefore, due to chronic antigenic stimulation, T cells may undergo a process of differentiation/exhaustion, leading to the accumulation of memory cells specific to previously encountered antigens which are no longer as effective as they were when first generated [25]. The best example of this process is persistent CMV infection, which drives the accumulation of late-differentiated $CD8^+$ T cells specific to CMV [12, 13, 59, 60]. These CMV-specific $CD8^+$ T cells help to prevent CMV reactivation by killing virus-infected cells, thereby controlling virus replication at the expense of immune exhaustion [19, 61]. Not only do these memory cells accumulate with aging and fill the 'immune space', but their specific functions, including clonal expansion, IL-2 production and their effector functions, are detrimentally altered. These functional changes are related to alterations in signaling pathways, including T cell receptor, CD28, and cytokine receptor signaling [62–64]. Such cells also produce excessive amount of IFNγ, have cytotoxic functions and accumulate in inflammatory lesions [65]. In addition to these differences, suppressive regulatory T cells seem to be more active in the elderly than in young individuals [66]. These alterations, together with the changes in the innate immune response, create a state of inflamm-aging [7–11, 67]. This state is a fertile soil for the development of chronic inflammatory diseases in relation to the aging process. Despite the compelling evidence that CMV can be a driving force for the adaptive immune changes with aging, it is still debated whether this is the cause of age-associated adaptive immune changes or just a coincidental finding [68, 69]. The fact that CMV induces similar changes in young subjects militates in favor of the hypothesis that this infection has little to do with the effect on the immune response per se. Interestingly, a recent study showed that CMV-specific late stage differentiated $CD8^+$ T cells express antigen receptors of low affinity and expand mostly in response to antigen-nonspecific cytokine stimulation [11]. Thus, the role of CMV-triggered memory expansion as a key stimulus for skewing the T cell repertoire is questionable and may be simply due to an inflammatory milieu widely observed with aging [61]. This situation may be at least partly maintained by the senescence associated secretory phenotype (SASP) [71–73]. This idea gains credibility with the acceptance of the notion that T cells may be a model for replicative senescence as described by Hayflick [65]. The problem is that it is still not known whether, despite their shortened telomere lengths, T cells reach the end of their potential clonal expansion capacity during the human lifespan. It is also of note that memory B cells show limited repertoire diversity, so that in elderly individuals the antibody response to new antigens is quantitatively decreased [74], less efficient, and of lower avidity. Furthermore, qualitative and quantitative changes may occur in T regulatory cells, which play a key role in controlling the host immune response [75].

Immune functions are mediated by the activation of cells following ligation of their membrane receptors, but the numbers of most of these receptors are not changed with aging. Thus, changes in signaling pathways have been described, explaining the functional alterations in the presence of unchanged receptor numbers [62–64]. Many signaling pathways, such as the Jak/STAT, PI3K and MAPK pathways, are altered under stimulatory conditions with aging and also explain the altered susceptibility to apoptosis. One of the most striking alterations in the innate immune system is the changes in TLR functions [33]. There is a decrease in TLR-1 expression with a concomitant decreased cytokine production. TLR-induced CD80 and CD86 expressions are also altered in aging. In contrast, the TLR4 stimulated in $CD14^{+}CD16^{+}$ inflammatory monocytes resulted in increased cytokine production, probably due to sustained NF-κB activity as seen in elderly hip fracture patients. In T cells, there is also an alteration in the signaling pathways, but especially in the very early stage resulting in the activation of Lck. There is disequilibrium between the tyrosine kinase stimulatory activity and the tyrosine phosphatase inhibitory activity (e.g., SHP-1) in favor of the latter [76]. This has also been observed for the regulation of Erk by dual specificity protein phosphatase [77]. Taken together, there is an altered intracellular signaling upon receptor stimulation in various immune cells with aging due to mostly intrinsic cell alterations resulting in an already activated status in the resting state.

### Effect of Aging on Inflammation

As a consequence of the continuous lifelong antigenic stimulation, these innate immune cells evolve in a proinflammatory environment that already exists at the quiescent state in aged individuals [42, 43]. This constant stimulation is accompanied by increases in the production of free radicals and proinflammatory cytokines, including TNF and IL-6, which may cause 'collateral damage' to host tissues. This basal activation further results in the dysregulation of other physiological systems, such as the musculoskeletal, cardiovascular, and neuroendocrine systems [78].

Other inflamm-aging influencing factors encompass changes occurring in the aging body such as increased cellular death, increased oxidative stress, nutritional status, microbiome changes related to intestinal leakage due to gut wall permeability increase, and to dysbiosis, hormone dysregulation, and latent co-morbidities including atherosclerosis and neurodegeneration [79]. All these factors may also contribute to inflamm-aging by a constant low grade activation of the cells of the innate immune system, most importantly of the tissue resident macrophages. This readiness of the innate system during challenge may rapidly result in excessive inflammation and tissue damage. Thus, this low grade inflammation may be the price to pay for a decreased adaptive immune response which, however, may still react even if at a different level to a new challenge.

Recently, a new phenomenon called trained memory has been described for the innate immune system [80]. This means that the innate immune response remembers the challenge even if the challenge is terminated. The many factors influencing lifelong activation of the innate immunity may result in continuous maintenance of the trained memory underlying the low grade inflammatory phenomenon. The underlying molecular pathway of the trained memory is driven by epigenetic changes in innate cells via the aerobic phosphorylation (Warburg effect) [81–84]. These new findings open future perspective in our understanding of the low grade inflammation in aging and provide targets for interventions.

Recently, the role of senescent cells in inflamm-aging is increasingly accepted. Once considered as metabolically inert, the senescent cells acquire SASP, leading to uncontrolled secretion of different proinflammatory molecules such as chemokines and other cytokines [71–73]. This phenotype, which can be beneficial in some physiologic circumstances as in wound healing, may become largely detrimental in the older organism. Destruction of SASP cells in a mouse model was beneficial for the aging process, but we do not have any data in human subjects.

### Effect of HIV on the Immune System

HIV-1 infection causes systemic immune activation fostered by a complex array of insults. As a consequence, there is an increased frequency of memory $CD4^+CD45RA^-CD45RO^+$ T cells and the so called 'senescent' $CD4^+CD57^+$ and $CD8^+CD57^+$ cells, which could also represent activated T cell subtypes [85–88]. Moreover, these T cells due to the chronic HIV infection or concomitant infections with other viruses such as CMV are undergoing several rounds of proliferation and reach a replicative limit, further characterized by the loss of the costimulatory receptor CD28 and shortened telomere length [61, 65]. Analysis of telomere length in HIV infection showed that $CD28^-$ T cells of 40-year-old HIV-infected individuals have identical telomere length compared to that of centenarians, suggesting that the patients' $CD8^+$ T cells that have undergone considerable proliferation resemble those that are found in healthy older adults [60, 65]. Moreover, a longitudinal study in young HIV-infected individuals showed a decrease in telomere length in $CD8^+$ T cells over time, which became progressively more oligoclonal [60, 85]. These cells are highly dysfunctional (e.g., they cannot proliferate), and besides being unable to clear the infection, have a unique inflammatory senescent phenotype characterized by producing a large amount of TNFα. They are also further characterized by their shortened telomeres and lack of substantial telomerase activity. This smoldering inflammation, resulting from persistent immune activation and immune senescence, characterizes the systemic milieu of chronic HIV infection [89].

During the acute and chronic phases of HIV infection, T cells demonstrate elements of immune cell aging with features of both senescence and activation. Early studies of the T cell response to HIV found that during acute infection, both HIV-specific $CD8^+$ T cells and the overall $CD8^+$ cell population were highly activated, as measured by the expression of CD38 and Ki-67 [19, 48, 65, 85, 90]. These activated T cells have a tendency to decrease in number when the infection becomes more chronic, with the concomitant decrease in their cytotoxic activity and when replaced by the above mentioned senescent $CD28^-$ T cells which show signs of exhaustion [19, 51, 70]. In persons with chronic HIV infections, it was shown that in both the $CD4^+$ and $CD8^+$ compartments an abnormal immune activation persists even in individuals with sustained viral suppression on HAART [90–93]. This signifies that factors other than viral load may maintain the activation of T cells in HIV infection. $CD4^+$ T cells show similar dysfunctional alterations in HIV infections, which further decrease the $CD8^+$ T cell functions.

In addition to the increase in senescent cell numbers, HIV infection is also characterized by accelerated thymic involution, reduced circulating naïve T cells, and decreased CD4/CD8 ratios. Thymic involution impairs naïve T cell production and limits regeneration of the naïve T cell pool [18, 61, 94]. Accelerated immune aging in HIV patients is certainly multifactorial. Treated HIV patients need to rebuild their T cell repertoire at an age when the thymic involution has already compromised thymic function, which has been further decreased and impaired by the HIV infection itself. Even if normal $CD4^+$ lymphocyte numbers are being reached as a function of ART treatment, T cell diversity and subset distribution may be compromised. Homeostatic proliferation to rebuild the repertoire will not only increase replicative stress to the system, but will also be associated with proliferation-induced differentiation even in the absence of antigen recognition.

The innate immune system in younger HIV-positive patients demonstrates similar changes as in healthy elderly. These changes include a higher baseline activation of dendritic cells and monocytes/macrophages, altered TLR functions, and decreased effector functions such as phagocytosis and cytotoxicity. Moreover, these cells (mainly monocytes) may serve as peripheral reservoir for the virus and convey their dissemination to various organs such as brain [47, 48, 50, 51, 95].

Taken together, these changes in the immune system due to chronic HIV infections were linked to premature aging of the immune response and to the appearance of chronic inflammatory diseases such as cardiovascular diseases seen normally in elderly individuals [96]. It has been hypothesized that non-immune organs sustain collateral damage due to the systemic inflammatory state either via circulating cytokines or from more direct insults when activation and senescent T cells are recruited to these organs at the site of infection or other injuries.

## Effect of HIV on Inflammation

Chronic inflammation, as also potentiated by HAART, is almost always present in HIV-infected patients over 50. Within a few weeks of infection, there is a massive depletion of $CD4^+$ T cells, mainly of the activated effector memory $CD4^+$ T cell subset and Th17 cells from the gastrointestinal (GI) associated lymphoid tissue (GALT)

[48, 51]. Could these early immune system changes influence later chronic inflammation? These changes in the GI tract lead to a breakdown of follicle-associated epithelial tight junctions and continual systemic leakage of microbial products (i.e., leaky gut), creating an antigenic burden that induces chronic immune activation and inflammation. It is presently thought that lipopolysaccharides (LPS) originating from the leaky gut result in the activation of the innate immune system, especially monocytes and macrophages [21, 97]. This can be measured in the circulation by assessing sCD14 levels, which has been suggested as a biomarker of non-AIDS mortality in HIV patients. Other inflammatory markers are also increased as a consequence of chronic activation by HIV such as IL-6, IL-1β, TNFα and CRP, which can also serve as biomarkers of non-AIDS mortality [50, 53]. Furthermore, other markers such as D-dimer, ICAM-1, and VCAM-1 are related to the cardiovascular risk [21, 86, 98, 99], while monocyte chemotactic protein osteopontin is related to the risk of dementia [100]. Other potential sources of chronic antigenic stimulation include co-infections such as HCV, HBV and CMV, thymic dysfunction, and adaptive immune dysregulation through impaired Treg function [48, 101, 102].

Interestingly, it is well established that the measures of T cell activation and inflammation predict morbidity and mortality in both treated and untreated HIV individuals independent of other factors. Many chronic inflammatory conditions such as cardiovascular diseases, neurodegenerative diseases, cancer, and frailty develop earlier in HIV-infected patients compared to controls [21]. Such disease development, especially cardiovascular disease, may not be simply explained by the traditional risk factors, such as dyslipidemia, hypertension, and/or obesity [50]. Evidence suggests that HIV itself predisposes to the accelerated development of atherosclerosis [96, 98, 99]. Because HIV induces chronic inflammation, immune activation and hypercoagulability, the endovascular microenvironment in HIV-infected patients tends to be pro-atherogenic. The T cell changes – mainly $CD8^+$ T cell senescence – are associated with atherosclerosis. It is of note that although HAART use is associated with improved endothelial function, HAART itself may predispose to cardiovascular events by increased dyslipidemia and insulin resistance. Cancers and neurocognitive disorders are also increased in HIV patients by the same multifactorial mechanisms, but especially by increased inflammation [21]. Osteoporosis, the underlying abnormality in patients with fragility fractures, is up to four times more prevalent in HIV-infected patients than in the general population [21].

## Is There Any Relationship between HIV and Immunosenescence Mediated by Inflammation?

The immune activation markers that are detected in HIV-1 infection are also elevated with increased age [18, 21, 47, 87]. One other common feature is that HIV infection similar to the aging process is associated with the premature development of cardiovascular disease, thromboembolic disease, type 2 diabetes, cancer, neurodegenerative diseases, end-organ disease, and frailty [21, 86, 103, 104]. It is of note that these diseases also develop even when HAART is effective [21, 87, 90–92].

The inflammation described above in HIV patients may mirror the low grade inflammatory process occurring with 'normal' aging or in frailty related to aging. In these conditions, an increase of some proinflammatory cytokines (mostly IL-6, TNFα) and SASP-associated factors may be detected [21, 22, 48, 50, 51, 105].

## Effect of Antiretroviral Treatment

Although HAART leads to a significant reduction of multiple markers of immune activation (CD38, HLA-DR, Ki-67), immune activation following HAART still remains significantly elevated compared with uninfected individuals [21, 92, 103]. The same effects were observed in the GALT. Initiation of HAART during primary HIV infection may limit the establishment of viral reservoirs, and very early HAART limits the seeding of the HIV reservoir in long-lived central memory CD4+ T cells [106–108]. Thus, it seems better to initiate ART therapy at higher CD4 T cell count. Antiretroviral treatment has dramatically increased life expectancy of HIV-infected individuals. As a result, over 50% of the HIV-infected population in the US is currently aged 50 or older [109]. Unfortunately, these gains in longevity have been accompanied by a growing burden of the so called age-related diseases, attributable both to the normal aging process and to the recently conceptualized HIV-induced accelerated cellular senescence, which may even potentiate the normal aging process. Diseases traditionally associated with aging have been identified in several organ systems such as cardiac, neurologic, hepatic, and renal at unexpected prevalence in cohorts of midlife HIV-infected patients. Finally, patients under HAART are usually administered one of 2 therapeutic regimens based on either a protease inhibitor or a non-nucleoside reverse transcriptase inhibitor (NNRTI). It has been reported that patients treated with NNRTI-based HAART for 16 weeks show a significantly higher level of MIP-1α and MIP-1β and this may be beneficial, as high β-chemokine levels have been associated with a slower disease progression [110]. Therefore, the drugs used during HAART could interfere with immune activation through modulation of chemokine production.

In the meantime, it was also shown that the modern HAART treatment of HIV infections also induces an increased susceptibility for diseases, such as type 2 diabetes. This could be by direct drug mitochondrial toxicity and also by lipoatrophy leading to insulin resistance [111]. Moreover, other conditions associated with aging, including chronic renal failure, bone fractures, frailty, and neurocognitive disorders, are increasingly important causes of HIV patient morbidity.

**Can HIV-Infection Be Considered as a 'Premature' State of Immunosenescence?**

The fact that HIV infection is associated with chronic diseases has given rise to the concern that HIV-1-infected individuals may suffer from premature or accelerated aging and neurocognitive impairment or comorbidities normally associated with advanced age much sooner than in the general population [19, 21]. One of the crucial questions is how the effect of HIV-1 infection, aging, and inflammation are interrelated and apparently converge on identical effects considering the disparate pathological consequences. In most of these cases, there are also confounding factors such as comorbidities, obesity or lifelong lifestyle differences, such as drug use, nutrition, social environment. Thus, the best way to dissect this potential intertwined relationship between aging and HIV infection, considering the inflammatory nature of both, is to compare, taking all the characteristics together, HIV-infected and non-infected subjects. It was found that in HIV-infected patients, both treated and not treated, plasma sCD14, CRP and IL-6 levels were significantly increased compared to controls. It is of note that the origin of the sCD14 is still controversial regarding whether they are mostly produced by circulating monocytes or tissue macrophages. Interestingly, the LPS levels were not different between the 2 groups, suggesting that aging and HIV may have the same effect on intestinal leakage [105].

As it is presently accepted, the inflammatory nature of aging is not only due to the activated innate immune system unbalancing the equilibrium with the adaptive immune response, but also due to the products of senescent cells, as mentioned above. One manifestation of this is the increase of $CD57^+$ T cells in aging and in HIV infection. This would suggest that in both cases a chronic viral infection may be in progress. Alternatively, this can be just the effect of the inflammatory milieu which triggers the differentiation of T cells to the senescent state.

Considering that from the immunological point of view, aging and HIV infection seem to have similar effects, and that HIV-infection was considered as a model for premature aging, the question arises whether immunosenescence may play any role in HIV infection? Considering the bulk of the experimental data, it can be said that HIV infection induced immune and inflammatory changes are much more marked than those associated with aging. Further evidence for this is that cardiovascular diseases, which occur in the general population with advancing age, seems to occur at an earlier age in HIV-infected patients [21]. The pathway hypothesized to lead to this apparent premature aging is the immune activation occurring in HIV infection and the consequent 'immunosenescence' being seemingly identical with the normal aging process, as reflected by decreased naïve T cells, increased memory $CD28^-CD4$ T cells, and increased proinflammatory cytokines even in HIV-positive subjects almost completely virologically suppressed [21]. Recent studies have introduced the hypothesis that chronic inflammation, immune activation, and immunosenescence might contribute to the development of concomitant chronic diseases such as atherosclerosis through endothelial activation. Thus, the question is: could HIV infection induce premature aging through immunosenescence? There is no clear cut answer. The age-related changes in the immune system are not unidirectional towards being only detrimental but there are also necessary changes setting an adequate threshold for maintaining the immune response.

Recently, in a 2015 paper published by Margolick and Ferrucci [112], the authors reviewed the criteria for diseases being considered as a model for premature or accelerated aging. This has important conceptual and therapeutic consequences. The reasons for including a disease or condition among those that accelerate aging are usually justified by the appearance of typical aging phenotypes at an earlier age than would normally be observed, and/or a delay in emergence of these phenotypes, including death, if the disease is cured or the condition moderated or reversed. The observed phenotypes may include straightforward features, such as a stooped posture or facial wrinkles, or biological features such as the reduction of naïve T lymphocytes, a proinflammatory gene expression profile, or shorter leukocyte telomeres. However, whether the resemblance of these changes to aging tells us anything important about the biological mechanisms of aging is questionable, as we do not presently understand all the mechanisms of the normal aging process.

The authors state that in theory any assertion of premature aging should meet 3 criteria: (1) the anatomic and functional manifestations seen must be the same as those seen in usual aging; (2) the mechanisms underlying these manifestations must be the same as in aging; and (3) both manifestations and mechanisms should be detected at a younger age than usual. Presently, no disease or condition has been studied with these criteria in mind, and none is currently known to really meet all 3 criteria [112].

Would the common criteria for a disease to be considered as premature aging, as defined by Margolick and Ferrucci [112], be met by the effectively treated HIV infection? This may be an interesting example, based on earlier-than-expected occurrence of aging-related diseases and enhanced immune senescence. There are also changes in body composition, that is, fat redistribution, sarcopenia, and loss of bone mass and architecture. Energy utilization has been reported to be less efficient, with higher resting oxygen consumption [113]. Treated HIV infection is still characterized by chronic low-level systemic inflammation. Life expectancy may be nearly normal or actually normal [114]. Thus, although treated HIV infection is one of the most-studied conditions claimed to accelerate aging [23], this claim may not yet be accepted as completely valid [115].

One other important difference between aging and the chronic antigenic stimulation is the induction of either senescent T cells or exhausted T cells, respectively [19]. The characteristic phenotype of exhausted T cells includes expression of TIM-3, PD-1, and LAG-3 [116], while senescent T cells express CD57, KLRG-1, ILT2, and KIRs [117]. In the former case, the surface markers are more functionally altered than in the latter case. Thus, T cell senescence is not exactly a reflection of chronic antigenic activation. These changes may also reflect that T cell repertoire changes related to age are distinct from those of chronic active viral diseases.

The presence of cells with the so-called senescent phenotype in the elderly has been associated with a decline in the functionality of these cells, reduced vaccine response and an increased risk of infection, neurodegeneration, and cardiovascular diseases [19, 70]. Interestingly, a similar signature of accelerated aging of the immune system has been recognized in individuals suffering from HIV infection. From this parallel, it is suggested that HIV infection accelerates aging and illnesses that are attributes of elderly are highly frequent among HIV-infected subjects, but develop at a much earlier age (10–15 years earlier), and even more so in HAART-treated patients [118]. Thus, to dissect and better understand their complex relationship we need to unravel the effect of aging per se on immune changes and inflammation, and their interrelation. A real differentiation of aging from the putative chronic antigenic stimulation, as was suggested by the acquisition of SASP, may in the future provide a better understanding of premature versus normal aging-induced immune changes. Furthermore, a better understanding of DNA repair and the metabolic pathways inside the cells and their epigenetic changes may provide further distinctive mechanisms distinguishing between these diseases and the aging process which cannot be considered as a disease.

## Conclusion

Aging in the context of HIV-1-infection is a complicated and expanding area of research. Age-related diseases such as bone disease, metabolic disorders, cardiovascular diseases, and immunologic dysregulation are linked to HIV-1 infection in several ways. HIV-1 infection can lead to the appearance of premature aging phenotypes and to chronic diseases, and treatment effects may be different in patients who are infected at older ages. The effects of age on HIV-1 infection and markers of HIV-1 disease progression remain controversial. More research is needed to elucidate the effects of age on HIV-1 diseases and vice versa, and how best to treat these patients. Studies on the impact of HIV-1 infection and age on each other have often been discrepant or did not account for possible confounding factors [119]. With regard to the effect of age on $CD4^+$ T cell count and viral load, comparing the overall mortality of older versus younger patients may be useful.

## Perspective

Understanding immune aging in HAART-treated HIV subjects is not only important to improve the quality of life and life expectancy in these patients, but may also provide a unique model to identify pathways that are central to normal immune aging.

Furthermore, the putative accelerated aging in treated HIV patients may provide an opportunity to understand how the senescent immune system contributes to major dysfunction in organ systems that are generally considered to be independent of immune function such as the cardiovascular and nervous system, lung, and kidneys. Constitutively increased production of proinflammatory mediators is likely to represent an important link between immunosenescence and accelerated age-associated dysfunction in several non-immune organ systems. The perspective for understanding these interrelations is exciting and may result in better interventions to increase quality of life of both the elderly and HIV-infected patients.


## Acknowledgments

This work was partly supported by grants from the Canadian Institutes of Health Research (Nos. 106634 and 106701), Canada Research Chairs (SCC), the Université de Sherbrooke, and the Research Center on Aging. Anis Larbi is funded by the Agency for Science Technology and Research. Georges Herbein is supported by grants from the University of Franche-Comté, the Région Franche-Comté (RECH-FON12-000013), the Agence Nationale de Recherche sur le SIDA (Nos. 13543 and 13544) and HIVERA 2013 (EURECA project). J.M.W. is funded by a statutory grant from Polish Ministry of Science and Higher Education 02-0058/07/262. The critical lecture on the manuscript by Prof. Victor Appay is greatly acknowledged.


## References


1 Department of Economic and Social Affairs Population Division: World Population Ageing. New York, United Nations, 2013.
2 Robert L, Fulop T (eds): Aging: Facts and Theories. Intrdisc Top Geriatr Gerontol. Basel, Karger, 2014, vol 39, pp 62–85.
3 López-Otín C, Blasco MA, Partridge L, Serrano M, Kroemer G: The hallmarks of aging. Cell 2013;153: 1194–1217.
4 Kennedy BK, Berger SL, Brunet A, Campisi J, Cuervo AM, Epel ES, Franceschi C, Lithgow GJ, Morimoto RI, Pessin JE, Rando TA, Richardson A, Schadt EE, Wyss-Coray T, Sierra F: Geroscience: linking aging to chronic disease. Cell 2014;159:709–713.
5 Pawelec G: T-cell immunity in the aging human. Haematologica 2014;99:795–797.
6 Solana R, Tarazona R, Gayoso I, Lesur O, Dupuis G, Fulop T: Innate immunosenescence: effect of aging on cells and receptors of the innate immune system in humans. Semin Immunol 2012;24:331–341.
7 Franceschi C, Bonafè M, Valensin S, Olivieri F, De Luca M, Ottaviani E, De Benedictis G: Inflamm-aging. An evolutionary perspective on immunosenescence. Ann N Y Acad Sci 2000;908:244–254.
8 Pawelec G, Goldeck D, Derhovanessian E: Inflammation, ageing and chronic disease. Curr Opin Immunol 2014;29:23–28.
9 Franceschi C, Campisi J: Chronic inflammation (inflammaging) and its potential contribution to age-associated diseases. J Gerontol A Biol Sci Med Sci 2014;69(suppl 1):S4–S9.
10 Howcroft TK, Campisi J, Louis GB, Smith MT, Wise B, Wyss-Coray T, Augustine AD, McElhaney JE, Kohanski R, Sierra F: The role of inflammation in age-related disease. Aging (Albany NY) 2013;5:84–93.
11 Pera A, Campos C, López N, Hassouneh F, Alonso C, Tarazona R, Solana R: Immunosenescence: implications for response to infection and vaccination in older people. Maturitas 2015;82:50–55.
12 Pawelec G, Akbar A, Caruso C, Solana R, Grubeck-Loebenstein B, Wikby A: Human immunosenescence: is it infectious? Immunol Rev 2005;205:257–268.

13 Solana R, Tarazona R, Aiello AE, Akbar AN, Appay V, Beswick M, Bosch JA, Campos C, Cantisán S, Cicin-Sain L, Derhovanessian E, Ferrando-Martínez S, Frasca D, Fulöp T, Govind S, Grubeck-Loebenstein B, Hill A, Hurme M, Kern F, Larbi A, López-Botet M, Maier AB, McElhaney JE, Moss P, Naumova E, Nikolich-Zugich J, Pera A, Rector JL, Riddell N, Sanchez-Correa B, Sansoni P, Sauce D, van Lier R, Wang GC, Wills MR, Zieliński M, Pawelec G: CMV and Immunosenescence: from basics to clinics. Immun Ageing 2012;9:23.
14 Kirk JB, Goetz MB: Human immunodeficiency virus in an aging population, a complication of success. J Am Geriatr Soc 2009;57:2129–2138.
15 Palella FJ Jr, Delaney KM, Moorman AC, Loveless MO, Fuhrer J, Satten GA, Aschman DJ, Holmberg SD: Declining morbidity and mortality among patients with advanced human immunodeficiency virus infection. HIV outpatient study investigators. N Engl J Med 1998;338:853–860.
16 Justice AC: HIV and aging: time for a new paradigm. Curr HIV/AIDS Rep 2010;7:69–76.
17 Rickabaugh TM, Jamieson BD: A challenge for the future: aging and HIV infection. Immunol Res 2010;48:59–71.
18 Appay V, Almeida JR, Sauce D, Autran B, Papagno L: Accelerated immune senescence and HIV-1 infection. Exp Gerontol 2007;42:432–437.
19 Le Saux S, Weyand CM, Goronzy JJ: Mechanisms of immunosenescence: lessons from models of accelerated immune aging. Ann N Y Acad Sci 2012;1247:69–82.
20 Ferrando-Martínez S, Ruiz-Mateos E, Romero-Sánchez MC, Muñoz-Fernández MÁ, Viciana P, Genebat M, Leal M: HIV infection-related premature immunosenescence: high rates of immune exhaustion after short time of infection. Curr HIV Res 2011;9:289–294.
21 Bhatia R, Ryscavage P, Taiwo B: Accelerated aging and human immunodeficiency virus infection: emerging challenges of growing older in the era of successful antiretroviral therapy. J Neurovirol 2012;18:247–255.
22 Nasi M, Pinti M, De Biasi S, Gibellini L, Ferraro D, Mussini C, Cossarizza A: Aging with HIV infection: a journey to the center of inflammAIDS, immunosenescence and neuroHIV. Immunol Lett 2014;162(1 pt B):329–333.
23 Pathai S, Bajillan H, Landay AL, High KP: Is HIV a model of accelerated or accentuated aging? J Gerontol A Biol Sci Med Sci 2014;69:833–842.
24 Lipsky MS, King M: Biological theories of aging. Dis Mon 2015;61:460–466.
25 Larbi A, Fulop T: From 'truly naïve' to 'exhausted senescent' T cells: when markers predict functionality. Cytometry A 2014;85:25–35.
26 Fulop T, Dupuis G, Baehl S, Le Page A, Bourgade K, Frost E, Witkowski JM, Pawelec G, Larbi A, Cunnane S: From inflamm-aging to immune-paralysis: a slippery slope during aging for immune-adaptation. Biogerontology 2016;17:147–157.
27 Franceschi C, Monti D, Barbieri D, Salvioli S, Grassilli E, Capri M, Troiano L, Guido M, Bonafè M, Tropea F, Salomoni P, Benatti F, Bellesia E, Macchioni S, Anderlini R, Sansoni P, Mariotti S, Wratten ML, Tetta C, Cossarizza A: Successful immunosenescence and the remodelling of immune responses with ageing. Nephrol Dial Transplant 1996;11(suppl 9):18–25.
28 Fulop T, Larbi A, Witkowski JM, Kotb R, Hirokawa K, Pawelec G: Immunosenescence and cancer. Crit Rev Oncog 2013;18:489–513.
29 Nilsson BO, Ernerudh J, Johansson B, Evrin PE, Löfgren S, Ferguson FG, Wikby A: Morbidity does not influence the T-cell immune risk phenotype in the elderly: findings in the Swedish NONA immune study using sample selection protocols. Mech Ageing Dev 2003;124:469–476.
30 Wikby A, Johansson B, Olsson J, Löfgren S, Nilsson BO, Ferguson F: Expansions of peripheral blood CD8 T-lymphocyte subpopulations and an association with cytomegalovirus seropositivity in the elderly: the Swedish NONA immune study. Exp Gerontol 2002;37:445–453.
31 Formiga F, Ferrer A, Padros G, Cintra A, Pujol R: Inverted CD4:CD8 ratio is not associated with three-year mortality in a sample of community-dwelling oldest old: the OCTABAIX immune study. J Nutr Health Aging 2014;18:425–428.
32 Montgomery RR, Shaw AC: Paradoxical changes in innate immunity in aging: recent progress and new directions. J Leukoc Biol 2015;98:937–943.
33 Shaw AC, Goldstein DR, Montgomery RR: Age-dependent dysregulation of innate immunity. Nat Rev Immunol 2013;13:875–887.
34 Tarazona R, Campos C, Pera A, Sanchez-Correa B, Solana R: Flow cytometry analysis of NK cell phenotype and function in aging. Methods Mol Biol 2015;1343:9–18.
35 Fortin CF, McDonald PP, Lesur O, Fülöp T Jr: Aging and neutrophils: there is still much to do. Rejuvenation Res 2008;11:873–882.
36 Juthani-Mehta M, Guo X, Shaw AC, Towle V, Ning Y, Wang X, Allore HG, Fikrig E, Montgomery RR: Innate immune responses in the neutrophils of community dwelling and nursing home elders. J Aging Sci 2014;pii:1000115.
37 Visan I: Aging neutrophils. Nat Immunol 2015;16:1113.

38 Baëhl S, Garneau H, Le Page A, Lorrain D, Viens I, Svotelis A, Lord JM, Phillips AC, Cabana F, Larbi A, Dupuis G, Fülöp T: Altered neutrophil functions in elderly patients during a 6-month follow-up period after a hip fracture. Exp Gerontol 2015;65:58–68.
39 Hazeldine J, Harris P, Chapple IL, Grant M, Greenwood H, Livesey A, Sapey E, Lord JM: Impaired neutrophil extracellular trap formation: a novel defect in the innate immune system of aged individuals. Aging Cell 2014;13:690–698.
40 Tseng CW, Liu GY: Expanding roles of neutrophils in aging hosts. Curr Opin Immunol 2014;29:43–48.
41 Qian F, Guo X, Wang X, Yuan X, Chen S, Malawista SE, Bockenstedt LK, Allore HG, Montgomery RR: Reduced bioenergetics and toll-like receptor 1 function in human polymorphonuclear leukocytes in aging. Aging (Albany NY) 2014;6:131–139.
42 Fortin CF, Larbi A, Lesur O, Douziech N, Fulop T Jr: Impairment of SHP-1 down-regulation in the lipid rafts of human neutrophils under GM-CSF stimulation contributes to their age-related, altered functions. J Leukoc Biol 2006;79:1061–1072.
43 Fülöp T, Fortin C, Lesur O, Dupuis G, Kotb JR, Lord JM, Larbi A: The innate immune system and aging: what is the contribution to immunosenescence? Open Longevity Science 2012;6:121–132.
44 Linton PJ, Thoman ML: Immunosenescence in monocytes, macrophages, and dendritic cells: lessons learned from the lung and heart. Immunol Lett 2014;162(1 pt B):290–297.
45 Nyugen J, Agrawal S, Gollapudi S, Gupta S: Impaired functions of peripheral blood monocyte subpopulations in aged humans. J Clin Immunol 2010;30:806–813.
46 Seidler S, Zimmermann HW, Bartneck M, Trautwein C, Tacke F: Age dependent alterations of monocyte subsets and monocyte-related chemokine pathways in healthy adults. BMC Immunol 2010;11:30.
47 Avelino-Silva VI, Ho YL, Avelino-Silva TJ, Santos Sde S: Aging and HIV infection. Ageing Res Rev 2011;10:163–172.
48 De Biasi S, Pinti M, Nasi M, Gibellini L, Bertoncelli L, Manzini S, Mussini C, Cossarizza A: HIV-1 infection and the aging of the immune system: facts, similarities and perspectives. J Exp Clin Med 2011;3:143–150.
49 Kedzierska K, Crowe SM: The role of monocytes and macrophages in the pathogenesis of HIV-1 infection. Curr Med Chem 2002;9:1893–1903.
50 Zapata HJ, Shaw AC: Aging of the human innate immune system in HIV infection. Curr Opin Immunol 2014;29:127–136.
51 Nasi M, Pinti M, Mussini C, Cossarizza A: Persistent inflammation in HIV infection: established concepts, new perspectives. Immunol Lett 2014;161:184–188.
52 Okazaki S, Sakaguchi M, Miwa K, Furukado S, Yamagami H, Yagita Y, Mochizuki H, Kitagawa K: Association of interleukin-6 with the progression of carotid atherosclerosis: a 9-year follow-up study. Stroke 2014;45:2924–2929.
53 Neuhaus J, Jacobs DR Jr, Baker JV, Calmy A, Duprez D, La Rosa A, Kuller LH, Pett SL, Ristola M, Ross MJ, Shlipak MG, Tracy R, Neaton JD: Markers of inflammation, coagulation, and renal function are elevated in adults with HIV infection. J Infect Dis 2010;201:1788–1795.
54 Zacca ER, Crespo MI, Acland RP, Roselli E, Núñez NG, Maccioni M, Maletto BA, Pistoresi-Palencia MC, Morón G: Aging impairs the ability of conventional dendritic cells to cross-prime CD8+ T cells upon stimulation with a TLR7 ligand. PLoS One 2015;10:e0140672.
55 Fülöp T, Larbi A, Pawelec G: Human T cell aging and the impact of persistent viral infections. Front Immunol 2013;4:271.
56 Palmer DB: The effect of age on thymic function. Front Immunol 2013;4:316.
57 Qi Q, Zhang DW, Weyand CM, Goronzy JJ: Mechanisms shaping the naïve T cell repertoire in the elderly – thymic involution or peripheral homeostatic proliferation? Exp Gerontol 2014;54:71–74.
58 Appay V, Sauce D: Naive T cells: the crux of cellular immune aging? Exp Gerontol 2014;54:90–93.
59 Pawelec G, McElhaney JE, Aiello AE, Derhovanessian E: The impact of CMV infection on survival in older humans. Curr Opin Immunol 2012;24:507–511.
60 van Baarle D, Tsegaye A, Miedema F, Akbar A: Significance of senescence for virus-specific memory T cell responses: rapid ageing during chronic stimulation of the immune system. Immunol Lett 2005;97:19–29.
61 Appay V, Fastenackels S, Katlama C, Ait-Mohand H, Schneider L, Guihot A, Keller M, Grubeck-Loebenstein B, Simon A, Lambotte O, Hunt PW, Deeks SG, Costagliola D, Autran B, Sauce D: Old age and anti-cytomegalovirus immunity are associated with altered T-cell reconstitution in HIV-1-infected patients. AIDS 2011;25:1813–1822.
62 Fulop T, Le Page A, Fortin C, Witkowski JM, Dupuis G, Larbi A: Cellular signaling in the aging immune system. Curr Opin Immunol 2014;29:105–111.
63 Larbi A, Pawelec G, Wong SC, Goldeck D, Tai JJ, Fülöp T: Impact of age on T cell signaling: a general defect or specific alterations? Ageing Res Rev 2011;10:370–378.
64 Goronzy JJ, Li G, Yu M, Weyand CM: Signaling pathways in aged T cells – a reflection of T cell differentiation, cell senescence and host environment. Semin Immunol 2012;24:365–372.
65 Dock JN, Effros RB: Role of CD8 T cell replicative senescence in human aging and in HIV-mediated immunosenescence. Aging Dis 2011;2:382–397.

66 Derhovanessian E, Chen S, Maier AB, Hähnel K, de Craen AJ, Roelofs H, Westendorp R, Pawelec G: CCR4+ regulatory T cells accumulate in the very elderly and correlate with superior 8-year survival. J Gerontol A Biol Sci Med Sci 2015;70:917–923.

67 Franceschi C, Bonafè M, Valensin S, Olivieri F, De Luca M, Ottaviani E, De Benedictis G: Inflamm-aging. An evolutionary perspective on immunosenescence. Ann N Y Acad Sci 2000;908:244–254.

68 Sansoni P, Vescovini R, Fagnoni FF, Akbar A, Arens R, Chiu YL, Cičin-Šain L, Dechanet-Merville J, Derhovanessian E, Ferrando-Martinez S, Franceschi C, Frasca D, Fulöp T, Furman D, Gkrania-Klotsas E, Goodrum F, Grubeck-Loebenstein B, Hurme M, Kern F, Lilleri D, López-Botet M, Maier AB, Marandu T, Marchant A, Matheï C, Moss P, Muntasell A, Remmerswaal EB, Riddell NE, Rothe K, Sauce D, Shin EC, Simanek AM, Smithey MJ, Söderberg-Nauclér C, Solana R, Thomas PG, van Lier R, Pawelec G, Nikolich-Zugich J: New advances in CMV and immunosenescence. Exp Gerontol 2014;55:54–62.

69 Pawelec G: Hallmarks of human 'immunosenescence': adaptation or dysregulation? Immun Ageing 2012;9:15.

70 Weyand CM, Yang Z, Goronzy JJ: T-cell aging in rheumatoid arthritis. Curr Opin Rheumatol 2014;26:93–100.

71 Laberge RM, Sun Y, Orjalo AV, Patil CK, Freund A, Zhou L, Curran SC, Davalos AR, Wilson-Edell KA, Liu S, Limbad C, Demaria M, Li P, Hubbard GB, Ikeno Y, Javors M, Desprez PY, Benz CC, Kapahi P, Nelson PS, Campisi J: MTOR regulates the pro-tumorigenic senescence-associated secretory phenotype by promoting IL1A translation. Nat Cell Biol 2015;17:1049–1061.

72 Van Deursen JM: The role of senescent cells in ageing. Nature 2014;509:439–446.

73 Tchkonia T, Zhu Y, van Deursen J, Campisi J, Kirkland JL: Cellular senescence and the senescent secretory phenotype: therapeutic opportunities. J Clin Invest 2013;123:966–972.

74 Tabibian-Keissar H, Hazanov L, Schiby G, Rosenthal N, Rakovsky A, Michaeli M, Shahaf GL, Pickman Y, Rosenblatt K, Melamed D, Dunn-Walters D, Mehr R, Barshack I: Aging affects B-cell antigen receptor repertoire diversity in primary and secondary lymphoid tissues. Eur J Immunol 2016;46:480–492.

75 Fessler J, Ficjan A, Duftner C, Dejaco C: The impact of aging on regulatory T-cells. Front Immunol 2013;4:231.

76 Le Page A, Fortin C, Garneau H, Allard N, Tsvetkova K, Tan CT, Larbi A, Dupuis G, Fülöp T: Downregulation of inhibitory SRC homology 2 domain-containing phosphatase-1 (SHP-1) leads to recovery of T cell responses in elderly. Cell Commun Signal 2014;12:2.

77 Li G, Yu M, Lee WW, Tsang M, Krishnan E, Weyand CM, Goronzy JJ: Decline in miR-181a expression with age impairs T cell receptor sensitivity by increasing DUSP6 activity. Nat Med 2012;18:1518–1524.

78 Cevenini E, Caruso C, Candore G, Capri M, Nuzzo D, Duro G, Rizzo C, Colonna-Romano G, Lio D, Di Carlo D, Palmas MG, Scurti M, Pini E, Franceschi C, Vasto S: Age-related inflammation: the contribution of different organs, tissues and systems. How to face it for therapeutic approaches. Curr Pharm Des 2010;16:609–618.

79 Castellani GC, Menichetti G, Garagnani P, Giulia Bacalini M, Pirazzini C, Franceschi C, Collino S, Sala C, Remondini D, Giampieri E, Mosca E, Bersanelli M, Vitali S, Valle IF, Liò P, Milanesi L: Systems medicine of inflammaging. Brief Bioinform 2016;17:527–540.

80 Netea MG, Quintin J, van der Meer JW: Trained immunity: a memory for innate host defense. Cell Host Microbe 2011;9:355–361.

81 Bekkering S, Joosten LA, van der Meer JW, Netea MG, Riksen NP: The epigenetic memory of monocytes and macrophages as a novel drug target in atherosclerosis. Clin Ther 2015;37:914–923.

82 Kyburz D, Karouzakis E, Ospelt C: Epigenetic changes: the missing link. Best Pract Res Clin Rheumatol 2014;28:577–587.

83 Ostuni R, Piccolo V, Barozzi I, Polletti S, Termanini A, Bonifacio S, Curina A, Prosperini E, Ghisletti S, Natoli G: Latent enhancers activated by stimulation in differentiated cells. Cell 2013;152:157–171.

84 Cheng SC, Quintin J, Cramer RA, Shepardson KM, Saeed S, Kumar V, Giamarellos-Bourboulis EJ, Martens JH, Rao NA, Aghajanirefah A, Manjeri GR, Li Y, Ifrim DC, Arts RJ, van der Veer BM, Deen PM, Logie C, O'Neill LA, Willems P, van de Veerdonk FL, van der Meer JW, Ng A, Joosten LA, Wijmenga C, Stunnenberg HG, Xavier RJ, Netea MG: mTOR- and HIF-1α-mediated aerobic glycolysis as metabolic basis for trained immunity. Science 2014;345:1250684.

85 Mohan T, Bhatnagar S, Gupta DL, Rao DN: Current understanding of HIV-1 and T-cell adaptive immunity: progress to date. Microb Pathog 2014;73:60–69.

86 D'Abramo A, Zingaropoli MA, Oliva A, D'Agostino C, Al Moghazi S, De Luca G, Iannetta M, Mastroianni CM, Vullo V: Immune activation, immunosenescence, and osteoprotegerin as markers of endothelial dysfunction in subclinical HIV-associated atherosclerosis. Mediators Inflamm 2014;2014:192594.

87 Deeks SG: HIV infection, inflammation, immunosenescence, and aging. Annu Rev Med 2011;62:141–155.

88 Fernandez S, French MA, Price P: Immunosenescent CD57+CD4+ T-cells accumulate and contribute to interferon-γ responses in HIV patients responding stably to ART. Dis Markers 2011;31:337–342.
89 Decrion AZ, Dichamp I, Varin A, Herbein G: HIV and inflammation. Curr HIV Res 2005;3:243–259.
90 Rajasuriar R, Wright E, Lewin SR: Impact of antiretroviral therapy (ART) timing on chronic immune activation/inflammation and end-organ damage. Curr Opin HIV AIDS 2015;10:35–42.
91 Deeks SG, Lewin SR, Havlir DV: The end of AIDS: HIV infection as a chronic disease. Lancet 2013;382:1525–1533.
92 Passaes CP, Sáez-Cirión A: HIV cure research: advances and prospects. Virology 2014;454–455:340–352.
93 Ipp H, Zemlin A: The paradox of the immune response in HIV infection: when inflammation becomes harmful. Clin Chim Acta 2013;416:96–99.
94 Perreau M, Levy Y, Pantaleo G: Immune response to HIV. Curr Opin HIV AIDS 2013;8:333–340.
95 Kumar A, Abbas W, Herbein G: HIV-1 latency in monocytes/macrophages. Viruses 2014;6:1837–1860.
96 Piconi S, Clerici M: HIV replication, inflammation and atherogenesis: dangerous liaisons. AIDS 2013;27:1521–1522.
97 Brenchley JM, Price DA, Schacker TW, Asher TE, Silvestri G, Rao S, Kazzaz Z, Bornstein E, Lambotte O, Altmann D, Blazar BR, Rodriguez B, Teixeira-Johnson L, Landay A, Martin JN, Hecht FM, Picker LJ, Lederman MM, Deeks SG, Douek DC: Microbial translocation is a cause of systemic immune activation in chronic HIV infection. Nat Med 2006;12:1365–1371.
98 Guaraldi G, Orlando G, Zona S, Menozzi M, Carli F, Garlassi E, Berti A, Rossi E, Roverato A, Palella F: Premature age-related comorbidities among HIV-infected persons compared with the general population. Clin Infect Dis 2011;53:1120–1126.
99 Guaraldi G, Zona S, Orlando G, Carli F, Ligabue G, Fiocchi F, Menozzi M, Rossi R, Modena MG, Raggi P: Human immunodeficiency virus infection is associated with accelerated atherosclerosis. J Antimicrob Chemother 2011;66:1857–1860.
100 Antinori A, Arendt G, Becker JT, Brew BJ, Byrd DA, Cherner M, Clifford DB, Cinque P, Epstein LG, Goodkin K, Gisslen M, Grant I, Heaton RK, Joseph J, Marder K, Marra CM, McArthur JC, Nunn M, Price RW, Pulliam L, Robertson KR, Sacktor N, Valcour V, Wojna VE: Updated research nosology for HIV-associated neurocognitive disorders. Neurology 2007;69:1789–1799.
101 Hunt PW, Martin JN, Sinclair E, Epling L, Teague J, Jacobson MA, Tracy RP, Corey L, Deeks SG: Valganciclovir reduces T cell activation in HIV-infected individuals with incomplete CD4+ T cell recovery on antiretroviral therapy. J Infect Dis 2011;203:1474–1483.
102 Appay V, Sauce D: Immune activation and inflammation in HIV-1 infection: causes and consequences. J Pathol 2008;214:231–241.
103 Pirrone V, Libon DJ, Sell C, Lerner CA, Nonnemacher MR, Wigdahl B: Impact of age on markers of HIV-1 disease. Future Virol 2013;8:81–101.
104 Tsoukas C: Immunosenescence and aging in HIV. Curr Opin HIV AIDS 2014;9:398–404.
105 Wallet MA, Buford TW, Joseph AM, Sankuratri M, Leeuwenburgh C, Pahor M, Manini T, Sleasman JW, Goodenow MM: Increased inflammation but similar physical composition and function in older-aged, HIV-1 infected subjects. BMC Immunol 2015;16:43.
106 Siliciano RF: Opening fronts in HIV vaccine development: targeting reservoirs to clear and cure. Nat Med 2014;20:480–481.
107 Chéret A, Bacchus-Souffan C, Avettand-Fenoël V, Mélard A, Nembot G, Blanc C, Samri A, Sáez-Cirión A, Hocqueloux L, Lascoux-Combe C, Allavena C, Goujard C, Valantin MA, Leplatois A, Meyer L, Rouzioux C, Autran B; OPTIPRIM ANRS-147 Study Group: Combined ART started during acute HIV infection protects central memory CD4+ T cells and can induce remission. J Antimicrob Chemother 2015;70:2108–2120.
108 Sáez-Cirión A, Bacchus C, Hocqueloux L, Avettand-Fenoel V, Girault I, Lecuroux C, Potard V, Versmisse P, Melard A, Prazuck T, Descours B, Guergnon J, Viard JP, Boufassa F, Lambotte O, Goujard C, Meyer L, Costagliola D, Venet A, Pancino G, Autran B, Rouzioux C; ANRS VISCONTI Study Group: Post-treatment HIV-1 controllers with a long-term virological remission after the interruption of early initiated antiretroviral therapy ANRS VISCONTI Study. PLoS Pathog 2013;9:e1003211.
109 Brooks JT, Buchacz K, Gebo KA, Mermin J: HIV infection and older Americans: the public health perspective. Am J Public Health 2012;102:1516–1526.
110 Burton CT, Hardy GA, Sullivan AK, Nelson MR, Gazzard B, Gotch FM, Imami N: Impact of NNRTI compared to PI-based highly active antiretroviral therapy on CCR5 receptor expression, beta-chemokines and IL-16 secretion in HIV-1 infection. Clin Exp Immunol 2002;130:286–292.

111 Jantarapakde J, Phanuphak N, Chaturawit C, Pengnonyang S, Mathajittiphan P, Takamtha P, Dungjun N, Pinyakorn S, Pima W, Prasithsirikul W, Phanuphak P: Prevalence of metabolic syndrome among antiretroviral-naive and antiretroviral-experienced HIV-1 infected Thai adults. AIDS Patient Care STDS 2014;28:331–340.
112 Margolick JB, Ferrucci L: Accelerating aging research: how can we measure the rate of biologic aging? Exp Gerontol 2015;64:78–80.
113 Fitch KV, Guggina LM, Keough HM, Dolan Looby SE, Hadigan C, Anderson EJ, Hubbard J, Liebau JG, Johnsen S, Wei J, Makimura H, Stanley TL, Lo J, Grinspoon SK: Decreased respiratory quotient in relation to resting energy expenditure in HIV-infected and noninfected subjects. Metabolism 2009; 58:608–615.
114 Wada N, Jacobson LP, Cohen M, French A, Phair J, Munoz A: Cause-specific life expectancies after 35 years of age for human immunodeficiency syndrome-infected and human immunodeficiency syndrome-negative individuals followed simultaneously in long-term cohort studies, 1984–2008. Am J Epidemiol 2013;177:116–125.
115 Martin J, Volberding P: HIV and premature aging: a field still in its infancy. Ann Intern Med 2010;153: 477–479.
116 Trautmann L, Janbazian L, Chomont N, Said EA, Gimmig S, Bessette B, Boulassel MR, Delwart E, Sepulveda H, Balderas RS, Routy JP, Haddad EK, Sekaly RP: Upregulation of PD-1 expression on HIV-specific CD8+ T cells leads to reversible immune dysfunction. Nat Med 2006;12:1198–1202.
117 Akbar AN, Henson SM: Are senescence and exhaustion intertwined or unrelated processes that compromise immunity? Nat Rev Immunol 2011; 11:289–295.
118 Althoff KN, McGinnis KA, Wyatt CM, Freiberg MS, Gilbert C, Oursler KK, Rimland D, Rodriguez-Barradas MC, Dubrow R, Park LS, Skanderson M, et al: Comparison of risk and age at diagnosis of myocardial infarction, end-stage renal disease, and non-AIDS-defining cancer in HIV-infected versus uninfected adults. Clin Infect Dis 2015;60:627–638.
119 Martin J, Volberding P: HIV and premature aging: a field still in its infancy. Ann Intern Med 2010;153: 477–479.

Tamàs Fülöp, MD, PhD
Research Center on Aging, Faculty of Medicine and Health Sciences
University of Sherbrooke, 3001
12th Avenue North, Sherbrooke, QC J1H 5N4 (Canada)
E-Mail Tamas.Fulop@Usherbrooke.ca

Brennan-Ing M, DeMarco RF (eds): HIV and Aging. Interdiscipl Top Gerontol Geriatr.
Basel, Karger, 2017, vol 42, pp 47–58 (DOI: 10.1159/000448543)

# Biomarkers and Clinical Indices of Aging with HIV

Kathleen V. Fitch • Meghan Noonan Feldpausch •
Sara E. Dolan Looby

Program in Nutritional Metabolism, Massachusetts General Hospital (KVF, MNF, SEDL), Yvonne L. Munn Center for Nursing Research and Harvard Medical School (SEDL), Boston, Mass., USA

**Abstract**

HIV infection may potentiate specific biomarkers that influence the development of premature clinical indices commonly associated with aging. Therefore, predicting mortality outcomes in people living with HIV is extremely important as this population ages. This chapter describes biomarkers associated with inflammation, coagulation, and immune activation in HIV, and reviews the association between specific biomarkers and the development of co-morbid conditions in individuals with HIV. Measures that incorporate specific biomarkers related to HIV infection, designed to predict mortality outcomes in individuals with HIV, are also discussed.


## Introduction

Emerging evidence suggests that HIV and/or antiretroviral therapy (ART) use may enhance the onset of aging and the development of co-morbid conditions commonly observed in non-HIV-infected individuals of advanced age. The onset of early aging in the HIV population has vast implications on morbidity and mortality, functional status, and quality of life. However, untangling the physiologic underpinnings of premature aging and associated co-morbid conditions in the HIV population is complex. Individual factors including older age at the time of HIV diagnosis and degree of viral suppression, coupled with HIV-specific factors such as chronic inflammation and immune dysfunction, may influence the development of clinical indices frequently observed in older persons [1]. Further, social and behavioral factors, in addition to modifiable risk factors such as substance abuse and smoking, may negatively impact an already precarious health state experienced by individuals with HIV.

Although standard biomarkers to characterize an aging phenotype among HIV-infected persons have not been formally established, recent studies have evaluated the role specific biomarkers may play in the premature development of clinical indices commonly associated with older age.

This chapter will:

- Provide an overview of biomarkers associated with inflammation, coagulation, and immune activation in HIV.
- Review prior studies evaluating the relationship between specific biomarkers and the development of clinical indices in HIV-infected individuals.
- Discuss measures that incorporate specific biomarkers and clinical indices to predict mortality outcomes in patients with HIV, such as the Veterans Aging Cohort Study (VACS) index.

## Immune Activation, Inflammation, and Development of Clinical Indices in HIV

A number of non-AIDS associated conditions such as cardiovascular disease (CVD), cancers, renal disease, and neurological disorders are increasingly prevalent among HIV-infected individuals, despite sustained viral suppression and restoration of the CD4 T-cell count [2–6]. In addition to the development of co-morbid conditions, HIV may be a predictor of frailty. To further explore this among individuals with HIV, investigators of the Multicenter AIDS Cohort Study (MACS) adapted a frailty-related phenotype (FRP), in which FRP was defined as experiencing at least 3 of the following variables: slowness, exhaustion, physical shrinking (weight loss), and decreased activity level. Increased FRP was found to be more prevalent among HIV-infected versus non-HIV-infected individuals, and was present approximately 10 years earlier among the HIV-infected subjects (HIV: age 55 years versus non-HIV: 65 years), indicating that signs of aging may occur earlier among individuals with HIV [7].

Early research suggested that more traditional factors explained the excessive rates of non-AIDS conditions observed in this population, including the effects of HIV on the immune system, side effects of ART, and personal factors such as family history and smoking. However, accumulating evidence supports a more physiologic hypothesis that abnormal and persistent immune activation experienced by HIV-infected individuals results in a chronic state of inflammation and associated abnormalities in coagulation that may contribute to excess morbidity and mortality, and the development of serious non-AIDS conditions [8–10].

One of the earliest cohort studies to expose the detrimental effects of persistent viral replication on the development of non-AIDS conditions was the Strategies for Management of ART (SMART) study. The SMART study evaluated among HIV-infected individuals, the effects of guided interruption of ART compared to continuous use of ART on the development of opportunistic infections or death (primary endpoint) and major CVD, renal or liver disease (secondary endpoint) [11]. The SMART study enrolled over 5,000 HIV-infected patients internationally and was conducted due to concerns over continued daily adherence to ART and development of several metabolic complications related to ART use. The ART interruption arm was discontinued after an average of 16-month follow-up, when an interim analysis revealed that treatment interruption was related to increased risk of all-cause mortality (hazard ratio (HR) 1.8, $p < 0.007$) and risk of death or development of opportunistic disease (HR 2.6, $p < 0.001$) [11]. Surprisingly, most deaths were attributed to non-AIDS conditions including cardiovascular, renal, and hepatic disease. The findings of the SMART study were unexpected, since the investigators initially hypothesized that ART was the source of many non-AIDS conditions observed in individuals with HIV infection; however, study findings showed that factors related to HIV may enhance the development of these conditions [11].

The etiology of persistent immune activation and inflammation in ART-treated HIV infection is multifactorial, and remains under investigation. Recently published review articles highlight several factors that may contribute to this perpetual inflammatory state including continuous viral replication, microbial translocation, and co-infection with chronic viruses such as cytomegalovirus and hepatitis C virus (HCV); as well as associated consequences of immune activation, including the development of atherosclerosis and other chronic conditions [12, 13]. Indeed, the collective burden of HIV-associated immune dysregulation on morbidity and mortality in HIV-infected individuals will present novel management challenges for clinicians caring for this population as they progress to advanced age.

## Biomarkers and Morbidity and Mortality in HIV

Persistent immune activation prompts an inflammatory response that can be measured by several biomarkers in the blood. Given the influx of aging HIV-infected individuals, the use of biomarkers to assess age-associated conditions may become an important strategy for HIV assessment and management. Cross-sectional studies have demonstrated that markers of immune activation (soluble CD163 (sCD163), soluble CD14 (sCD14)), inflammation (C-reactive protein (CRP), interleukin-6 (IL-6)), and coagulation (D-dimer) are altered in HIV infection [5, 14–17]. While altered levels of these biomarkers do not play a direct causal role in excess morbidity, mortality, and the development of non-AIDS conditions, measuring these biomarkers may provide important clues about immune system activity in individuals with HIV. These biomarkers may also provide signals regarding increased risk of serious non-AIDS related conditions, commonly associated with aging in the general population, including CVD, neurocognitive dysfunction, osteoporosis, and non-AIDS cancers.

In follow-up to the findings of the initial SMART study described before, a secondary analysis was completed to further explore potential causes for the increased risk of death from non-AIDS conditions observed in the ART interruption arm of the study cohort [10]. Investigators of this analysis hypothesized that increased HIV viral load levels observed in the treatment interruption arm induced inflammatory changes including thrombosis and fibrinolysis that increase the risk of mortality in this population. This study determined that biomarkers including IL-6, a proinflammatory cytokine, and D-dimer were significantly increased during the first month following the interruption of ART. Additionally, baseline hsCRP, IL-6, and D-dimer levels were related to mortality among study participants in both the interrupted ART and continuous ART groups, demonstrating an effect of HIV, despite ART use, on inflammatory and coagulation pathways that relate to all causes of mortality [10]. Findings from this study were among the first to show that HIV induces activation of inflammatory and coagulation pathways that may enhance the development of comorbid conditions in this population [10].

Investigating the precise role specific biomarkers play in the development of age-associated non-AIDS conditions, and elucidating the prognostic value of biomarkers for determining morbidity and mortality in the HIV population are priority research areas for the National Institutes of Health, Office of AIDS Research [1]. Although many biomarkers are still in an investigational stage, an overview of biomarkers of inflammation, coagulation, and immune activation associated with mortality and the development of non-AIDS conditions is presented in table 1.

## Biomarkers of Inflammation

### *Interleukin-6*

IL-6 is both an acute phase reactant and a pro-inflammatory cytokine. In a state of chronic inflammation, IL-6 elicits mononuclear cell accumulation resulting in antiapoptotic functions on T-cells [18]. IL-6 has also been found to promote osteoclast formation [19, 20], and IL-6 production has been found to be an important component of the autocrine [21] and paracrine [22] processes that are related to growth of solid tumors.

Levels of IL-6 are increased in HIV infection [16], and IL-6 independently predicts the progression of primary HIV infection [23]. IL-6 has been related to an increased risk of all-cause mortality [10, 24] and death due to CVD in HIV-infected individuals [25]. With regard to non-AIDS defining illnesses, a sub-analysis of the SMART study demonstrated that IL-6 is related to CVD events [2], and among 3

Table 1. Overview of biomarkers and associations with morbidity/mortality in HIV

| Biomarker | Biomarker classification | Associated with increased mortality | Associated with non-AIDS conditions |
|---|---|---|---|
| IL-6 | Proinflammatory | Yes [10, 24] | CVD [2, 25]<br>BMD [27]<br>Cancer [26] |
| CRP | Proinflammatory | Yes [8, 10] | CVD [2, 4] |
| D-dimer | Coagulation | Yes [10, 33] | CVD [34, 35] |
| sCD14 | Immune activation | Yes [9] | CVD [41–43]<br>Neuro [44] |
| sCD163 | Immune activation | Unknown | CVD [45, 46] |

BMD = Bone mineral density; Neuro = neurological function. Numbers in the table correspond to the appropriate reference.

pooled cohorts of HIV-infected individuals, IL-6 was associated with an increased risk of cancer (HIV-associated or non-HIV associated) [26]. In a prospective study to evaluate bone loss in HIV, Hileman et al. [27] determined that higher IL-6 at baseline was independently associated with progression of osteopenia or osteoporosis.

*C-Reactive Protein*

CRP is a pro-inflammatory marker that is produced predominantly in hepatocytes, and is regulated by IL-6 [28]. CRP is present in atherosclerotic lesions, where it binds to various unmodified and modified LDL particles, and is utilized by macrophages and ultimately involved in foam cell formation [29].

CRP levels have been shown to be elevated in HIV-infected individuals compared with non-HIV-infected individuals [15, 30]. CRP was also assessed in the SMART main study and sub-analyses, and similar to IL-6, was found to be related to all-cause mortality [10] and CVD events in HIV-infected individuals [2]. Similarly, in The Study of Fat Redistribution and Metabolic Change, higher CRP was related to higher adjusted odds of death among HIV-infected individuals [8], and a cross-sectional analysis from the MACS cohort determined that elevated CRP was associated with more rapid progression to AIDS compared to HIV-infected individuals with lower CRP levels [31]. Furthermore, in an analysis from the Partners HealthCare System of 487 HIV and 69,870 non-HIV infected individuals, Triant et al. [4] found that HIV and elevated CRP levels were associated with an increased risk of acute myocardial infarction (AMI), and HIV-infected individuals with elevated CRP had an increased relative risk of AMI compared to non-HIV-infected individuals.

## Biomarkers of Coagulopathy

*D-Dimer*

D-dimer level is a measure of clot formation resulting from the degradation of fibrin following blood clots [32]. Clots form in blood vessels during CVD and may be facilitated by inflammatory cytokines. The VACS further validated the value of D-dimer in predicting mortality in HIV-infected patients [33], as did the SMART study [10]. D-dimer levels have also been associated with venous thromboembolic events [34] and cardiovascular events [35] in 2 retrospective case control studies among HIV-infected individuals. These findings demonstrate a strong relationship between D-dimer and vascular events in HIV-infection.

In a more detailed analysis to characterize the effects of HIV replication and ART on coagulation biology, Baker et al. [36] measured pro- and anticoagulation factors within the extrinsic (tissue factor) pathway. Findings from this investigation demonstrated that while untreated HIV infection led to some short-term increases in some pro-coagulation measures, the net effect of HIV replication was increased coagulation potential, suggesting that HIV infection may upregulate pathways related to clotting [36].

More recently, Green et al. [37] investigated the interaction between coagulation, platelets, and the adaptive immune system in HIV-infected individuals compared with healthy controls. Platelets of the HIV-infected participants formed conjugates with T cells and were observed in CD4+ and CD8+ T cell subsets; these conjugates were composed of activated platelets and were significantly associated with D-dimer levels [37]. These platelet–monocyte conjugates may have an effect on maintaining inflamed tissues by way of increasing T-cell trafficking.

## Markers of Immune Activation

*Soluble CD14*

Immune activation is altered in HIV disease, and this is partially due to rapid CD4 T-cell depletion that takes place within weeks of infection [38]. T-cell depletion occurs mainly in the gastrointestinal tract, and has a deleterious effect on the mucosal lining that in turn allows for translocation of microbes, ultimately resulting in systemic immune activation [38]. Soluble sCD163, sCD14, and IL-6 are biomarkers released by activated monocytes and macrophages. sCD14 and lipopolysaccharide (LPS) are commonly used biomarkers to measure microbial translocation [38]. LPSs are the major components of the cell wall in gram-negative bacteria and are strong stimulators of immune responses through their interaction with the membrane receptor CD14 to induce cytokines such as tumor necrosis factor-α and IL-6 [39]. Levels of LPS were observed to be predictive of HIV progression by Marchetti et al. [40], such that LPS was an indicator of microbial translocation. However, a relationship between LPS and clinical outcomes among SMART study participants was not observed by Sandler et al. [9], though investigators determined that sCD14 levels were significantly related to all-cause mortality in this cohort of HIV-infected individuals [9]. Plasma levels of sCD14 also correlate with measures of subclinical atherosclerosis among individuals with HIV [41, 42] and LPS, and sCD14 has been shown to predict increased carotid intima media thickness, a measure of subclinical atherosclerosis, in HIV-infected individuals [43]. In addition to CVD, increased plasma levels of sCD14 have been associated with neurological dysfunction in HIV-infected individuals as assessed by formal neurological testing [44].

*Soluble CD163*

CD163 is a hemoglobin scavenger receptor expressed on monocytes and macrophages. Activation of monocytes and macrophages with LPS and other factors causes CD163 to shed from the cell surface in a soluble form, referred to as sCD163 [14]. sCD163 is elevated in acute and chronic HIV infections and is linked with viral replication as well as monocyte and macrophage immune responses [14]. Elevated levels of sCD163 are associated with the presence of CVD among HIV-infected patients. In studies exploring subclinical atherosclerosis among HIV-infected individuals compared with HIV-negative individuals with similar CVD risk factors, plasma sCD163 was related to increased prevalence of atherosclerotic plaques among those with HIV [45, 46]. In a more recent study, levels of sCD163 correlated with arterial inflammation in individuals receiving ART as determined by PET scan [47].

In summary, there is evidence of both increased inflammation and coagulation in HIV infection. These processes do not likely occur independently. HIV infection may lead to activation of inflammatory markers, thereby stimulating the coagulation cascade, and this in turn can substantially stimulate inflammatory activity and perpetuate a persistent state of inflammation and increased coagulation in HIV [48]. Large clinical trials are needed to determine if the relationship between inflammation, coagulation, and immune activation does in fact increase the mortality as well as non-AIDS illnesses. Effective therapies that target these processes will likely increase the life span and reduce the incidence of non-AIDS conditions in individuals living with HIV.

## Measures to Predict Mortality in HIV-Infected Individuals

In addition to biomarkers, assessment of clinical indices that predict mortality and risk for development of conditions linked to mortality is important for optimal clinical management of the aging HIV population. Indeed, clinical calculators to determine the risk for development of specific conditions, such as CVD, exist and include the Framingham risk calculator (http://cvdrisk.nhlbi.nih.gov/) and the Atherosclerotic Cardiovascular Disease (ASCVD) risk calculator (http://tools.acc.org/ASCVD-Risk-Estimator/). However, these measures comprise traditional CVD risk factors, commonly observed in non-HIV-infected individuals and do not consider non-traditional risk factors known to associate with mortality in HIV infection including HIV viral load, CD4 count, and AIDS defining illnesses [49, 50].

As HIV-infected individuals continue to advance in age, measures to determine the risk for morbidity and mortality that are sensitive to the clinical characteristics and unique risk factors experienced by this population are needed. A recent study evaluated the use of a clinical risk calculator to predict the CVD risk using data from the Data-Collection on Adverse Effects of Anti-HIV Drugs study [51]. Although useful, this risk calculator focuses only on one measure of morbidity and mortality related to aging, CVD, and may not be generalizable to all-cause mortality in this population. Alternatively, the Veterans Aging Cohort Study (VACS) index was established to create a mortality risk assessment tool specific to HIV-infected individuals, and was developed and validated using data from this cohort [52] (http://medicine.yale.edu/intmed/vacs/). The VACS index score is a calculated, weighted score that estimates all-cause mortality in HIV-infected individuals using carefully selected measures including: markers of HIV disease and non-HIV-associated biomarkers indicative of anemia, renal, and liver dysfunction. The overarching goal was to create a risk prediction calculator to capture the burden of HIV disease, markers of chronic inflammation, and subsequent organ dysfunction thought to be related to the risk of all-cause mortality in the HIV population.

The original VACS index, which was tested and validated in HIV-positive veterans initiating treatment with ART, utilized the following variables to calculate the mortality risk: age, CD4 count, HIV viral load, AIDS-defining illness, estimated glomerular filtration rate (calculated imputing creatinine, age, gender, race), liver fibrosis (FIB4 index, calculated using ALT, AST, platelets, age), hemoglobin, HCV, hepatitis B virus (HBV), and substance abuse. This index was validated in 6 additional VACS cohorts and also among subgroups of individuals with HCV co-infection, women, and those with a HIV viral load <500 copies/ml [52]. The VACS index has since been modified to calculate the mortality risk among HIV-infected individuals who have received ART for at least 1 year [53]. When the modified VACS index was created, 3 variables were removed from the original index: (1) AIDS defining illness, as this was rarely observed in individuals on ART, (2) HBV, as data was not always available, and HBV associated with HCV, and (3) substance abuse, as these data were not collected in a standard fashion [53] (fig. 1).

The VACS index has been formally evaluated in a number of clinical trials among HIV-infected individuals, and was shown to be a strong predictor of 5-year mortality among HIV-infected individuals receiving 1–5 years of ART [54]. The VACS index has been associated with mortality in younger, healthy HIV populations [55] and in older, multi-ART-regimen resistant HIV-infected individuals [56]. Furthermore, the VACS index has also been shown to correlate with rates and severity of hospitalization in HIV-infected individuals. In this regard, elevated VACS scores correlated with hospitalization in HIV-infected patients, and more specifically, predicted increased admission rates to the medical intensive care unit [57]. In addition to mortality, VACS index scores correlate with various co-morbidities associated with aging, including

| Component | Level | Points |
|---|---|---|
| Age (years) | <50 | 0 |
| | 50 to 64 | 12 |
| | ≥65 | 27 |
| CD4 (cells/mm³) | ≥500 | 0 |
| | 350 to 499 | 6 |
| | 200 to 349 | 6 |
| | 100 to 199 | 10 |
| | 50 to 99 | 28 |
| | <50 | 29 |
| HIV-1 RNA (copies/ml) | <500 | 0 |
| | 500 to 99.999 | 7 |
| | $\geq 1 \times 10^5$ | 14 |
| Hemoglobin (g/dl) | ≥14 | 0 |
| | 12 to 13.9 | 10 |
| | 10 to 11.9 | 22 |
| | <10 | 38 |
| FIB-4 | <1.45 | 0 |
| | 1.45 to 3.25 | 6 |
| | >3.25 | 25 |
| eGFR (ml/min) | ≥60 | 0 |
| | 45 to 59.9 | 6 |
| | 30 to 44.9 | 8 |
| | <30 | 26 |
| Hepatitis C co-infection | | 5 |

**Fig. 1.** The VACS index. http://medicine.yale.edu/intmed/vacs/welcome/vacsindexinfo.aspx.

frailty, fragility fracture, disability, and community acquired pneumonia [58–61]. The VACS index has also been shown to associate with the presence of HIV-associated neurocognitive impairment when controlling other psychological and psychosocial factors, including depressed mood and substance abuse [62].

Correlations have also been observed between the VACS index and various biomarkers affiliated with immune activation, inflammation, aging, and HIV. Williams et al. [63] demonstrated among HIV patients described as 'immunologic non-responders' (e.g. undetectable viral load and concurrent CD4 count less than 250 cells/mm$^3$), elevated sCD14 and sCD163 levels associated with higher VACS index scores, HCV, and FIB 4. Among the participants in the VACS cohort receiving ART, the VACS index correlated with biomarkers of coagulopathy and inflammation including D-dimer, IL-6, and sCD14, 3 biomarkers shown to associate with mortality [33]. In an analysis controlling the VACS index, D-dimer and sCD14 remained associated with mortality, whereas IL-6 was not [33]. This finding suggests that D-dimer and sCD14 are markers associated with mortality independent of the VACS score, which may be valuable in predicting the mortality risk in the clinical setting [33].

Limitations to the VACS index have also been cited in the literature, and include potential over-prediction of mortality in HIV-infected individuals [64], and limited generalizability for use in HIV-infected women. Indeed, the VACS index was developed among a cohort largely comprised of men, and although it has been validated among women, tailoring the data collected in the VACS index to include more gender-specific markers may increase the accuracy of calculating the risk of mortality in HIV-positive women [65].

In summary, emerging data illustrating the relationship of the VACS index with multiple factors affecting aging and risk of morbidity and mortality in HIV-infected individuals suggest that the VACS index may be a useful measure to improve patient care and enhance preventative health in the clinical setting. Furthermore, there is great potential to utilize the VACS index in future research trials related to HIV, aging, and mortality.

## Conclusion

This chapter highlights several tremendous breakthroughs regarding the identification and investigation of biomarkers associated with the development of clinical indices commonly observed with aging and mortality that may be potentiated by HIV infection. However, as individuals with HIV live longer, more research is needed to further define HIV-specific characteristics of existing biomarkers; identify novel biomarkers that may have prognostic value to HIV-infected individuals; and enhance the current understanding of the link between persistent immune activation and inflammation, and the contribution of these processes to morbidity and mortality in this population. Additionally, further evaluation of existing measures that predict outcomes including all-cause and cause-specific mortality, which are unique to HIV-infected individuals are needed, such as the VACS index. These priority research areas are supported by the Office of AIDS Research [1] and are critical to the overall health and well-being of individuals living with HIV. Importantly, early identification of burdensome co-morbid conditions through the use of biomarkers and clinical calculators will provide both patients and clinicians an opportunity to engage in a discussion around education and supportive strategies to reduce modifiable risk factors, and address psycho-social factors that influence health outcomes and quality of life.

## References


1 High KP, et al: HIV and aging: state of knowledge and areas of critical need for research. A report to the NIH office of AIDS research by the HIV and aging working group. J Acquir Immune Defic Syndr 2012; 60(suppl 1):S1–S18.
2 Duprez DA, et al: Inflammation, coagulation and cardiovascular disease in HIV-infected individuals. PLoS One 2012;7:e44454.
3 Silverberg MJ, et al: Risk of cancers during interrupted antiretroviral therapy in the SMART study. AIDS 2007;21:1957–1963.
4 Triant VA, et al: Increased acute myocardial infarction rates and cardiovascular risk factors among patients with human immunodeficiency virus disease. J Clin Endocrinol Metab 2007;92:2506–2512.
5 Schouten J, et al: Cross-sectional comparison of the prevalence of age-associated comorbidities and their risk factors between HIV-infected and uninfected individuals: the AGEhIV cohort study. Clin Infect Dis 2014;59:1787–1797.

6 Vivithanaporn P, et al: Neurologic disease burden in treated HIV/AIDS predicts survival: a population-based study. Neurology 2010;75:1150–1158.
7 Desquilbet L, et al: HIV-1 infection is associated with an earlier occurrence of a phenotype related to frailty. J Gerontol A Biol Sci Med Sci 2007;62:1279–1286.
8 Tien PC, et al: Inflammation and mortality in HIV-infected adults: analysis of the FRAM study cohort. J Acquir Immune Defic Syndr 2010;55:316–322.
9 Sandler NG, et al: Plasma levels of soluble CD14 independently predict mortality in HIV infection. J Infect Dis 2011;203:780–790.
10 Kuller LH, et al: Inflammatory and coagulation biomarkers and mortality in patients with HIV infection. PLoS Med 2008;5:e203.
11 Strategies for Management of Antiretroviral Therapy (SMART) Study Group, El-Sadr WM, et al: CD4+ count-guided interruption of antiretroviral treatment. N Engl J Med 2006;355:2283–2296.
12 Hunt PW: HIV and inflammation: mechanisms and consequences. Curr HIV/AIDS Rep 2012;9:139–147.
13 Zanni MV, Grinspoon SK: HIV-specific immune dysregulation and atherosclerosis. Curr HIV/AIDS Rep 2012;9:200–205.
14 Burdo TH, et al: Soluble CD163 made by monocyte/macrophages is a novel marker of HIV activity in early and chronic infection prior to and after antiretroviral therapy. J Infect Dis 2011;204:154–163.
15 Dolan SE, et al: Increased cardiovascular disease risk indices in HIV-infected women. J Acquir Immune Defic Syndr 2005;39:44–54.
16 Breen EC, et al: Infection with HIV is associated with elevated IL-6 levels and production. J Immunol 1990;144:480–484.
17 Jong E, et al: The effect of initiating combined antiretroviral therapy on endothelial cell activation and coagulation markers in South African HIV-infected individuals. Thromb Haemost 2010;104:1228–1234.
18 Gabay C: Interleukin-6 and chronic inflammation. Arthritis Res Ther 2006;8(suppl 2):S3.
19 Ishimi Y, et al: IL-6 is produced by osteoblasts and induces bone resorption. J Immunol 1990;145:3297–3303.
20 Kwan Tat S, et al: IL-6, RANKL, TNF-alpha/IL-1: interrelations in bone resorption pathophysiology. Cytokine Growth Factor Rev 2004;15:49–60.
21 Dougan M, et al: A dual role for the immune response in a mouse model of inflammation-associated lung cancer. J Clin Invest 2011;121:2436–2446.
22 Stone RL, et al: Paraneoplastic thrombocytosis in ovarian cancer. N Engl J Med 2012;366:610–618.
23 Hamlyn E, et al: Interleukin-6 and D-dimer levels at seroconversion as predictors of HIV-1 disease progression. AIDS 2014;28:869–874.
24 French MA, et al: Plasma levels of cytokines and chemokines and the risk of mortality in HIV-infected individuals: a case-control analysis nested in a large clinical trial. AIDS 2015;29:847–851.
25 Borges AH, et al: Determinants of IL-6 levels during HIV infection. J Int AIDS Soc 2014;17(4 suppl 3): 19482.
26 Borges ÁH, et al: Predicting risk of cancer during HIV infection: the role of inflammatory and coagulation biomarkers. AIDS 2013;27:1433–1441.
27 Hileman CO, et al: Is bone loss linked to chronic inflammation in antiretroviral-naive HIV-infected adults? A 48-week matched cohort study. AIDS 2014;28:1759–1767.
28 Heinrich PC, Castell JV, Andus T: Interleukin-6 and the acute phase response. Biochem J 1990;265:621–636.
29 Zimmermann O, et al: C-reactive protein in human atherogenesis: facts and fiction. Mediators Inflamm 2014;2014:561428.
30 Sundaram M, Anitha JC, Srinivas CN, Sunil SS, Ashwin N, Balakrishnan P, Muragavel KG, Suniti S, Kumarasamy N: C-Reactive Protein in HIV-Infected Patients – Could It Be a Marker of Immunosuppression? Toronto, XVI International AIDS Conference, 2006.
31 Lau B, et al: C-reactive protein is a marker for human immunodeficiency virus disease progression. Arch Intern Med 2006;166:64–70.
32 Eisenberg PR, et al: Validity of enzyme-linked immunosorbent assays of cross-linked fibrin degradation products as a measure of clot lysis. Circulation 1990;82:1159–1168.
33 Justice AC, et al: Does an index composed of clinical data reflect effects of inflammation, coagulation, and monocyte activation on mortality among those aging with HIV? Clin Infect Dis 2012;54:984–994.
34 Musselwhite LW, et al: Markers of endothelial dysfunction, coagulation and tissue fibrosis independently predict venous thromboembolism in HIV. AIDS 2011;25:787–795.
35 Ford ES, et al: Traditional risk factors and D-dimer predict incident cardiovascular disease events in chronic HIV infection. AIDS 2010;24:1509–1517.
36 Baker J, et al: Monocyte Activation, but Not T cell Activation, Predicts Progression of Coronary Artery Calcium in a Contemporary HIV Cohort. Atlanta, CROI, 2013, p 66 LB.
37 Green SA, et al: Activated platelet-T-cell conjugates in peripheral blood of patients with HIV infection: coupling coagulation/inflammation and T cells. AIDS 2015;29:1297–1308.
38 Brenchley JM, et al: Microbial translocation is a cause of systemic immune activation in chronic HIV infection. Nat Med 2006;12:1365–1371.
39 Alexander C, Rietschel ET: Bacterial lipopolysaccharides and innate immunity. J Endotoxin Res 2001;7: 167–202.

40 Marchetti G, et al: Microbial translocation predicts disease progression of HIV-infected antiretroviral-naive patients with high CD4+ cell count. AIDS 2011;25:1385–1394.
41 Merlini E, et al: T-cell phenotypes, apoptosis and inflammation in HIV+ patients on virologically effective cART with early atherosclerosis. PLoS One 2012; 7:e46073.
42 McKibben RA, et al: Elevated levels of monocyte activation markers are associated with subclinical atherosclerosis in men with and those without HIV infection. J Infect Dis 2015;211:1219–1228.
43 Kelesidis T, et al: Biomarkers of microbial translocation and macrophage activation: association with progression of subclinical atherosclerosis in HIV-1 infection. J Infect Dis 2012;206:1558–1567.
44 Fischer-Smith T, et al: CNS invasion by CD14+/CD16+ peripheral blood-derived monocytes in HIV dementia: perivascular accumulation and reservoir of HIV infection. J Neurovirol 2001;7:528–541.
45 Burdo TH, et al: Soluble CD163, a novel marker of activated macrophages, is elevated and associated with noncalcified coronary plaque in HIV-infected patients. J Infect Dis 2011;204:1227–1236.
46 Fitch KV, et al: Noncalcified coronary atherosclerotic plaque and immune activation in HIV-infected women. J Infect Dis 2013;208:1737–1746.
47 Subramanian S, et al: Arterial inflammation in patients with HIV. JAMA 2012;308:379–386.
48 Levi M, van der Poll T, Büller HR: Bidirectional relation between inflammation and coagulation. Circulation 2004;109:2698–2704.
49 May M, et al: Prognosis of HIV-1-infected patients up to 5 years after initiation of HAART: collaborative analysis of prospective studies. AIDS 2007;21: 1185–1197.
50 May MT, et al: HIV treatment response and prognosis in Europe and North America in the first decade of highly active antiretroviral therapy: a collaborative analysis. Lancet 2006;368:451–458.
51 Friis-Møller N, et al: An updated prediction model of the global risk of cardiovascular disease in HIV-positive persons: the data-collection on adverse effects of anti-HIV drugs (D:A:D) study. Eur J Prev Cardiol 2016;23:214–223.
52 Justice AC, et al: Towards a combined prognostic index for survival in HIV infection: the role of 'non-HIV' biomarkers. HIV Med 2010;11:143–151.
53 Tate JP, et al: An internationally generalizable risk index for mortality after one year of antiretroviral therapy. AIDS 2013;27:563–572.
54 Justice AC, et al: Predictive accuracy of the veterans aging cohort study index for mortality with HIV infection: a North American cross cohort analysis. J Acquir Immune Defic Syndr 2013;62:149–163.
55 Bebu I, et al: The VACS index predicts mortality in a young, healthy HIV population starting highly active antiretroviral therapy. J Acquir Immune Defic Syndr 2014;65:226–230.
56 Brown ST, et al: The VACS index accurately predicts mortality and treatment response among multi-drug resistant HIV infected patients participating in the options in management with antiretrovirals (OPTIMA) study. PLoS One 2014;9:e92606.
57 Akgün KM, et al: Risk factors for hospitalization and medical intensive care unit (MICU) admission among HIV-infected veterans. J Acquir Immune Defic Syndr 2013;62:52–59.
58 Oursler KK, et al: Association of the veterans aging cohort study index with exercise capacity in HIV-infected adults. AIDS Res Hum Retroviruses 2013; 29:1218–1223.
59 Escota GV, et al: Short communication: the veterans aging cohort study index is an effective tool to assess baseline frailty status in a contemporary cohort of HIV-infected persons. AIDS Res Hum Retroviruses 2015;31:313–317.
60 Barakat LA, et al: Comparing clinical outcomes in HIV-infected and uninfected older men hospitalized with community-acquired pneumonia. HIV Med 2015;16:421–430.
61 Womack JA, et al: Physiologic frailty and fragility fracture in HIV-infected male veterans. Clin Infect Dis 2013;56:1498–1504.
62 Marquine MJ, et al: The veterans aging cohort study index is associated with concurrent risk for neurocognitive impairment. J Acquir Immune Defic Syndr 2014;65:190–197.
63 Williams B, et al: Short communication: SCD14 and SCD163 levels are correlated with VACS index scores: initial data from the blunted immune recovery in CORE patients with HIV (BIRCH) cohort. AIDS Res Hum Retroviruses 2016;32:144–147.
64 Furuya-Kanamori L, Kelly MD, McKenzie SJ: Comorbidity, ageing and predicted mortality in antiretroviral treated Australian men: a quantitative analysis. PLoS One 2013;8:e78403.
65 Cohen MH, et al: Gender-related risk factors improve mortality predictive ability of VACS index among HIV-infected women. J Acquir Immune Defic Syndr 2015;70:538–544.

Kathleen Fitch, MSN, FNP-BC
Program in Nutritional Metabolism
Massachusetts General Hospital
55 Fruit Street, 5 LON 207, Boston, MA 02114 (USA)
E-Mail kfitch@partners.org

Brennan-Ing M, DeMarco RF (eds): HIV and Aging. Interdiscipl Top Gerontol Geriatr.
Basel, Karger, 2017, vol 42, pp 59–73 (DOI: 10.1159/000448544)

# Multimorbidity and Burden of Disease

Todd T. Brown[a] · Giovanni Guaraldi[b]

[a]Division of Endocrinology, Diabetes, and Metabolism, Johns Hopkins University, Baltimore, Md., USA;
[b]Department of Medical and Surgical Sciences for Children and Adults, University of Modena and Reggio Emilia, Modena, Italy

**Abstract**

With effective antiretroviral therapy, HIV has become a chronic disease, and life expectancy among HIV-infected persons is approaching that of HIV-uninfected persons. Despite this success, epidemiologic evidence suggests that the burden of multiple aging-related diseases, including cardiovascular disease, liver disease, metabolic abnormalities, chronic kidney disease, cognitive dysfunction, and osteoporosis, is higher in HIV-infected persons compared to their HIV-uninfected peers. These comorbid diseases tend to cluster in a single person, leading to multimorbidity and polypharmacy. Emerging evidence suggests that multimorbidity among HIV-infected persons results in functional decline, reduced quality of life, and increased mortality. In this review, we examine the epidemiology, risk factors, etiologies, and potential consequences of multimorbidity in aging HIV-infected persons. With aggressive risk factor management for comorbidities and less toxic antiretroviral medications, the burden of multimorbidity in HIV-infected persons can be reduced



## Epidemiology of Aging in HIV

With the introduction of effective combination antiretroviral therapy (ART) nearly 20 years ago, morbidity and mortality related to opportunistic infections and other AIDS-related conditions has plummeted, and mortality among HIV-infected individuals is approaching that of HIV-uninfected populations [1–3]. As a consequence, the median age of HIV-infected persons has been increasing steadily. It is estimated that in 2015, approximately half of HIV-infected persons were over 50 years in the USA [4]. In the Netherlands, for example, the proportion of HIV-infected persons over 50 years will increase from 28% in 2010 to 73% in 2030 [5]. Similarly, in the developing world, where ART use is becoming widespread the HIV-infected population is also aging [6, 7]. In addition to successful treatment of HIV, another contributor to the 'graying' of the HIV-infected population is the number of new HIV infections among older persons. In 2013, 17% of the new HIV infections were diagnosed in those older than 50 years, according to the US Centers for Disease Control and Prevention [8].

### Comorbidity among Older HIV-Infected Persons

With the aging of the HIV population, the burden of comorbid medical conditions, also referred to as non-communicable diseases or HIV-associated non-AIDS (HANA) conditions, has also been increasing steadily [9]. From 2003 to 2013 in the USA Medicaid Database, increasing prevalence was observed for cardiovascular disease (CVD; 3–7%), renal impairment (5–11%), osteoporosis (4–6%), and diabetes mellitus (9–19%) [10]. Also in this period, non-AIDS mortality was increased, and has eclipsed AIDS-related mortality as the major cause of death in population with widespread access to ART [11–13].

In addition to the effects of increasing age on the incidence of medical conditions, there is mounting evidence that the prevalence of these comorbidities may be higher in HIV-infected population than in their uninfected counterparts, related to the effects of chronic HIV infection, contributions of some ART, and a higher burden of behavior risk factors, such as smoking in HIV-infected populations [14].

The increasing burden of comorbid conditions among HIV-infected persons provides a challenge in the medical management of HIV, at a time when HIV therapy has become less toxic and easier to take. Multiple comorbidities in the same patient have increased the demand for sub-specialist care and has led to polypharmacy in many HIV-infected persons, increasing the risk of drug–drug interaction and non-compliance. Comorbid conditions are also a major driver of hospitalizations in HIV-infected persons [15]. Importantly, as in the general population, multimorbidity places patients at an increased risk of functional decline and disability [16, 17]. Oftentimes, comorbidity and its risk factors can be managed effectively at an early stage, thereby reducing the incidence of end-organ dysfunction. It is imperative, therefore, for clinicians to screen for comorbid conditions and intervene to prevent long-term complications, which pose a major threat to health of the aging HIV-infected patient, as was suggested by the HIV and Aging Consensus Project (http://www.aahivm.org/hivandagingforum).

### Burden of Multimorbidity in HIV-Infected Populations

Multimorbidity is the accumulation of multiple serious chronic health conditions that occur in older people and threaten their functional and/or cognitive status [16]. It is common for these debilitating conditions to interact to amplify their impact on morbidity and mortality. In the general population, the definition and assessment methods of multimorbidity have not been clearly delineated.

Chronic health conditions are very common in the general population and increase in frequency with greater age. In a very large cross-sectional study from the general population in Scotland, the mean number of morbid conditions was 0.5 in young adults (ages 25–44 years), 1.2 in middle-aged adults (45–64 years), 2.6 in adults 65–84 years, and 3.6 in adult 85 years and older [18]. Among older people in this sample, 65% of those 65–84 years and 82% of those ≥85 years had multimorbidity, defined as the presence of 2 or more of 40 targeted health conditions. Of note, the frequency of multimorbidity was highest in those with the lowest socioeconomic status and in those with concomitant psychiatric disease.

The age distribution in HIV-infected populations differs from the general population in that there are relatively few HIV-infected persons 65 and older. In the Dutch ATHENA cohort, for example, the median age in 2010 was 43.9 years with 28% over 50 years and 8% over 60 years [5]. As a result, in many studies examining aging in HIV, the age of 50 has been used as a cutoff point to define an older population; however, there is no clear biologic rationale for this age. Understanding health changes in HIV-infected persons as they age past their sixth decade is a critical goal of HIV comorbidity research, especially with the anticipated change in the age distribution of HIV-infected persons over the next 20 years. In the ATHENA cohort, it is expected that by 2030, the percentage of HIV-infected persons 60 years and older will be 39% and those 70 years and older will be 12% [5]. With the increasingly widespread availability of effective ART, similar trends are expected in resource limited settings, where the majority of HIV individuals live [19].

Multiple studies have demonstrated that the comorbidity burden among HIV-infected persons is higher than expected based on age alone. In the $AGE_hIV$ cohort study, a large cohort of older HIV-infected persons ≥45 years in Amsterdam and demographically similar HIV-uninfected persons, the prevalence of comorbid conditions was assessed [20]. In this population, with a mean age of 52 years, the number of comorbid conditions was higher in HIV-infected individuals compared to the HIV-uninfected controls (1.3 vs. 1.0, $p < 0.001$). As expected, the prevalence of comorbid conditions increased with increasing age. In those 65 and older, the prevalence of comorbid conditions was 1.96 in the HIV-infected group and 1.51 in the HIV-uninfected group. Of note, the number of comorbid conditions in the 60–64 years HIV-infected individuals was nearly identical to the number of comorbid conditions in the HIV-uninfected group ≥65 years (i.e., 5 years older).

Similar findings were also observed in a large HIV clinic population in Modena, Italy [21]. Compared to a demographically matched control population, HIV-infected individuals were more likely to have multimorbidity (≥2 comorbid conditions). Among those >60 years, the prevalence of multimorbidity was 47% in the HIV-infected individuals compared to 19% in the HIV-uninfected individuals. Similarly, the prevalence of multimorbidity in the HIV-infected persons 41–50 years (9%) was similar to that of the HIV-uninfected control group a decade older (7% in those 51–60 years; fig. 1).

With the aging of the HIV population compounded by the increasing frequency of most comorbid conditions with advancing age, the burden of multimorbidity among

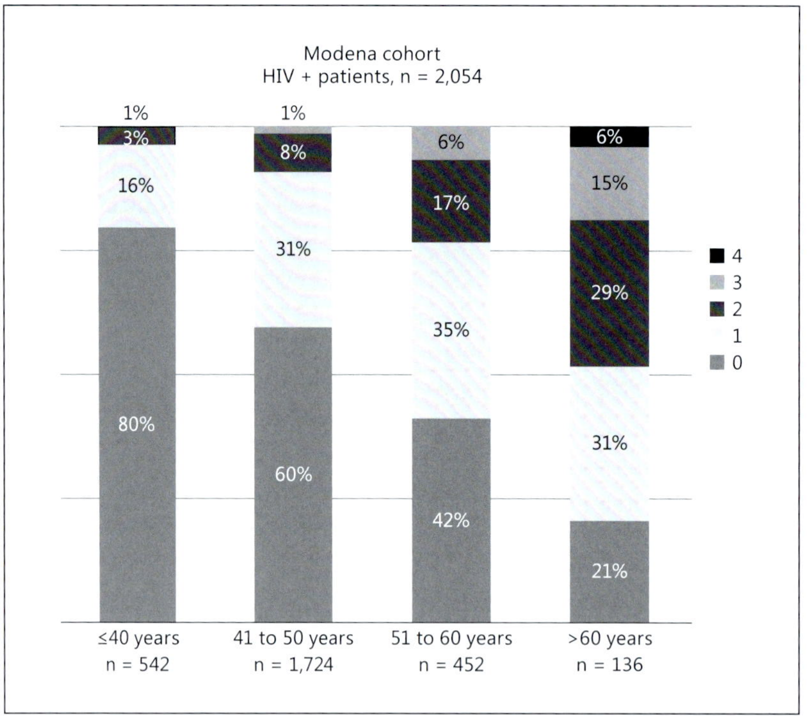


**Fig. 1.** Prevalence of comorbidities with increasing age from the Modena Metabolic Clinic. Adapted from Guaraldi et al. [21].

HIV-infected persons is expected to increase dramatically over the next 12–20 years. In the ATHENA cohort in 2030, 27% of HIV-infected persons will have 3 or more comorbid conditions compared to 19% of HIV-uninfected persons [5]. Approximately 55% of HIV-infected persons over 65 years in the ATHENA cohort will have ≥3 comorbid conditions, compared to 40% of HIV-uninfected individuals in the same age range. In modelling of the ATHENA population in 2030, it is predicted that 78% of HIV-infected persons will be diagnosed with CVD, 17% with diabetes, and 17% with malignancy. The prevalence of multimorbidity is expected to be similar to HIV-uninfected persons 15 years older. This increase in multimorbidity burden is anticipated to have a marked impact on health care utilization, quality of life, functional status, and caregiving needs among older HIV-infected persons.

## Pathways to Multimorbidity in HIV

The pathogenesis of comorbid conditions in HIV-infected persons is multifactorial, with contributions for the effects of chronic HIV infection/co-infections, antiretroviral exposures, and behavioral risk factors.

*Immune Activation*
HIV infection is a chronic inflammatory disease. Whereas immunodeficiency characteristic of advanced HIV disease will lead to opportunistic infections, concomitant immune dysregulation results in the activation of the innate immune system and the production of inflammatory cytokines. Successful ART leading to an undetectable viral load decreases the levels of inflammatory cytokines, such as tumor necrosis factor α (TNF-α) and interleukin (IL)-6, but these levels remain elevated compared to matched HIV-uninfected persons [22, 23]. Chronic inflammation has, therefore, been implicated in the pathogenesis of multiple comorbid conditions in HIV-infected persons, such as CVD [24], diabetes mellitus [25], cognitive dysfunction [26], osteoporosis [27], and chronic kidney disease [28], and there is an intense effort to find therapies that may decrease systemic inflammation, with the goal of decreasing the frequency of these comorbidities.

The drivers of systemic inflammation in chronic HIV infection have not been clearly elucidated. With acute HIV infection, there is a profound and rapid loss of gut lymphocytes which disrupt the gut immune barrier, resulting in microbial translocation and systemic inflammation (sometimes known as 'leaky gut') [29]. It is hypothesized that these gut lymphocytes are not adequately restored even with effective ART, and microbial translocation continues with chronic treated HIV infection [30]. Another hypothesized source of inflammation is chronic low-level HIV replication, in areas such as the gut and lymphoid tissue [29]. The degree of replication is not sufficient to lead to detectable viremia, but may lead to activation of the innate immune system.

Co-infections may also contribute to immune activation. Cytomegalovirus (CMV) infection is very common in HIV-infected populations, but generally does not cause clinical disease in an immunocompetent host. However, even among HIV-infected persons without immunodeficiency, the immune system remains activated against CMV and large proportion of T-cells react to CMV antigens [31]. The chronic inflammation resulting from CMV-directed immune activation contributes to the overall systemic inflammation [32]. This hypothesis is further supported by a CMV treatment study, which showed significant decreases in immune activation with valganciclovir treatment [33].

Other co-infections, such as chronic hepatitis C virus (HCV) may also contribute to systemic inflammation in HIV-infected persons [34]. Chronic HCV has been independently associated with multiple comorbidities including CVD, osteoporosis, cognitive dysfunction, and kidney disease [35]. Recently available, highly effective oral HCV therapies will help to determine whether HCV eradication will decrease systemic inflammation among HIV/HCV co-infected persons and decrease the incidence of end-organ disease. If HCV therapy does decrease the risk of extra-hepatic disease, there would be additional justification for the more widespread use of this effective, yet expensive treatment.

The degree of immune activation in HIV-infected persons is heterogeneous. One consistent risk factor for immune activation in successfully treated patients is a low nadir CD4 cell count or poor immunologic recovery despite ART, which suppresses HIV RNA [34, 36]. In these patients, the immune dysfunction appears to be more profound [37]. With initiation of ART earlier in the disease course (i.e., at a higher CD4 cell count), as is currently recommended, some of the chronic systemic inflammation may be mitigated.

*Antiretroviral Therapy*

Highly active ART was introduced in 1996–1997 and transformed HIV into a chronic disease for the majority of patients for whom the medications were accessible. Although effective against HIV, many early ART had multiple metabolic toxicities, including marked dyslipidemia, glucose dysregulation, subcutaneous lipoatrophy, and central fat accumulation. Chief among these were thymidine analogue nucleoside reverse transcriptase inhibitors (NRTIs), such as stavudine, and early protease inhibitors (PIs), such as indinavir. Stavudine, and to a lesser extent zidovudine, lead to mitochondrial dysfunction and adipocyte apoptosis which resulted in subcutaneous fat wasting [38]. Early NRTIs also led to peripheral neuropathy and lactic acidosis [39]. Early PIs were associated with dramatic increases in triglycerides and peripheral and hepatic insulin resistance. These metabolic abnormalities have been implicated in multiple comorbidities, including diabetes mellitus, CVD, and cognitive dysfunction, and also have a significant effect on the functional status and aging-related quality of life [40, 41].

In the last 20 years, major progress has been made in the development of antiretroviral medications with fewer metabolic toxicities. As a result, stavudine, a major driver of lipoatrophy and to a lesser extent, dyslipidemia and insulin resistance, for example, is used very infrequently at present [42]. However, the effects of previous exposure persist in many patients many years after discontinuation. Switch studies examining the effects of stavudine substitution show convincingly that subcutaneous lipoatrophy improves after discontinuation [43, 44]. However, these changes are relatively modest and may not be perceptible to the patient. The negative consequences of previous exposures (i.e., a legacy effect) may contribute to end-organ disease. In the Multicenter AIDS Cohort Study (MACS), subcutaneous fat was markedly lower among HIV-infected men compared to HIV-uninfected despite the fact that very few men were receiving thymidine analogue NRTIs at the time of assessment [45]. Moreover, lower subcutaneous fat among HIV-infected men was related to lower adiponectin levels, which were significantly associated with subclinical CVD, even after adjustment for traditional cardiovascular risk factors. These findings suggest that fat atrophy and hypoadiponectinemia persist even after thymidine analogues are discontinued, and may contribute to cardiovascular risk.

Perhaps because of the legacy effect of more metabolically toxic ART regimen, longer duration of HIV infection has also been associated with increased prevalence of multimorbidity. In a case control study from the Modena cohort, the prevalence of multimorbidity in HIV-infected persons with a long duration of HIV infection was compared to HIV-infected persons with a shorter duration of HIV infection and matched with HIV-uninfected controls [46]. The prevalence of multimorbidity was 5-fold higher in people aging with a longer duration of HIV infection compared to people without HIV, while HIV-infected individuals who seroconverted at an older age had an intermediate risk. Comparing the 2 HIV-infected groups, the prevalence of multimorbidity was significantly higher in those with longer duration of HIV (OR 1.92, 95% CI 1.03–3.56, $p = 0.04$) after multivariable adjustment. The reasons underlying these differences in multimorbidity by HIV duration are unclear, but may be due to an increased exposure to more metabolically toxic regimens or more advanced disease at ART initiation. The group with longer duration of HIV infection was more likely to have lipohypertrophy, lipoatrophy, insulin resistance, and dyslipidemia.

In addition to legacy effects of previous exposure to metabolically toxic ART, currently used ART may also contribute to the risk of multimorbidity. Tenofovir disoproxil fumarate, the most widely used NRTI, is associated with renal and bone toxicities [47, 48], whereas even the most contemporary PIs, such as darunavir and atazanavir, are associated with dyslipidemia and bone loss, compared to non-NRTIs and integrase inhibitors [49, 50]. Abacavir, another commonly used NRTI medication, has been associated with the risk of CVD in some, but not all studies [51, 52]. A new generation of ART regimens, including regimens without NRTIs, use of a new preparation of tenofovir, and decreasing reliance on PIs, may mitigate the impact of ART on the risk of comorbid conditions in the next decade.

*Behavioral Factors*

The burden of multimorbidity in HIV-infected population is also impacted by behavioral risk factors. Smoking has a major effect on multiple health outcomes and is more common in HIV-infected populations than in the general population. In the Swiss cohort study, 68% of HIV-infected persons reported having smoked and 37% reported current smoking [53]. These prevalences were higher than an HIV-uninfected reference population (60 and 22%, respectively). Smoking has been associated with incident and prevalent multimorbidity. In the Swiss cohort, the prevalence of CVD, stroke, hypertension, kidney disease, and liver disease were all higher compared to a Swiss reference population [54]. Interestingly, the differences in the rates of CVD by HIV-serostatus were no longer present, after taking smoking into consideration in the statistical models, suggesting that smoking, rather than HIV status, was the primary driver of CVD in this population. As an important mode of HIV transmission, injection drug use is also more common in HIV-infected populations compared to the general population. In addition, non-injection illicit drug use, such as cocaine, is highly prevalent in some HIV-infected populations [55]. Both heroin and cocaine use have independent effects on cardiac and endothelial function and contribute to cardiovascular morbidity and mortality [56, 57]. Physical inactivity contributes to the risk of diabetes mellitus, cognitive dysfunction, CVD, and multiple other conditions [58]. In the $AGE_hIV$ cohort with an average age of 52 years, only 44% of HIV-infected persons reported adequate physical activity according to Dutch National Guidelines, compared to 53% of the matched HIV-uninfected controls [20]. Since physical activity generally decreases with age, the disparities may even have a larger impact on multimorbidity as the HIV-infected population ages.

## Consequences of Multimorbidity

*Frailty and Functional Decline*

One of the major consequences of multimorbidity is a hastened decline in physical function with aging and the development of frailty. There is mounting evidence that aging HIV-infected persons have an accelerated decline in physical function and a premature development of frailty. In the MACS cohort, gait speed measured by a 4 m walk declined after about age 45 in both HIV-uninfected men, but the decline in gait speed was more than 2-fold faster in the HIV-infected men, who were 57% more likely to develop a gait speed <1.0 m/s, a level of performance that has been linked to an increased mortality in the general population [59]. Similarly, as described below, multiple cohorts have described higher prevalences of frailty in HIV-infected persons compared to HIV-uninfected controls. Accelerated functional decline may underlie the higher prevalence of geriatric syndromes in older HIV-infected persons [60].

In addition to the effects of multimorbidity on the pathogenesis of functional decline and frailty in HIV-infected population, immune activation and immune senescence, even among treated HIV-infected persons, have been hypothesized to be a major driver of reduced physical function in older HIV-infected person. In a clinical study from the University of Colorado, functional impairment was associated with both immune activation (e.g., soluble CD14 and CD163, CD16+ monocytes, HLA-DR+/CD38+ CD8+ T cells) and immune senescence markers (e.g., terminally differentiated CD45RA+, CCR7–, and CD4+ T cells), as well as inflammatory circulating cytokines (e.g., IL-6, TNF-α) [61]. Frailty among HIV-infected persons has also been associated with lower CD4 cell count and uncontrolled HIV viral replication [62, 63]. These findings support the hypothesis that functional decline in aging HIV-infected persons maybe driven in part by immune dysregulation, or 'inflamm-aging' [64, 65]. Other comorbid conditions, co-infections, and behavioral risk factors may amplify this process, as depicted in figure 2.

## Frailty in HIV-Infected Populations

Frailty is defined as a physiologic state of increased vulnerability to stressors that results from decreased physiologic reserves and deregulation of multiple physiological systems [66]. In the general population, even relatively minor insults among frail

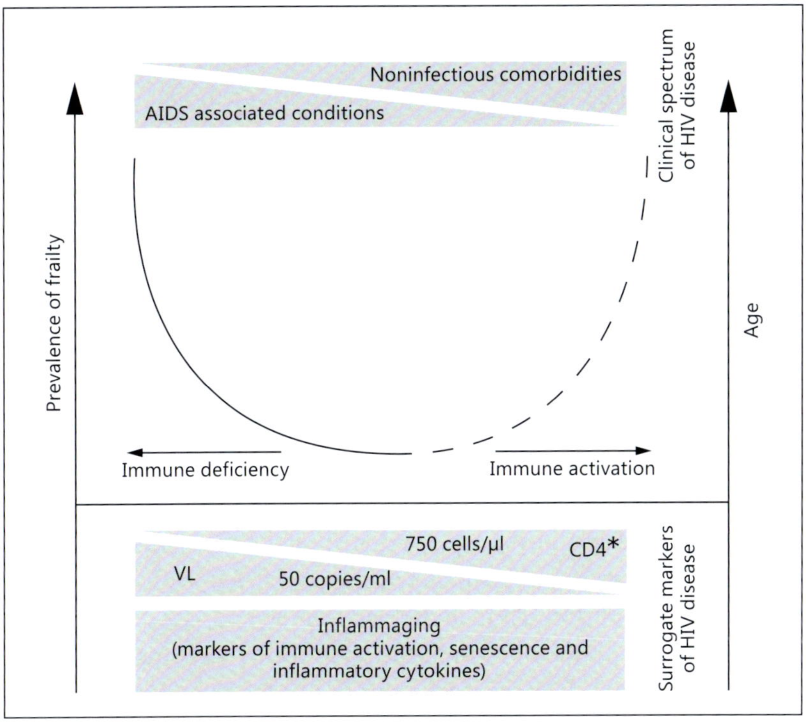


**Fig. 2.** Hypothetical association between frailty prevalence, HANA conditions, and immune system dysregulation. Adapted from Brothers et al. [67].

persons can accelerate functional decline, due to impaired homeostatic responses. In HIV populations, frailty is increasingly recognized and is hypothesized to be a major threat to physical health and quality of life with aging [67].

As in the general population, there is no universally accepted definition of frailty among HIV-infected persons [66]. Two different conceptual models have been borrowed from the geriatric literature and applied to HIV-infected populations: the phenotype model [68] and the cumulative deficit model [69]. These models, as well as other instruments, have different strengths and limitations, as reviewed elsewhere [70, 71].

The most commonly used frailty phenotype measurement instrument was proposed by Fried et al. [68] in 2001, and defines frailty as the presence of 3 or more of the following 5 characteristics; slowness, weight loss, impaired strength, exhaustion, and low physical activity/energy expenditure. Subsequent research in the general population has demonstrated that this phenotype is highly predictive of reduced quality of life, incident disability, and mortality, among other health outcomes [72]. Among HIV-infected populations, the reported prevalence of frailty has ranged from 7–29%, and is generally higher than in age-matched control groups or prevalence rates expected in the background populations [73]. In the $AGE_hIV$ cohort study, the prevalence of frailty using the Fried criteria among the HIV-infected individuals was 10.6% compared to 2.7% in HIV-uninfected group, and was over 2-fold more common after adjustment for demographic factors, smoking, HCV coinfection, and comorbidities [74]. In the developing world, frailty is also increasingly recognized. In a study from South Africa, frailty was identified in 19% of HIV-infected persons compared to 13% of HIV-uninfected controls [75]. The frailty phenotype in HIV-infected persons has also been shown to be associated with hospitalizations, falls, reduced quality of life, and mortality [76, 77].

In the frailty phenotype model, comorbidities are considered either confounders or mediators of frailty. In the deficit accumulation model, frailty is considered a health state, rather than a specific clinical syndrome, and frailty is hypothesized to arise from the cumulative impact of age-related health deficits. A frailty index, first proposed in 2001, calculates the ratio of health deficits present within an individual out of a number of pre-specified health variables [78]. The frailty index includes a minimum of 30 health variables that cover multiple physiologic systems; each deficit must be associated with adverse health outcomes and have increasing prevalence with age [79]. In studies on the general population, which includes between 30 and 100 variables, the frailty index has been a potent predictor of multiple poor health outcomes [80].

In HIV-infected populations, data regarding the frailty index are beginning to emerge. In the Modena HIV Metabolic Clinic cohort, a 38-item frailty index predicted incident multimorbidity, independent of age, gender, CD4 cell count, and injection drug use [81]. In a recent analysis of the Modena cohort [82], the frailty phenotype and the frailty index were compared; 10% of participants were frail, 30% were prefrail, and 60% were robust; the mean frailty index score was 0.30 ± 10. With both frailty instruments, frailty tended to increase with age, did not differ by gender, and was associated with nadir CD4 cell count and a history of AIDS. Frailty index, and not frailty phenotype, was associated with the duration of HIV infection, duration of ART, and current CD4 cell count. Interestingly, higher frailty index scores were associated with hypertension, diabetes, liver cirrhosis, osteoporosis/osteopenia, renal insufficiency, dyslipidemia, sarcopenia, and multimorbidity, whereas the frailty phenotype was not associated with any comorbidity. Further work is needed to better understand the differences in these 2 models of frailty in HIV-infected persons, such that the most appropriate population can be identified for interventions that prevent functional decline.

### Polypharmacy

Another major consequence of multimorbidity is polypharmacy, generally defined as taking 5 or more different medications on a daily basis [83]. Among HIV population, polypharmacy is particularly a problem given the medications needed to treat HIV infection, in addition to medications required to treat non-AIDS comorbidities [84].

In the Swiss cohort study, 14% of patients over 65 were taking 4 or more non-ART drugs, most of which were either vitamins, supplements, or drugs for cardiovascular or neurologic disorders [53]. In the ATHENA cohort, it is predicted that with the aging of the Dutch HIV population, 20% of patients will be prescribed 3 or more medications in addition to their antiretrovirals, compared to 5% in 2010 [5]. With the increases in polypharmacy, the probability of drug–drug interactions and adverse drug reactions will increase, potentially compounding the impact of multimorbidity on poor health outcomes and geriatric syndromes. In the Colorado cohort, polypharmacy and specifically antihypertensives, antidepressants, sedatives, and opiates were strongly associated with fall frequency [85].

## Clinical Recommendations to Reduce Multimorbidity and Its Consequences

Clinicians should take a multifaceted approach to reduce the burden of multimorbidity in HIV-infected persons. Risk factors for comorbid diseases should be identified and treated aggressively. At the same time, consideration needs to be given to risks, benefits, and costs of additional medications. Recommendations regarding screening for comorbid conditions in HIV-infected populations are available from the Infectious Disease Society of America [86] and the European AIDS Clinical Society (http://www.eacsociety.org/guidelines/eacs-guidelines/eacs-guidelines.html). In addition to screening for comorbid conditions that may be clinically silent (e.g., dyslipidemia, diabetes mellitus, osteoporosis), clinicians should provide support to help patients stop smoking, reduce heavy alcohol intake, stop illicit drug use, increase exercise, and reduce sedentary behavior. Dietary habits should be reviewed and referrals should be made to nutrition support services when needed. Treatment for coinfection, such as hepatitis C, should be sought. Older patients may benefit from a comprehensive geriatric assessment and physical therapy interventions to improve mobility, balance, and strength. Consideration should be given to switching patients to antiretroviral regimens that are easy to take with a low toxicity profile. While multiple interventions are being evaluated in clinical trials to decrease inflammation and immune activation in HIV-infected persons, none are currently recommended for this purpose.

## Conclusions

Non-AIDS comorbidities in HIV-infected persons are common and have eclipsed AIDS conditions as the most frequent cause of hospitalization and mortality among HIV-infected populations. At a time when HIV management has been simplified, the care of aging HIV-infected persons has increased in complexity, driven by the presence of multimorbidity. Multimorbidity is also likely a major determinant of functional decline and the development of frailty in HIV-infected populations, and will increase markedly in the coming decades with the aging of the HIV population. Research to understand the factors contributing to multimorbidity, which are unique to or are more pronounced in HIV-infected people, such as immune activation and immune senescence will help to prevent or minimize the impact of multimorbidity on the heath of the aging HIV population.

## References


1 Mocroft A, Vella S, Benfield TL, Chiesi A, Miller V, Gargalianos P, D'Arminio Monforte A, Yust I, Bruun JN, Phillips AN, et al: Changing patterns of mortality across Europe in patients infected with HIV-1. EuroSIDA study group. Lancet 1998;352:1725–1730.

2 Helleberg M, Kronborg G, Larsen CS, Pedersen G, Pedersen C, Gerstoft J, Obel N: Causes of death among Danish HIV patients compared with population controls in the period 1995–2008. Infection 2012;40:627–634.

3 Lohse N, Hansen AB, Pedersen G, Kronborg G, Gerstoft J, Sørensen HT, Vaeth M, Obel N: Survival of persons with and without HIV infection in Denmark, 1995–2005. Ann Intern Med 2007;146:87–95.

4 High KP, Brennan-Ing M, Clifford DB, Cohen MH, Currier J, Deeks SG, Deren S, Effros RB, Gebo K, Goronzy JJ, et al: HIV and aging: state of knowledge and areas of critical need for research. A report to the NIH office of AIDS research by the HIV and aging working group. J Acquir Immune Defic Syndr 2012; 60(suppl 1):S1–S18.

5 Smit M, Brinkman K, Geerlings S, Smit C, Thyagarajan K, Sighem Av, De Wolf F, Hallett TB: Future challenges for clinical care of an ageing population infected with HIV: a modelling study. Lancet Infect Dis 2015;15:810–818.

6 Cardoso SW, Torres TS, Santini-Oliveira M, Marins LM, Veloso VG, Grinsztejn B: Aging with HIV: a practical review. Braz J Infect Dis 2013;17:464–479.

7 Narayan KM, Miotti PG, Anand NP, Kline LM, Harmston C, Gulakowski R 3rd, Vermund SH: HIV and noncommunicable disease comorbidities in the era of antiretroviral therapy: a vital agenda for research in low- and middle-income country settings. J Acquir Immune Defic Syndr 2014;67(suppl 1):S2–S7.

8 Centers for Disease Control and Prevention. http://www.cdc.gov/hiv/group/age/olderamericans/index.html (accessed January 26, 2016).

9 Goulet JL, Fultz SL, Rimland D, Butt A, Gibert C, Rodriguez-Barradas M, Bryant K, Justice AC: Aging and infectious diseases: do patterns of comorbidity vary by HIV status, age, and HIV severity? Clin Infect Dis 2007;45:1593–1601.

10 Meyer N, Gallant JE, Hsue P, Song X: Comorbidities of Patients with Human Immunodeficiency Virus (HIV) in the USA – A Longitudinal Analysis of Prevalent HIV Patients Over 11 Years. San Diego, ICAAC/ICC, 2015.

11 Alejos B, Hernando V, López-Aldeguer J, Segura F, Oteo JA, Rubio R, Sanvisens A, Sobrino P, Del Amo J, Coris C: Overall and cause-specific mortality in HIV-positive subjects compared to the general population. J Int AIDS Soc 2014;17(4 suppl 3):19711.

12 Morlat P, Roussillon C, Henard S, Salmon D, Bonnet F, Cacoub P, Georget A, Aouba A, Rosenthal E, May T, et al: Causes of death among HIV-infected patients in France in 2010 (national survey): trends since 2000. AIDS 2014;28:1181–1191.

13 Miller CJ, Baker JV, Bormann AM, Erlandson KM, Huppler Hullsiek K, Justice AC, Neuhaus J, Paredes R, Petoumenos K, Wentworth D, et al: Adjudicated morbidity and mortality outcomes by age among individuals with HIV infection on suppressive antiretroviral therapy. PLoS One 2014;9:e95061.

14 Effros RB, Fletcher CV, Gebo K, Halter JB, Hazzard WR, Horne FM, Huebner RE, Janoff EN, Justice AC, Kuritzkes D, et al: Aging and infectious diseases: workshop on HIV infection and aging: what is known and future research directions. Clin Infect Dis 2008;47:542–553.

15 Berry SA, Fleishman JA, Moore RD, Gebo KA: Trends in reasons for hospitalization in a multisite United States cohort of persons living with HIV, 2001–2008. J Acquir Immune Defic Syndr 2012;59: 368–375.

16 Guaraldi G, Silva AR, Stentarelli C: Multimorbidity and functional status assessment. Curr Opin HIV AIDS 2014;9:386–397.

17 Althoff KN, Jacobson LP, Cranston RD, Detels R, Phair JP, Li X, Margolick JB: Age, comorbidities, and AIDS predict a frailty phenotype in men who have sex with men. J Gerontol A Biol Sci Med Sci 2014;69: 189–198.

18 Barnett K, Mercer SW, Norbury M, Watt G, Wyke S, Guthrie B: Epidemiology of multimorbidity and implications for health care, research, and medical education: a cross-sectional study. Lancet 2012;380:37–43.

19 Report on the Global AIDS Epidemic. UNAIDS. 2013. http://www.unaids.org/sites/default/files/en/media/unaids/contentassets/documents/epidemiology/2013/gr2013/UNAIDS_Global_Report_2013_en.pdf (accessed January 26, 2016).
20 Schouten J, Wit FW, Stolte IG, Kootstra NA, van der Valk M, Geerlings SE, Prins M, Reiss P: Cross-sectional comparison of the prevalence of age-associated comorbidities and their risk factors between HIV-infected and uninfected individuals: the AGEhIV cohort study. Clin Infect Dis 2014;59:1787–1797.
21 Guaraldi G, Orlando G, Zona S, Menozzi M, Carli F, Garlassi E, Berti A, Rossi E, Roverato A, Palella F: Premature age-related comorbidities among HIV-infected persons compared with the general population. Clin Infect Dis 2011;53:1120–1126.
22 Wada NI, Jacobson LP, Margolick JB, Breen EC, Macatangay B, Penugonda S, Martínez-Maza O, Bream JH: The effect of HAART-induced HIV suppression on circulating markers of inflammation and immune activation. AIDS 2015;29:463–471.
23 Neuhaus J, Jacobs DR Jr, Baker JV, Calmy A, Duprez D, La Rosa A, Kuller LH, Pett SL, Ristola M, Ross MJ, et al: Markers of inflammation, coagulation, and renal function are elevated in adults with HIV infection. J Infect Dis 2010;201:1788–1795.
24 Shaked I, Hanna DB, Gleißner C, Marsh B, Plants J, Tracy D, Anastos K, Cohen M, Golub ET, Karim R, et al: Macrophage inflammatory markers are associated with subclinical carotid artery disease in women with human immunodeficiency virus or hepatitis C virus infection. Arterioscler Thromb Vasc Biol 2014;34:1085–1092.
25 Brown TT, Tassiopoulos K, Bosch RJ, Shikuma C, McComsey GA: Association between systemic inflammation and incident diabetes in HIV-infected patients after initiation of antiretroviral therapy. Diabetes Care 2010;33:2244–2249.
26 Lake JE, Vo QT, Jacobson LP, Sacktor N, Miller EN, Post WS, Becker JT, Palella FJ Jr, Ragin A, Martin E, et al: Adiponectin and interleukin-6, but not adipose tissue, are associated with worse neurocognitive function in HIV-infected men. Antivir Ther 2015;20:235–244.
27 Yin MT, McMahon DJ, Ferris DC, Zhang CA, Shu A, Staron R, Colon I, Laurence J, Dobkin JF, Hammer SM, et al: Low bone mass and high bone turnover in postmenopausal human immunodeficiency virus-infected women. J Clin Endocrinol Metab 2010;95:620–629.
28 Abraham AG, Darilay A, McKay H, Margolick JB, Estrella MM, Palella FJ Jr, Bolan R, Rinaldo CR, Jacobson LP: Kidney dysfunction and markers of inflammation in the multicenter AIDS cohort study. J Infect Dis 2015;212:1100–1110.
29 Hunt PW: HIV and inflammation: mechanisms and consequences. Curr HIV/AIDS Rep 2012;9:139–147.
30 Lederman MM, Funderburg NT, Sekaly RP, Klatt NR, Hunt PW: Residual immune dysregulation syndrome in treated HIV infection. Adv Immunol 2013;119:51–83.
31 Li H, Margolick JB, Bream JH, Nilles TL, Langan S, Bui HT, Sylwester AW, Picker LJ, Leng SX: Heterogeneity of CD4+ and CD8+ T-cell responses to cytomegalovirus in HIV-infected and HIV-uninfected men who have sex with men. J Infect Dis 2014;210:400–404.
32 Freeman ML, Mudd JC, Shive CL, Younes SA, Panigrahi S, Sieg SF, Lee SA, Hunt PW, Calabrese LH, Gianella S, et al: CD8 T-cell expansion and inflammation linked to CMV coinfection in ART-treated HIV infection. Clin Infect Dis 2016;62:392–396.
33 Hunt PW, Martin JN, Sinclair E, Epling L, Teague J, Jacobson MA, Tracy RP, Corey L, Deeks SG: Valganciclovir reduces T cell activation in HIV-infected individuals with incomplete CD4+ T cell recovery on antiretroviral therapy. J Infect Dis 2011;203:1474–1483.
34 Borges ÁH, O'Connor JL, Phillips AN, Rönsholt FF, Pett S, Vjecha MJ, French MA, Lundgren JD: Factors associated with plasma IL-6 levels during HIV infection. J Infect Dis 2015;212:585–595.
35 Soriano V, Berenguer J: Extrahepatic comorbidities associated with hepatitis C virus in HIV-infected patients. Curr Opin HIV AIDS 2015;10:309–315.
36 Ghislain M, Bastard JP, Meyer L, Capeau J, Fellahi S, Gérard L, May T, Simon A, Vigouroux C, Goujard C: Late antiretroviral therapy (ART) initiation is associated with long-term persistence of systemic inflammation and metabolic abnormalities. PLoS One 2015;10:e0144317.
37 Lederman MM, Calabrese L, Funderburg NT, Clagett B, Medvik K, Bonilla H, Gripshover B, Salata RA, Taege A, Lisgaris M, et al: Immunologic failure despite suppressive antiretroviral therapy is related to activation and turnover of memory CD4 cells. J Infect Dis 2011;204:1217–1226.
38 de Waal R, Cohen K, Maartens G: Systematic review of antiretroviral-associated lipodystrophy: lipoatrophy, but not central fat gain, is an antiretroviral adverse drug reaction. PLoS One 2013;8:e63623.
39 Margolis AM, Heverling H, Pham PA, Stolbach A: A review of the toxicity of HIV medications. J Med Toxicol 2014;10:26–39.
40 Scherzer R, Heymsfield SB, Lee D, Powderly WG, Tien PC, Bacchetti P, Shlipak MG, Grunfeld C: Decreased limb muscle and increased central adiposity are associated with 5-year all-cause mortality in HIV infection. AIDS 2011;25:1405–1414.
41 Erlandson KM, Reynolds SM, Cox C, Palella FJ, Witt MD, Kingsley LA, Brown TT, Plankey M: Self-reported body fat change in HIV-infected men is a marker of decline in physical health-related quality of life with aging, independent of co-morbidity. PLoS One 2014;9:e114166.

42 Slama L, Li X, Brown T, Jacobson LP, Pialoux G, Macatangay B, Bolan RK, Phair J, Palella FJ Jr: Increases in duration of first highly active antiretroviral therapy over time (1996–2009) and associated factors in the multicenter AIDS cohort study. J Acquir Immune Defic Syndr 2014;65:57–64.
43 Martin A, Smith DE, Carr A, Ringland C, Amin J, Emery S, Hoy J, Workman C, Doong N, Freund J, et al: Reversibility of lipoatrophy in HIV-infected patients 2 years after switching from a thymidine analogue to abacavir: the MITOX extension study. AIDS 2004;18:1029–1036.
44 McComsey GA, Ward DJ, Hessenthaler SM, Sension MG, Shalit P, Lonergan JT, Fisher RL, Williams VC, Hernandez JE: Improvement in lipoatrophy associated with highly active antiretroviral therapy in human immunodeficiency virus-infected patients switched from stavudine to abacavir or zidovudine: the results of the TARHEEL study. Clin Infect Dis 2004;38:263–270.
45 Ketlogetswe KS, Post WS, Li X, Palella FJ Jr, Jacobson LP, Margolick JB, Kingsley LA, Witt MD, Dobs AS, Budoff MJ, et al: Lower adiponectin is associated with subclinical cardiovascular disease among HIV-infected men. AIDS 2014;28:901–909.
46 Guaraldi G, Zona S, Brothers TD, Carli F, Stentarelli C, Dolci G, Santoro A, Beghetto B, Menozzi M, Mussini C, et al: Aging with HIV vs. HIV seroconversion at older age: a diverse population with distinct comorbidity profiles. PLoS One 2015;10:e0118531.
47 Cooper RD, Wiebe N, Smith N, Keiser P, Naicker S, Tonelli M: Systematic review and meta-analysis: renal safety of tenofovir disoproxil fumarate in HIV-infected patients. Clin Infect Dis 2010;51:496–505.
48 Powderly WG: Osteoporosis and bone health in HIV. Curr HIV/AIDS Rep 2012;9:218–222.
49 Ofotokun I, Na LH, Landovitz RJ, Ribaudo HJ, McComsey GA, Godfrey C, Aweeka F, Cohn SE, Sagar M, Kuritzkes DR, et al: Comparison of the metabolic effects of ritonavir-boosted darunavir or atazanavir versus raltegravir, and the impact of ritonavir plasma exposure: ACTG 5257. Clin Infect Dis 2015;60:1842–1851.
50 Brown TT, Moser C, Currier JS, Ribaudo HJ, Rothenberg J, Kelesidis T, Yang O, Dubé MP, Murphy RL, Stein JH, et al: Changes in bone mineral density after initiation of antiretroviral treatment with tenofovir disoproxil fumarate/emtricitabine plus atazanavir/ritonavir, darunavir/ritonavir, or raltegravir. J Infect Dis 2015;212:1241–1249.
51 Cruciani M, Zanichelli V, Serpelloni G, Bosco O, Malena M, Mazzi R, Mengoli C, Parisi SG, Moyle G: Abacavir use and cardiovascular disease events: a meta-analysis of published and unpublished data. AIDS 2011;25:1993–2004.
52 Marcus JL, Neugebauer RS, Leyden WA, Chao CR, Xu L, Quesenberry CP Jr, Klein DB, Towner WJ, Horberg MA, Silverberg MJ: Use of abacavir and risk of cardiovascular disease among HIV-infected individuals. J Acquir Immune Defic Syndr 2016;71:413–419.
53 Hasse B, Ledergerber B, Furrer H, Battegay M, Hirschel B, Cavassini M, Bertisch B, Bernasconi E, Weber R: Morbidity and aging in HIV-infected persons: the Swiss HIV cohort study. Clin Infect Dis 2011;53:1130–1139.
54 Hasse B, Tarr PE, Marques-Vidal P, Waeber G, Preisig M, Mooser V, Valeri F, Djalali S, Andri R, Bernasconi E, et al: Strong impact of smoking on multimorbidity and cardiovascular risk among human immunodeficiency virus-infected individuals in comparison with the general population. Open Forum Infect Dis 2015;2:ofv108.
55 The NSDUH Report: HIV/AIDS and Substance Use Rockville, 2010. http://www.samhsa.gov/data/2k10/HIV-AIDS/HIV-AIDs.htm. 2010 (updated January 12, 2010; cited January 29, 2016).
56 Lai S, Gerstenblith G, Li J, Zhu H, Bluemke DA, Liu CY, Zimmerman SL, Chen S, Lai H, Treisman G: Chronic cocaine use and its association with myocardial steatosis evaluated by 1H magnetic resonance spectroscopy in African Americans. J Addict Med 2015;9:31–39.
57 Dettmeyer R, Friedrich K, Schmidt P, Madea B: Heroin-associated myocardial damages – conventional and immunohistochemical investigations. Forensic Sci Int 2009;187:42–46.
58 Kruk J: Health and economic costs of physical inactivity. Asian Pac J Cancer Prev 2014;15:7499–7503.
59 Schrack JA, Althoff KN, Jacobson LP, Erlandson KM, Jamieson BD, Koletar SL, Phair J, Ferrucci L, Brown TT, Margolick JB: Accelerated longitudinal gait speed decline in HIV-infected older men. J Acquir Immune Defic Syndr 2015;70:370–376.
60 Greene M, Covinsky KE, Valcour V, Miao Y, Madamba J, Lampiris H, Cenzer IS, Martin J, Deeks SG: Geriatric syndromes in older HIV-infected adults. J Acquir Immune Defic Syndr 2015;69:161–167.
61 Erlandson KM, Allshouse AA, Jankowski CM, Lee EJ, Rufner KM, Palmer BE, Wilson CC, MaWhinney S, Kohrt WM, Campbell TB: Association of functional impairment with inflammation and immune activation in HIV type 1-infected adults receiving effective antiretroviral therapy. J Infect Dis 2013;208:249–259.
62 Desquilbet L, Margolick JB, Fried LP, Phair JP, Jamieson BD, Holloway M, Jacobson LP: Relationship between a frailty-related phenotype and progressive deterioration of the immune system in HIV-infected men. J Acquir Immune Defic Syndr 2009;50:299–306.
63 Piggott DA, Muzaale AD, Mehta SH, Brown TT, Patel KV, Leng SX, Kirk GD: Frailty, HIV infection, and mortality in an aging cohort of injection drug users. PLoS One 2013;8:e54910.

64 Guaraldi G, Prakash M, Moecklinghoff C, Stellbrink HJ: Morbidity in older HIV-infected patients: impact of long-term antiretroviral use. AIDS Rev 2014; 16:75–89.
65 Franceschi C, Campisi J: Chronic inflammation (inflammaging) and its potential contribution to age-associated diseases. J Gerontol A Biol Sci Med Sci 2014;69(suppl 1):S4–S9.
66 Clegg A, Young J, Iliffe S, Rikkert MO, Rockwood K: Frailty in elderly people. Lancet 2013;381:752–762.
67 Brothers TD, Kirkland S, Guaraldi G, Falutz J, Theou O, Johnston BL, Rockwood K: Frailty in people aging with human immunodeficiency virus (HIV) infection. J Infect Dis 2014;210:1170–1179.
68 Fried LP, Tangen CM, Walston J, Newman AB, Hirsch C, Gottdiener J, Seeman T, Tracy R, Kop WJ, Burke G, et al: Frailty in older adults: evidence for a phenotype. J Gerontol A Biol Sci Med Sci 2001; 56:M146–M156.
69 Rockwood K, Song X, MacKnight C, Bergman H, Hogan DB, McDowell I, Mitnitski A: A global clinical measure of fitness and frailty in elderly people. CMAJ 2005;173:489–495.
70 Theou O, Brothers TD, Peña FG, Mitnitski A, Rockwood K: Identifying common characteristics of frailty across seven scales. J Am Geriatr Soc 2014;62:901–906.
71 Walston JD, Bandeen-Roche K: Frailty: a tale of two concepts. BMC Med 2015;13:185.
72 Chang SF, Lin PL: Frail phenotype and mortality prediction: a systematic review and meta-analysis of prospective cohort studies. Int J Nurs Stud 2015;52: 1362–1374.
73 Erlandson KM, Schrack JA, Jankowski CM, Brown TT, Campbell TB: Functional impairment, disability, and frailty in adults aging with HIV-infection. Curr HIV/AIDS Rep 2014;11:279–290.
74 Kooij KW, Wit FW, Schouten J, van der Valk M, Godfried MH, Stolte IG, Prins M, Falutz J, Reiss P: HIV infection is independently associated with frailty in middle-aged HIV type 1-infected individuals compared with similar but uninfected controls. AIDS 2016;30:241–250.
75 Pathai S, Lawn SD, Gilbert CE, McGuinness D, McGlynn L, Weiss HA, Port J, Christ T, Barclay K, Wood R, et al: Accelerated biological ageing in HIV-infected individuals in South Africa: a case-control study. AIDS 2013;27:2375–2384.
76 Akgün KM, Tate JP, Crothers K, Crystal S, Leaf DA, Womack J, Brown TT, Justice AC, Oursler KK: An adapted frailty-related phenotype and the VACS index as predictors of hospitalization and mortality in HIV-infected and uninfected individuals. J Acquir Immune Defic Syndr 2014;67:397–404.
77 Piggott DA, Varadhan R, Mehta SH, Brown TT, Li H, Walston JD, Leng SX, Kirk GD: Frailty, inflammation, and mortality among persons aging with HIV infection and injection drug use. J Gerontol A Biol Sci Med Sci 2015;70:1542–1547.
78 Mitnitski AB, Mogilner AJ, Rockwood K: Accumulation of deficits as a proxy measure of aging. ScientificWorldJournal 2001;1:323–336.
79 Searle SD, Mitnitski A, Gahbauer EA, Gill TM, Rockwood K: A standard procedure for creating a frailty index. BMC Geriatr 2008;8:24.
80 Rockwood K, Mitnitski A: Frailty defined by deficit accumulation and geriatric medicine defined by frailty. Clin Geriatr Med 2011;27:17–26.
81 Guaraldi G, Brothers TD, Zona S, Stentarelli C, Carli F, Malagoli A, Santoro A, Menozzi M, Mussi C, Mussini C, et al: A frailty index predicts survival and incident multimorbidity independent of markers of HIV disease severity. AIDS 2015;29:1633–1641.
82 Guaraldi G, Torelli R, Malagoli A, Brothers TD, Wallace L, Garlassi S, Santoro A, Theou O, Kirkland S, Rockwood K: Two Methods of Measuring Frailty among People Aging with HIV. Washington, 6th International Workshop on HIV and Aging, 2015.
83 Gnjidic D, Hilmer SN, Blyth FM, Naganathan V, Waite L, Seibel MJ, McLachlan AJ, Cumming RG, Handelsman DJ, Le Couteur DG: Polypharmacy cutoff and outcomes: five or more medicines were used to identify community-dwelling older men at risk of different adverse outcomes. J Clin Epidemiol 2012; 65:989–995.
84 Gleason LJ, Luque AE, Shah K: Polypharmacy in the HIV-infected older adult population. Clin Interv Aging 2013;8:749–763.
85 Erlandson KM, Allshouse AA, Jankowski CM, Duong S, MaWhinney S, Kohrt WM, Campbell TB: Risk factors for falls in HIV-infected persons. J Acquir Immune Defic Syndr 2012;61:484–489.
86 Aberg JA, Gallant JE, Ghanem KG, Emmanuel P, Zingman BS, Horberg MA: Primary care guidelines for the management of persons infected with HIV: 2013 update by the HIV medicine association of the infectious diseases society of America. Clin Infect Dis 2014;58:e1–e34.

Todd T. Brown, MD, PhD
Division of Endocrinology, Diabetes, and Metabolism
Johns Hopkins University, 1830 East Monument Street
Suite 333, Baltimore, MD 21287 (USA)
E-Mail tbrown27@jhmi.edu

Brennan-Ing M, DeMarco RF (eds): HIV and Aging. Interdiscipl Top Gerontol Geriatr.
Basel, Karger, 2017, vol 42, pp 74–84 (DOI: 10.1159/000448545)

# Polypharmacy, Using New Treatments to Customize Care for Aging Patients and Adherence Present and Future

Leonard H. Alberts

College of Nursing and Health Science, University of Massachusetts, Boston, Mass., USA

**Abstract**

Nearly 50% of HIV patients in the US are now over 50, and the problem of comorbidities associated with the aging process is becoming increasingly complicated. In this chapter, we will review the challenge of polypharmacy and suggest ways of minimizing drug–drug interactions. Newer medications and combinations that reduce the pill burden, and allow the healthcare provider to customize HIV treatment while remaining mindful of other medical issues will be addressed. Adherence to medication schedules and possible future alternative drug delivery systems will also be presented.



## Polypharmacy

Polypharmacy is an unavoidable consequence of aging [1]. Older individuals develop health conditions associated with aging, and many, if not all of these conditions require pharmacologic intervention [2]. The experience with multimorbidity related to aging is further complicated with the need for HIV treatment, which requires a minimum of 3 effective antiviral drugs taken consistently as directed [3]. To complicate things further, HIV-associated conditions may demand even more drugs against infections that begin evolving as the immune system tries to fight off microbes that ordinarily would be non-threatening.

Polypharmacy is defined as the need for 5 or more medications, whatever the condition [4]. While prescriptions for drugs for aging patients is increasing, antiretroviral treatment (ART) considerably adds to the burden of medication intake because even though the amounts (pill count) of these medications have diminished, they are known to have negative interactive and adverse effects that are accentuated due to the changing function of aging organ systems such as kidney and liver metabolism [5]. We know that HIV itself may accelerate the aging process, and many non-HIV diseases may appear earlier than in the general population [6]. Those with HIV are more susceptible to age-related conditions that are at least plausibly related to the chronic inflammation associated with direct viral effects. Due to the increasing prevalence of renal and hepatic diseases, particularly in aging HIV patients, medications must be selected with great care because of the risk of exacerbating end-organ damage [7].

Polypharmacy is associated with adherence challenges as well; as the medication regimens become increasingly complex and difficult for many patients to manage, as does the ability to take medications as prescribed. The greater number of pills and the complexity of the pill-taking schedule can become extremely confusing and riddled with potential unintentional errors [8]. In addition, the universal challenge of patients taking independent and intentional long or short drug holidays is problematic. Drug holidays are often taken for relief from the negative side effects that cause patients distress. Obesity, lipoatrophy, lipodystrophy, and fatigue, for example, are some problems that people living with HIV experience and dislike. Many of these side effects, whether from HIV or from the interaction of HIV and other medications leads to stigma, negative self-image, and depression [9].

Medications are also a large part of the ongoing therapeutic course for people living with HIV. There are many challenges with coordination of care, particularly in the area of medication management. Health professionals with prescriptive authority may prescribe a medication in the domain of their specialty without completely understanding the risks and side effects of many of the newer ART medications [10]. The need for a primary care provider and/or a skilled case manager to maintain a complete and up-to date list of all medications is essential. An involved and dedicated pharmacist, who keeps an updated list, is often critically helpful as a member of the care team, especially in the era of evolving electronic medical records.

Transitions between different levels of care can also cause challenges within polypharmacy. Going from hospital to nursing home to home often results in disruption of medication schedules. Most studies of transition have been completed following the release of inmates from a prison setting. Almost 20% of people living with HIV in their catchment area transition through the prison system every year [11]. A large retrospective study of 882 HIV-positive prisoners was carried out using multiple databases. They found a significant increase in the maintenance of viral suppression after release. They attributed this to newer medications with lower pill burden and fewer adverse medication effects, and an effective case management system that tracked the released prisoners, and helped them stay in care during their transition [12].

Use of over-the-counter and recreational drugs must also be considered when addressing polypharmacy, aging, and interaction effects. Of more than 100 patients surveyed in Canada, only 18% of the medications taken per patient were ART meds, while 25% were OTC, 22% were complementary and alternative, and 13% were non-medical (presumably recreational) [13]. Even when drugs taken for non-medical uses were excluded, the range of drugs taken was from 6 to 32 separate medications per day. Complementary and alternative medications include many vitamins, supplements, herbal products, homeopathic medications, and others. Many of these have not been studied as sources of possible adverse drug interactions in persons aging and living with HIV [14].

Only a few studies have shown the effect of polypharmacy and comorbidities as a detriment to the patient's quality of life. A recently published report shows that in a group of 262 people living with HIV in the San Diego area, polypharmacy and comorbidity burden adversely affects the health-related quality of life, as measured using the Charlson Co-morbidity Index (CCI) [15]. The CCI is a widely used measure, cited in many comorbidity studies. The CCI, with some modifications, can be used to predict the 10-year mortality for a patient who may have a range of comorbid conditions, such as heart disease, AIDS, or cancer (a total of 22 conditions). Each condition is assigned a score of 1, 2, 3, or 6, depending on the risk of dying associated with each one. Scores are summed to provide a total score to predict mortality over a 10-year follow-up period. In considering CCI scores relative to age, HIV status, and comorbidity, this chapter emphasizes the relationship between these variables. Younger AIDS patients (age <50) only have a slight increase in their CCI score, but older patients have a CCI score that is 4 times greater than their matched HIV-negative cohort. These scores indicate that the morbidity risk is significantly affected when age, HIV status, and comorbidity interact.

A Swiss study, underway with recruitment of participants and primary care providers, demonstrates the efforts being taken with particular interventions being tested to improve the accuracy of medication regimen adherence in a world of polypharmacy. This Swiss study is using an algorithm to assess and reassess each individual medication, with a goal of simplifying medication regimens [16]. This is a study with the goal of reducing polypharmacy as much as is safely possible, and will be prospective and randomized. The researchers plan to recruit about 35 primary healthcare practices, and subsequently have one cohort use a new algorithm to prioritize the medication list for its patients. The control cohort will hear a discussion about the problem of comorbidity, but will not use the algorithm. Decision points in the algorithm include:

(1) The indication for the prescribed medication seems valid and relevant. If not, stop using the drug.

(2) Do the known possible adverse reactions of the drug outweigh the possible benefits? If not, stop the drug.

(3) Can the dosage be reduced with no significant risk to the patient? If yes, reduce the dose.

(4) Is there another drug that might be superior to the drug in question? If yes, switch to the other drug.

While this analysis may seem obvious, the hope is that by raising consciousness of the provider by using the algorithm, comorbidity will decrease. Results will be evaluated every 6 months for at least 2 years.

Clearly, polypharmacy is becoming a more urgent concern as the population of those with HIV increases. Not only are those who have been infected earlier in their life living longer, but also older people are more sexually active, and new cases are also being discovered in those over 50. Careful coordination of care and thoughtful assessment are key to managing these patients in the future.

## Newer Treatment Guidelines

We know that ART causes side effects, which include hyperlipidemia, diabetes, body morphology, and lactic acidosis [17]. One of the benefits of newer ARTs, particularly medication regimens that are able to avoid the use of protease inhibitors, is that many of these experiences can be avoided [18]. Concern is now heightened regarding long-term cardiovascular mortality in patients who experience dyslipidemia, and/or glucose intolerance, as well as other common comorbidities associated with age [19]. In general, it appears that the benefits of ART used in accordance with published guidelines outweigh the risk of cardiovascular disease and other comorbidities associated with long-term exposure.

What is critical is that as we come to know more and more about drug interactions and adverse reactions, healthcare providers need to take the time or create an accessible system that allows them to easily find resources to guide their practice with patients who are aging, living with HIV and coming to see them for multiple reasons (multiple comorbidities).

Useful resources for providers to assess the potential of drug–drug interactions as they individualize patient regimens include:

- DHHS Guidelines for the Use of Antiretroviral agents (htpps://aidsinfo.nih.gov);
- University of California San Francisco HIVInSite Database of Drug interactions (http://arv.ucsf.edu);
- The Toronto General Hospital Immunodeficiency Clinic Drug Interaction Tables (http://www.hivclinic.ca/main/drugsinteract.html).

In the most recent guidelines for the Use of Antiretroviral Agents in HIV-1 Infected Adults, produced by the United States Department of Health and Human Services Panel on Antiretroviral guidelines, there is a major change in treatment options. There are now 5 recommended combinations for the antiretroviral naïve patient, consisting of 4 integrase strand transfer inhibitors (INSTIs), and one boosted protease-based combination. Two previously recommended treatment combinations have been switched to 'alternative' regimens, with the non-nuclear reverse transcriptase efavirenz downgraded because of tolerance issues in many studies. Another previously preferred option, combining boosted atazanavir with tenofovir (TFV) and FTC (emtricitabine) has also been downgraded because of a greater rate of discontinuance due to toxicities of atazanavir. As there is a wide variety of drugs available, there are important caveats for the use of many of these treatment plans [20].

To determine which of the medication combinations are best suited for an individual patient, a baseline evaluation is recommended. Aside from including the usual markers (HIV antibody, CD4 count, plasma viral load, complete blood count, chemistries, liver function tests, kidney function tests, serology for hepatitis A, B, and C, and fasting glucose and lipids), a genotypic resistance test is also recommended [21]. This test determines the genotype of the predominant virus that has infected the patient, and if there is resistance to a certain drug. Some patients are infected with a virus that has already acquired resistance to some medications, which must be avoided if possible. They also recommend evaluation of the patient's psychological readiness to begin ART, an assessment for high risk behaviors, substance abuse, presence of adequate social support, active or past mental illness, medical comorbidities, economic factors, insurance and financial status, and any other factors that have been historically shown to impair adherence in the experience of the provider in his or her home area [20].

Other specific tests may be indicated, for example, if a CCR5 co-receptor antagonist will be part of the plan, a co-receptor tropism assay should be done [22]. CCR5 is one of the receptors on the surface of the CD4 cell that is necessary to bind the virus in the early stage of infection. If the patient is a candidate for this type of drug (the CCR5 antagonist), this test will assure the prescriber that this drug will be useful.

If abacavir is used, a test to screen for the presence of HLA-B*5701 (human lymphocyte antigen), an inherited marker, must be done to reduce the risk of a life-threatening hypersensitivity reaction. A negative test for this antibody is about 95% accurate to avoid this reaction [23].

The current guidelines recommend treatment for all HIV-infected persons, regardless of the CD4 level. There are no longer differences in the guidelines for any variation of age of the patient. The presence of HIV-associated nephropathy, co-infection with hepatitis B and/or hepatitis C or other liver diseases may necessitate alterations in the regimen, and influence the choices made by the provider. Presence of other HIV-associated comorbidities, such as diabetes, hypertension, cardiovascular disease, lipid abnormalities, and many others may often direct the provider to change the therapy. Careful consideration of drug interactions must be thoughtfully considered.

### Drug–Drug Interactions

The IDSA, HHS, and European guidelines for the older HIV-infected patients are no longer different from those for younger patients, other than cautioning about the increased risk of drug–drug interactions. The guidelines go on to state that '...data that would favor the use of any of the...regimens on the basis of age are not available'. The choice of regimen should be based on a comprehensive review of the patient's other medical conditions and medications. A noteworthy limitation of currently available information is the lack of data on the long-term safety of specific antiretroviral drugs in older patients [20]. Most previous studies have excluded patients over 50, except the ongoing Veteran's Administration cohort.

The guidelines also caution about the uncertainty of dosage levels because of the lack of systemic studies: focusing on the efficacy, pharmacokinetics, adverse effects, and drug interaction potential of HIV medication in the older adult. It is well known that the main routes of drug clearance are hepatic and renal; but function of both of these organs often deteriorate with age. This can presumably result in impaired drug elimination, and consequent drug accumulation. Whether drug accumulation in the older patient may lead to a greater incidence and severity of adverse events is yet to be studied [24].

## Future Treatment Options

### *Reformulation of Drugs*

One of the goals, both to increase adherence and to minimize drug resistance, is to combine several medications in one tablet. Without getting into an inclusive list of the rapidly evolving armamentarium, the reader is urged to use current sources of drug information to keep abreast of the situation. Some examples of approved 'all-in-one' medications are:

- Complera (emtricitibine, rilpivirine, TFV);
- Atripla (efavirenz, TFV, emtricibine);
- Stribild (elvitegravir, cobicistat, TFV, emtricitibine);
- Genvoya (elvitegravir, cobicistat, TFV alafenamide, emtricibine);
- A new formulation of TFV.

There are also several 2-drug combinations that can be used with a third and/or fourth agent. Many other combinations are in development. A useful chart of current medications, including actual photographs of the medications and simple guidelines for their use is maintained by AIDSWeb, an American non-profit organization [25]. Another source is supported by the US government [26]. A source for current drugs approved in the European Union is maintained by AIDSMap [27].

TFV has been and is currently the backbone of many of the recommended drug combinations, but there is increasing evidence that its long-term use may be associated with bone and renal toxicities; problems that are exacerbated with age [28, 29]. A new formulation of TFV, TFV alafenamide, has been designed and is currently in Phase 3 clinical trials. It was approved by the US Food and Drug Administration in November 2015 for use in a combination drug, but would not be available as a single agent until sometime in 2016 [30]. It is a novel TFV prodrug with a 90% reduction of plasma TFV concentration, which maintains therapeutic intranuclear drug levels. These regimens can have increased renal and bone safety when compared with the old TFV disoproxil fumarate preparation. This may hopefully decrease some of the long-term toxicities of TFV [10].

Asensi et al. [32] ask if antiretroviral therapy can be tailored to each human immunodeficiency virus-infected individual [31]. This work discusses whether the growing field of pharmacogenomics might help clinicians increase the efficacy of antiretroviral drugs by improving their pharmacokinetics and pharmacodynamics, and by decreasing their side effects. Single nucleotide polymorphisms (SNPs) may be isolated but have an effect on drug metabolism. Unfortunately, it is concluded that 'much more effort needs to be devoted to complete large prospective studies with multiple SNPs genotyping to reveal more clues'.

## Adherence

The World Health Organization describes adherence as the extent to which a person's behavior – taking medication, following a specific diet, and/or managing lifestyle changes – that correspond to the negotiated recommendations from their healthcare provider [33]. They go on to subdivide adherence problems into those related to:

- Social and economic factors. Poverty, homelessness, solitary existence without support structure.
- Health system-related, including the patient–provider interaction, the follow-up care from the provider's team, and fragmentation of care. Personal, friendly, and consistent care from the team is vital.
- Condition-related, including characteristics of the disease and its severity and chronicity. Patients in more advanced stage of their HIV may require more complex interventions. Other significant comorbidities must also be considered.
- Patient-related, including the patient's own understanding of the treatment, the patient's level of cognitive function, health literacy, motivation, and social support.
- Therapy-related; including polypharmacy, complexity of administration schedules, adverse drug reactions, and duration of therapy [34].

One would intuitively think that the combination of multiple ARTs in one tablet, decreasing the pill burden and frequency of administration of medications would increase adherence, but a study in Canada in aging patients shows otherwise [35]. While only one or 2 pills needed to be taken for HIV treatment, the number of pills needed to treat comorbid conditions increased with the patient's age. The decrease in HIV medication-related pill burden, indicate a decrease in the number of HIV pills taken per day from 1990 to 2010 and the upward change in the total pill burden.

On average, the frequency of dosing of antiretrovirals on a daily basis in 1990 was 3 times a day. By 2000, most patients were able to switch to twice daily medication, and by 2010, almost 70% of patients were only required to take pills once a day.

However, as patients aged (by living longer with their HIV infection), they acquired multiple comorbidities. The average total pill burden in 1990 was 4–5 tablets per day. With the onset of highly active ART in 1996, the pill burden increased to 10–12 pills per day, with most of them being HIV medications. As better combinations became available, the HIV medication aspect of the pill burden decreased, but the average patient in this study was still taking 7–8 pills per day.

Hence, there was actually no real change in the need for adherence to a multiple medication schedule, as the decreased HIV pill burden was confounded by the need for other medications to treat the comorbidities. The reasons for these findings may be that patients are living longer.

Other factors that may influence adherence are the active use of opiates. Several studies have shown that some sort of opiate maintenance program has a somewhat beneficial effect on adherence [36]. In a study of 557 HIV-positive adults in the greater New York City area, the subjects were sorted into days any HIV medication was missed, and the number of days the participants used alcohol, marijuana, cocaine/crack cocaine, opiates, and other drugs. Poorest adherence was reported in groups using alcohol combined with marijuana, those using alcohol and cocaine, and those using multiple substances. It was concluded that the type of substance(s) used matters when assessing the health of older adults living with HIV, and that multiple substance use implies greater problems and more urgent need for intervention.

Springer et al. [37] found that in a study of 295 opioid-dependent patients with HIV on ART, a significant improvement in adherence and long-term control of the virus was associated with buprenorphine and/or naloxone maintenance therapy. The longer duration of this therapy was not shown to have any detrimental effect on HIV markers. Most of those who failed in the study were those who had comorbid substance use disorders and/or mental health problems.

The primary care guidelines directly address the maximization of adherence, and the most salient recommendations are summarized here:

- All HIV-infected patients should be offered timely access to routine and urgent care.
- HIV care sites should provide care that is linguistically and culturally appropriate.
- HIV sites, even those using a multidisciplinary model, should identify a primary care provider and support the development of a trusting relationship.
- All patients should be evaluated for depression and substance abuse, and if present, an appropriate management plan should be developed.
- An HIV team that includes an involved case manager has been found to be helpful.
- Social services should be involved to help with inadequate access to food and/or safe housing [38].

## The Future

Several pharmaceutical companies are researching long-acting (LA) ART medications, some given by injection, but no product has entered wide clinical trials yet [39]. Cabotegravir (CAB, GSK744) is an HIV integrase strand inhibitor under development as both an oral and LA injectable. At the 2015 Conference on Retroviruses and Opportunistic Infections meeting in Boston, a report was presented on a Phase II clinical trial showing efficacy in a 2-drug combination. There is speculation that it may be potent enough to be used as long-term injectable monotherapy [40]. A vaginal ring that dispenses TFV in low doses over a 3-month span has been studied in animals and shows pharmacologic efficacy in sheep [41]. Further development is still pending, although a new study is currently enrolling, and a recent report online, from PR (Public Relations) Newsletter, details a new study of this technique.

The study, which will be funded by the US Agency for International Development (USAID) and the US President's Emergency Plan for AIDS Relief (PEPFAR), plans to examine a multipurpose prevention technology (MPT) ring that contains TFV, an antiretroviral that has been shown to prevent HIV replication in susceptible cells and also provide some protection against HSV-2 (herpes) infection, plus levonorgestrel (LNG), an established hormonal contraceptive.

The study plans to enroll a total of 50 women at Eastern Virginia Medical School (EVMS), the parent organization of CONRAD, and at Profamilia, a clinical site in the Dominican Republic. Subjects enrolled will be randomly assigned to 3 different groups: one group will use a ring containing TFV plus LNG, another group will use a ring containing TFV only, and a third group will use a placebo ring. The active product rings are designed to be effective for up to 3 months. Each woman will participate in the study for approximately 2–3 months, and use her assigned ring for up to 3 weeks. Participants began using study products for this Phase I study, which assesses safety, acceptability, and pharmacokinetics/pharmacodynamics (looking at drug concentrations in the body and the effects of drugs and how they work in the body) of the TFV/LNG ring and TFV-only ring [42]. Enrollment for this study is in progress, and preliminary reports are expected at the next international meeting in 2016.

## Summary

Even though the possibility of a cure for HIV is still not on the horizon, future improvements in treatments will continue to provide a nearly normal lifespan. However, as our patient's age, they will assume the burden of those comorbidities associated with normal aging, as well as the chronic low-grade inflammation caused by the virus. Continued attempts at treatment simplification and management of the complexities of drug–drug interaction will require ongoing surveillance. However, the many newer drug options and combinations, and the increasingly positive results from the use of the INSTI drugs allow some optimism. These INSTIs have less toxicity, less likelihood for interactions with the drugs used to treat comorbid conditions, and greater durability and higher genetic resistance to mutations. However, the sociological problems that still do not assure access to competent care will continue to

Brennan-Ing M, DeMarco RF (eds): HIV and Aging. Interdiscipl Top Gerontol Geriatr.
Basel, Karger, 2017, vol 42, pp 85–100 (DOI: 10.1159/000448546)

# Behavioral Health

David W. Pantalone[a, b] • Stephanie E. Czajkowski[b] • S. Wade Taylor[b, c]

[a]Department of Psychology, University of Massachusetts Boston, [b]The Fenway Institute, Fenway Health, and [c]Department of Social Work, Wheelock College, Boston, Mass., USA

**Abstract**

In this chapter, we will describe the state of the literature on behavioral health, which includes mental health and substance use problems, and the available treatment interventions to ameliorate these problems, for older adults living with HIV (OALH). The scientific literature on the behavioral health of OALH is highly underdeveloped, especially in terms of the creation of empirically supported interventions to alleviate psychological distress. From the literature that does exist, there are a number of salient factors that emerge, including stereotypes (i.e., older adults are not sexually active), stigmatization (of those who are HIV-positive), social isolation, unique psychosocial needs for newly-infected OALH, and elevated rates of emotional distress and concomitant disorders – especially, depression. These factors persist alongside findings that OALH have fewer sources of social or institutional support, fewer surviving peers, and a lack of family to care for them. Additionally, many OALH report problems with substance use, both as a function of their 'baby-boomer' generational status (i.e., people born between 1946 and 1964) and in terms of the life experiences associated with their HIV-positive status. Overall, it is unclear how mental health and substance use problems affect combination antiretroviral therapy adherence, multimorbidity, polypharmacy, or treatment outcomes in this population, and further study is needed. 

## Overview and Definitions

In this chapter, we will describe the state of the literature on behavioral health among older adults living with HIV (OALH). We conceptualize behavioral health as including mental health and substance use problems faced by OALH, and treatment interventions that are available to ameliorate these problems. We begin by providing a brief overview of some social and biological factors that help in understanding the behavioral health of OALH. Then, we discuss the phenomenology of mental health and substance use problems affecting this population. We describe the extant literature on service utilization and treatment approaches designed to address the behavioral health challenges of OALH. Finally, we end by highlighting some open questions in the field that, if addressed, would greatly improve the health and well-being of OALH.

With effective treatment, OALHs live longer and healthier lives. According to a recent report on HIV and aging that was prepared by the National Institutes of Health (NIH) Office of AIDS Research (OAR) [1], effective treatment may help HIV-infected individuals to live well into their 70s. In this chapter, we define OALH as those individuals whose chronological age is 50 or greater. Using age 50 as a cutoff is not necessarily supported by the gerontology literature at large. However, age 50 is a commonly used convention for dichotomously splitting the HIV-positive population, likely because of historical features of the epidemic, that is, for so long it was a 'young man's disease' [2]. In this chapter, we will use the term OALH intentionally to represent those people aged 50 and older who are currently living with the virus, to match best the published literature in this area.

It bears mention, before addressing the major findings from the literature, that behavioral health among OALH is a highly underdeveloped topic. There are countless studies on the behavioral health of people living with HIV generally, but not enough attention has been paid to OALH specifically, in terms of their mental health and substance use problems, and even less attention has been paid to the development of interventions to ameliorate their psychological distress. The literature that does exist, across topics, investigates predictors and outcomes inconsistently across studies, which hampers direct comparisons. However, we are undaunted in our charge: to expose readers of this volume to a high-level summary of the literature on behavioral health and OALH.

### Factors Affecting the Behavioral Health of OALH

In the US, HIV/AIDS has become a chronic condition that can often be managed long-term, resulting in an aging cohort of people living with HIV, bringing with it a new set of research questions for the field to answer [3]. There is generally little consideration in the literature given to OALH, since the behaviors implicated in HIV transmission – sex and drug use – are not expected of older people [4]. Despite expectations, by 2015, people aged 50 and over are expected to comprise approximately 50% of HIV/AIDS cases in the US [5]. Thus, older adults represent a sizeable and growing segment of the population of people living with the virus.

Why is there a growing proportion of the population of HIV-infected adults who are over 50? There are many social and biological factors associated with the increasing burden of HIV on older adults, and this impacts their behavioral health. Arguably the most significant factor contributing to the increasing proportion of OALH is the effectiveness and widespread availability of combination antiretroviral therapy (cART), which has facilitated this growth in 2 ways [3]. Indeed, there is a need to differentiate between 2 populations in HIV and aging research, including those older adults who acquired the virus in later life, and those older adults who have successfully survived a longstanding infection into older age. The former group may have been infected with HIV through sexual contact with the latter group, which is made possible by the increased lifespan and general overall health – which contributes to maintaining an active sex life. According to data findings, over 50% of OALH are sexually active [6], with 33–42% reporting having engaged in condomless anal or vaginal sex [7], which might further explain these HIV infection rates.

Consideration of the current behavioral health status of OALH requires an explicit acknowledgement of the heterogeneity of life history and experiences inherent in any present-day snapshot of these individuals. OALH who have more recently acquired the virus will have some unique psychosocial needs, such as coping with a new infection, adjusting to the demands of treatment, and learning to navigate disclosure to family, friends, and sex partners [8]. These factors may be present for newly-infected older adults, in addition to the general factors affecting all OALH, including fear of death, social isolation, neurological changes, fatigue, changes in appearance, and financial distress [9]. These unique experiences, often co-occurring over time, remain unexplored in the behavioral health literature on OALH. Also, addressing multiple behavioral health targets in interventions might help to increase the overall health profiles for diverse groups of OALH.

Other factors affecting the lives of OALH may be elevated rates of emotional distress and concomitant disorders. For example, they have fewer sources of social or institutional support, fewer surviving peers, lack of family to care for them, and their HIV-uninfected peers may consider their HIV-positive status as more stigmatizing than do the peers of younger adults living with the virus [10]. According to the CDC, 99% of new diagnoses aged 20–24 survived over a year after their diagnosis compared with rates of 73–89% for OALH [11]. Furthermore, because of being less attuned to the risk of infection, older people may be diagnosed later in the course of their HIV illness, making successful treatment more difficult, and reducing the time between diagnosis and death [10]. Indeed, there is evidence that many older adults receive a 'delayed diagnosis', that is, at the time of their first HIV-positive test result they already meet criteria for AIDS [12]. In this same study, several sobering statistics emerge: older (>50) late presenters were 14 times more likely to die within a year of diagnosis compared with older adults who were not diagnosed late (14 vs. 1%, $p < 0.001$) and had 2.4 times the risk of dying than younger (<50) late presenters.

Given that the domestic US HIV epidemic is still one primarily fueled by condomless sex, the widespread availability of erectile-enhancing medications [13] likely played a role in the shifting burden of HIV to older adults. Many adults over 50, especially heterosexual individuals (particularly postmenopausal women), may harbor outmoded misconceptions about HIV being a 'gay disease' and may not think about their sex lives in terms of the risk of acquiring other sexually transmitted infections (STIs). The frame has been one of pregnancy prevention, and they may eschew barrier protection once it is biologically impossible [4]. With population-level trends, such as increases in the mean lifespan of the general population, divorce becoming more widespread, and the rise of the internet as a means of connecting people who are not (or even who are, in the case of extra-dyadic sex) already in relationships, we should expect more HIV infections among older adults [4]. This is further compounded by society's misguided expectation that older adults do not engage in sexual activity [4] and, as a result, HIV prevention campaigns are infrequently tailored specifically to this demographic. Pre-exposure prophylaxis or PrEP, a daily anti-HIV medication regimen has been shown to be highly effective in preventing HIV acquisition in MSM [14]. However, we could not locate any published empirical data about the frequency of PrEP prescriptions among older sexually active adults (especially for those <65 with no history of kidney disease), and it could provide a helpful adjunctive HIV prevention strategy in this population.

Social factors, also, are likely to contribute to the mental health problems, for example, depression and substance use of OALH. Social participation, which decreases with age in the general population, may be especially limited for OALH. Removal from the workforce plays a role in increasing social isolation, as well as decreasing availability of informal support networks like family and friends [9]. Again, some amount of social withdrawal is expected, given the age-related social network changes in the general population, due to retirement, illness, relocation, or death – along with ageism [9]. However, OALH face the additional stigma of living with the virus and, potentially, a higher burden of physical health problems that could limit mobility and curtail independence, impacting the ability to maintain social relationships over time [9]. These social stressors – along with the burden of living with potentially multiple comorbid health conditions to manage – is the most probable cause for the high burden of behavioral health challenges facing OALH. The complex and dynamic interactions between these psychosocial and medical factors conspire to mark OALH as an especially vulnerable population.

In addition to the social and biological factors that influence HIV epidemiology and the psychological experience of living with the virus for OALH, there are also medical factors to consider. Aging with HIV is linked with multimorbidity, which includes managing multiple chronic conditions concurrently, and polypharmacy, comprising the numerous treatments to manage or alleviate those conditions [9]. For OALH, there is a significant burden on their physical health from HIV and other health problems, including the HIV-associated non-AIDS or 'HANA' conditions. HANA are increasingly common and associated with both aging and chronic inflammation, including cardiovascular disease, infectious and noninfectious cancers, osteopenia/osteoporosis, liver cirrhosis, and renal disease [9]. Some evidence has been reported, indicating that the progress of these conditions is accelerated for OALH [9]. Disentangling the relative contributions of these factors to the mental health and substance use problems of HIV infection, HIV treatment, other comorbid health conditions, and typical aging processes is one of the primary challenges to the current literature.

In summary, there are multiple, overlapping social, biological, and medical factors operating in the background as we approach the study of mental health and substance use problems of OALH. Indeed, these factors – those that, for our purposes, are in the 'background' – have actually been the subject of significant research attention, while our interest, behavioral health, has not. There is much published work that aims to explicate the associations among, for example, biological aging, long-term cART use, and enduring HIV infection; however, there has been relatively little written about the role of mental health and substance use as they relate to those areas [2]. Despite the limited literature, in the ensuing sections of the chapter, we report on what has been published in these areas: first mental health symptoms, then substance use problems, and finally interventions to address them in OALH.

## Mental Health of OALH

There is limited research on the mental health status of OALH. Here, under the umbrella of 'mental health', we include both traditional psychiatric symptoms, such as depression and anxiety, that would be seen in the DSM-5 [15], as well as other psychosocial stressors that may not fit within the parameters of a strict definition – such as loneliness, stigma, and coping. There is significant literature on HIV-related cognitive impairments; this will be addressed comprehensively in another chapter. Despite the relative dearth of empirical studies in this area, the published findings are unequivocal: OALH appear to be vulnerable to psychological distress, especially depression.

There are several recent review articles that summarize the extant findings. In the most comprehensive paper on this topic, Chambers et al. [9] performed a systematic review of 13 databases and consulted with 45 experts, eventually identifying 204 studies on 'aging and health' of OALH. Among those studies identified, 59 focused on psychological factors related to aging; however, the majority were concerned with HIV-associated neurocognitive disorders; only 17 focused on other mental health concerns. Among those, most studies focused on depression (12/17) or psychological well-being (12/17), through quantitative or qualitative designs, with a significant minority addressing resilience (7/17). This chapter details the burden of mental health symptoms on OALH. The literature overwhelmingly reported on relatively recent (2007 and later) findings from studies conducted in the US, using clinical samples, and disproportionately focused on sexual minority men (SMM) or MSM [9]. This focus on SMM/MSM is reasonable because they are the demographic group in the US with the greatest prevalence; however, this literature does not take into account the prevalence (due to increasing incidence) of HIV among women and especially heterosexually identified women of color [11].

In another systematic review, the focus was more specifically on social and behavioral research (more health behaviors than mental health, specifically) on HIV and aging. Sankar et al. [2] identified 58 research papers that address the interaction of HIV and age. They noted that there were fewer clear age-related differences than they expected. However, they did observe significant differences in terms of disclosure and stigma, with OALH less likely to reveal their HIV status and to report more HIV stigma than younger adults. Also, differences emerged among OALH when groups were defined by mode of transmission (e.g., IDU vs. sex), as well as notable racial/ethnic differences. Ethnic minority OALH had smaller social networks, and they were more likely to feel isolated. In some studies, social support served as a buffer – those with more medical problems had more support – and more support was associated with better psychological functioning. These authors note, further, that a life course perspective may provide insight into the high burden of mental health problems reported by OALH. That is, because of deviations from the expected life course, such as living with an incurable STI later in life – which requires explanations and justifications, and may be seen as evidence of incompetence, irresponsibility, or carelessness – OALH may have a strongly and chronically increased allostatic load, physiological degradation of the body resulting from a chronic illness, that is, HIV.

Given these qualifications and caveats, as one might predict, mental health symptoms appear to be a significant concern for OALH, across studies. Most of the published findings are focused on depression and related symptoms, such as loneliness (which could be a cause of depression) and suicidal ideation (which could be a result). In between-group comparisons, depressive symptoms were typically higher in OALH compared to age-matched HIV-negative peers or younger adults living with HIV. Depression appears to be the most common psychological mental health problem of OALH [16]. OALH are more likely to live alone and are at a higher risk of social isolation, depression, and loneliness [17]. Depression was found in OALH at rates of 25–39% of the samples with some association with loneliness and HIV stigma [2]. The severity of depression in OALH appears to be positively associated with stigma and negatively associated with social support and self-reported social problem-solving skills [18]. Engagement with behavioral health care was associated with less depressive symptoms [19], and a greater number of medical comorbidities was associated with greater depressive symptoms [20]. Notably, depressive symptoms were significantly correlated with decreased physical functioning as well as vision and hearing loss, skin problems, heart and respiratory conditions, broken bones and fractures, erectile dysfunction, and neuropathy [20, 21]. In one study, they found that depression, combined with a higher number of medical problems, was associated with a decrease in life expectancy [22]. Similar findings emerged for psychosocial distress and suicidal ideation [9].

Social support was well-represented in the behavioral health literature on OALH. In several studies, various forms of psychosocial distress were associated with each other, or loneliness or lack of social support was associated with such distress. As people age, they tend to seek and receive social support less frequently, which contributes to having greater distress [23]. Also, according to the socioemotional selectivity theory, as people age, their perceived time becomes constrained, so their focus shifts to emphasize emotional satisfaction over information-gathering; this change in motivation leads to less-informed decisions which can be detrimental to their health when compared to younger populations who are more likely to seek a second opinion, gather additional information, and take more time to make to a decision [24]. In a study of 95 African American OALH [25], investigators found that greater perceived support was associated with better overall health and, as perceived support decreased, depressive symptoms, trait anger, and other psychosocial stressors increased. One finding from the general psychology literature was replicated for OALH: lower social support was associated with increased suicidality [26]. Social support and its converse, loneliness, as discussed below, should remain the focus of future research on mental health of OALH.

Finally, a number of studies on the mental health of OALH deal with the topic of stigma. Generally, authors found that stigma was associated with more psychological symptoms, such as social isolation and depression [27]. For example, Grov et al. [28] found a positive correlation between stigma and depression, loneliness, poor perceived health, decreased cognitive functioning, and low energy levels. In addition, perceived stigma corresponded to a higher HIV-related life-stressor burden, decrease in support from friends, and less access to healthcare and social services [29]. Stigma is an important area for future research on OALH, including the various areas that are relevant: HIV stigma and age-stigma, of course, but also the intersectional stigmas based on other identities, including race/ethnicity, sexual orientation, and ability/disability.

Overall, it appears from the limited available literature on the mental health of the ever-growing population of OALH that there are many unanswered questions, and the evidence that does exist shows that this is a population of concern in terms of mental health. A chief concern is why we see high levels of depressive symptoms in OALH, despite their ongoing engagement with medical care for their HIV treatment. Having a better understanding of the etiology of depression in OALH is specifically needed, and depression prevention or reduction strategies are also needed for OALH to ameliorate the potential negative impact of depression on HIV disease management, cART adherence, and engagement with care [30].

## Substance Use of OALH

Substance use is an emerging public health concern for the 'baby-boom' generation (i.e., people born between 1946 and 1964), and regardless of their HIV status, substance use in older adults seems to be rising. Adults who use illegal drugs earlier in life often continue the behavior into older age. In 2009, Han et al. [31] estimated that the number of adults 50 years and older with a substance use disorder will more than double, to approximately 5.7 million, by 2020. Indeed, a systematic review of the literature [32] revealed that substance use disorders were common among older adults, and that treatment admissions for both illegal and prescription drug abuse in this population have been increasing in the US. It is clear that substance abuse is an ongoing – or, perhaps, growing – problem for older adults.

Despite the robust literature on behavioral aspects of HIV over the past 30 years, there have been relatively few studies focused specifically on substance use of OALH [33–35]. In 2012, the OAR of the NIH convened a Working Group on HIV and Aging, and one product of the group was a paper based on their published report to NIH that outlined specific knowledge gaps and priority research areas to be addressed [1]. These areas include how substance use might influence HIV transmission in older adults, medication adherence, comorbidities, and treatment outcomes. Some research on OALH has identified relationship between substance use, comorbidities and HIV/AIDS [10, 36, 37]. However, ongoing substance use in the context of comorbid illnesses and understanding these relationships is a major concern for individuals living with HIV, especially OALH [38]. Data suggest that, compared to older HIV-negative people, OALH will more likely continue using substances throughout their lives [39]. This presents a unique challenge for HIV prevention efforts: substance use is highly associated with HIV transmission risk behavior across populations and, thus, fine-grained evaluation of these relationships in OALH sub-groups is greatly needed. In addition, experts noted that the lack of social networks in this at-risk group might be associated with alcohol, tobacco, psychoactive drug use, as well as misuse of prescription medications. Furthermore, the group recommended observational studies and randomized clinical trials to characterize, and ameliorate, the effect of substance use on OALH mental health and HIV transmission [1].

These concerns are notable, especially, since some published studies suggest that rates of substance use in OALH are similar to their HIV-uninfected peers. For example, using longitudinal data (6,351 HIV-infected and uninfected adults) from the 8-site Veterans Aging Cohort Study [40], authors discovered that there was no significant difference in the past year alcohol use between HIV-negative older adults and OALH (approximately 68% for each) [33]. A similar pattern emerged for drug abuse and drug dependence: no significant differences emerged for OALH compared to their HIV-negative peers (25% for each group). However, OALH reported a significantly greater frequency of drug use [33]. Our ability to present descriptive data for OALH substance use is limited by the scarce epidemiologic research on this topic. It is important to note that, given other published data on substance use and veterans, we would expect higher rates among this group due to common comorbidities within the said population.

Green et al. [33] suggest that their data support the need for physicians and caregivers to continue screening OALH for substance use and dependence. Other researchers have provided data to support this need to screen OALH, who use and misuse substances [41] and to develop effective healthcare models for this population [32]. Alternatively, others claim that OALH have a greater risk for mental health and substance use problems, including alcohol and substance abuse and dependence, when compared to their HIV-negative counterparts [16].

Recent surveillance data collected by the CDC [42] suggests that nearly two-thirds of US adults consume alcohol. Some research suggests alcohol consumption is lower in older adults compared to younger adults [43, 44]. However, only a few studies provide evidence about alcohol consumption and older persons living with HIV. For example, in a study to understand alcohol use in OALH who are on antiretroviral therapy, Williams et al. [45] found in a sample of 447 participants 50 or over, 57% reported drinking alcohol in the past year and 22% presented with unhealthy alcohol use. They noted that this finding is similar to the prevalence of the entire US population (22.6%) identified by Dawson et al. [43]. In addition, Gongvatana [75] (2014) identified that alcohol negatively affects neurocognitive deficits in HIV-infected persons 60 and older. More studies are needed to address alcohol use and its effects on health behaviors and HIV management in OALH.

Evidence suggests that alcohol use accelerates HIV progression [46–48] and might accentuate comorbidities such as functional decline and organ system failure that advances clinical diseases [49]. There is some indication that both alcohol use [50] and drug use [51, 52] may be associated with poorer cART adherence, which might be a pathway through which substance use indirectly affects disease progression. Furthermore, evidence suggests across several studies that substance use is associated with engagement in condomless vaginal or anal sex. For example, Lovejoy et al. [53] sampled older HIV-infected adults (n = 290) from 3 USA AIDS service organizations and found that in the past 3 months 38% were sexually active. Furthermore, of those sexually active 33% reported at least one condomless sex act in the same time period. Similarly, Golub et al. [7] surveyed 328 sexually active OALH in New York City and identified that psychological well-being was associated with protected sex practices. Not surprisingly, condomless sex acts might place individuals and their partners at risk for STI acquisition – which can draw on immune system resources and negatively impact HIV health. More secondary HIV preventions are needed to address multiple behavioral health targets (e.g., sexual risk behavior, psychological well-being, and HIV disease management).

In a thorough literature review, Edelman et al. [38] identified the substances most commonly used by OALH: tobacco, non-opioid prescription medications, heroin and prescription opioids, marijuana, and stimulants. Paying attention to prescription drug abuse (and drug–drug interactions, including interactions between illicit drugs and prescription drugs) seems important for this group, given the multimorbidity and ensuing polypharmacy that are so common for OALH. In addition, Edelman et al. [38] noted that alcohol use appears in this population at a rate that is similar to that of younger HIV-uninfected patients. In one study, in a sample of 239 HIV-positive gay and bisexual men over 50, Brennan-Ing et al. [54] found that bisexual men were more likely to use tobacco, cocaine, crack and heroin, compared to gay men – but were less likely to use crystal methamphetamine. Siconolfi et al. [55] found, in a diverse sample of OALH in New York City (n = 914), that the most commonly used substances were cigarettes (57.2%) and alcohol (38.8%), but generally drug use differed by gender and sexual orientation; that is, gay and bisexual male OALH were more likely to report using alcohol and poppers, while heterosexual OALH were more likely to report tobacco use. Taken together, research in this area indicates that, in understanding the patterns of substance use in OALH, we need to be mindful of potentially reliable differences across demographic subgroups. More studies are needed that address substance use in older HIV-infected SMM, in particular.

Tobacco use plays a major role in negative health outcomes in people living with HIV; approximately between 31 and 84% of HIV-infected patients identify as smokers [56, 57]. However, Edelman et al. [38] noted that little attention has been given to understand tobacco smoking in older HIV-infected adults. A cross-sectional study conducted by Mdodo et al. [57] found that older age was associated with greater smoking prevalence, while Fredriksen-Goldsen et al. [58] determined that lesbian, gay, bisexual, and transgender older HIV-infected adults used much more tobacco than their un-infected peers. More recently, in a sample of 199 HIV-infected SMM, Ompad et al. [59] identified that current smokers were less likely to report an undetectable HIV viral load, and suggested that tobacco smoking might be related to poorer HIV clinical indicators. However, more empirical studies, with larger samples that ensure greater generalizability, are needed to better understand and contextualize the effects of all substances of use on health outcomes and functional impairment in OALH.

Although sparse, emerging literature points to psychosocial correlates of substance use in older HIV-infected adults. Parsons et al. [60] reported on data from a sample of 557 HIV-infected older adults recruited in New York City, to better understand the psychosocial and behavioral correlates of substance use. These authors identified 4 distinct latent-class patterns of substance use: 'excessive alcohol use', 'alcohol and marijuana', 'alcohol and cocaine/crack', and 'multiple substance use'. They found that gay and bisexual OALH were overly represented in the class of multiple substance users, and heterosexual participants were overly represented in the class of alcohol and cocaine/crack users. Participants in all of these classes reported higher rates of HIV cART non-adherence compared to participants in 'no use' or 'exclusive alcohol use' classes. There is also evidence of comorbidity between mental health and substance use in OALH. For example, in one study of 301 depressed OALH, Skalski et al. [61] found that substance use was positively associated with self-destructive avoidance. Hence, further research on drinking and substance use motives of OALH is needed.

Older women who live with HIV/AIDS have received little attention in the empirical literature and in the development of relevant interventions. Durvasula [62] suggests that 'drug or alcohol use may be less prevalent in older women, and the potential augmentation of the impact of drug and alcohol use in older women reveals that the assessment of substance use in older women must be conducted in a contextualized manner (and mindful of sexual orientation, ethnic minority status, and trauma history)'. Indeed, there are a few studies which suggest that a large proportion of female OALH have histories of substance use and dependence [63, 64], highlighting this as an important area for future research and intervention development.

For OALH and substance use, as with mental health, there is a significantly underdeveloped scientific literature. Here, too, it seems that OALH might be at increased risk for having substance use at present, or in their past, especially for some demographic groups, such as women and SMM. There are many questions that remain unanswered, including basic questions about prevalence, patterns, motives, and correlates of substance use and abuse across substances and across OALH demographic subgroups.

### Behavioral Health Treatment Approaches for OALH

A literature review of work that focuses solely on evidence-based treatments for the behavioral health problems of OALH reveals a program of research by Heckman et al. [65–67] as the best example of intervention development in this area. These investigators tested multiple intervention formats – individual, group, and telephone-delivered therapy – to decrease depression, improve adaptive coping, and decrease sexual risk behavior in OALH. Their work should serve as a model for future work in this area, in terms of designing culturally tailored and efficacious interventions for OALH. There are other publications that provide clinical or theoretical guidance about ways that clinicians might effectively treat OALH, such as using a strength-based perspective [68], although these have not been tested empirically.

Challenges have been identified for addressing the behavioral health needs of older adults generally. Indeed, health services researchers have been working hard to address some of these barriers, including the mismatch between the current system of care and the preferences/needs of older adults; a fragmented and poorly integrated system across sectors and settings (primary care, mental health care, nursing homes, hospital-based care, aging-network providers, family and peer providers, etc.); and a complicated payment system that was predicted on a model of inpatient, acute behavioral health treatment, among others [69]. Despite these problems, it appears that a sizable proportion of OALH are in need of behavioral health services.

In addition to specifically tailored interventions for OALH to meet their behavioral health needs, there has been a call within the literature to improve service provision for this population through existing healthcare and social service structures [70]. Authors observed that policies and programs for older adults (such as the Older Americans Act of 1965 and Medicaid), and those for people living with HIV (such as the Ryan White CARE Act of 1990 and the AIDS Drug Access Program), are not integrated and could result in OALH 'falling through the cracks'. Furthermore, there are few providers overall – including, especially, providers who have experience with and skills for working with OALH [71]. It appears that housing status is one important factor affecting the behavioral health of OALH and their ability to access needed services [72].

From the published literature, there are some reports that OALH who needed care were not receiving it [16, 73]. This seems consistent with the significant proportion of OALH who endorse loneliness, low social support, and depression. There is some evidence to support the notion that OALH with more severe (vs. less severe) psychological symptoms were more likely to be engaged with behavioral health care, including PTSD, mania, and psychosis [16]. Other works have shown that, in a sample of adults living with HIV, old age was not associated with higher service utilization [74]. Rather than feeling encouraged, concluding that this type of finding may indicate that OALH are not in need of services, we worry that it actually indicates that there are not well-tailored services available (i.e., measures of utilization of existing services would not provide us with information on this aspect). Alternately, it could be that, in some locations where culturally tailored services are available for OALH, there are other barriers to access that we have yet to discover.

## Future Directions

In summary, there is surprisingly little behavioral health research on OALH and, from the limited research that has been published, it appears that this is a population in need of further study, especially in terms of intervention development. There is limited research on OALH generally and, as an extension, even less research performed on demographic subgroups including women, sexual and gender minorities, racial and ethnic minorities, people with unstable housing, and people with mental health conditions other than depression. There are a few studies that address each of these topics but not nearly enough for us to feel confident about the reliability or validity of the findings. Many studies performed were small qualitative or cross-sectional quantitative designs and, therefore, are limited in their ability to describe causal associations. Furthermore, a majority of research relied solely on self-report measures that are susceptible to reporting and recall biases. Older adults face the task of distinguishing symptoms of HIV from those of aging and, in several studies, participants were more likely to attribute reported symptoms to HIV than aging; whether or not that was, indeed, the case is an area for further study [2].

Indeed, there are so many open questions in the field of behavioral health and OALH that an entire chapter could be dedicated to it. Since space precludes an exhaustive treatment of this topic, we will, instead, reflect some of the key future directions described by Stoff [3] on the needed basic research, and by the NIH OAR Working Group [1] on the treatment research that is needed. Stoff [3] highlights the need for prospective studies of epidemiologic comorbidity, to examine incidence and prevalence rates of psychiatric disorders and to determine whether the age-related decline in psychopathology in the general population holds for this group. Some evidence [10] holds that this might not be true, at least not for depression and substance use. Further, more information is needed about the temporal sequencing of co-occurring mental health and substance use problems. These data, in addition to answers to the following questions posed by the NIH OAR Working Group, are needed for future intervention development efforts:

- How do the common mental health problems in OALH impact physical health and functioning, including retention in care, medical compliance, and medication adherence? What about substance use problems?
- What interventions are effective in reducing mental health and substance use problems and, thus, increasing the functionality of OALH?
- From a health systems perspective, how can we help to meet the mental health and substance use treatment needs of OALH?
  - What barriers exist that prevent community-based providers from providing adequate mental health and substance use treatments?
  - What mental health and substance use service delivery formats are associated with more favorable clinical and psychosocial outcomes?

Thirty years into the epidemic, there is a great deal of knowledge about the areas related to the behavioral health situation and needs of people living with HIV. Hopefully in the next phase of the epidemic's history, we can bring some of that ingenuity and tenacity to the study of OALH.

## References


1 High KP, Brennan-Ing M, Clifford DB, Cohen MH, Currier J, Deeks SG, Deren S, Effros RB, Gebo K, Goronzy JJ, Justice AC, Landay A, Levin J, Miotti PG, Munk RJ, Nass H, Rinaldo CR Jr, Shlipak MG, Tracy R, Valcour V, Vance DE, Walston JD, Volberding P; OAR Working Group on HIV and Aging: HIV and aging: state of knowledge and areas of critical need for research. A report to the NIH office of AIDS research by the HIV and aging working group. J Acquir Immune Defic Syndr 2012;60(suppl 1):S1–S18.

2 Sankar A, Nevedal A, Neufeld S, Berry R, Luborsky M: What do we know about older adults and HIV? A review of social and behavioral literature. AIDS Care 2011;23:1187–1207.

3 Stoff DM: Mental health research in HIV/AIDS and aging: problems and prospects. AIDS 2004;18(suppl 1):S3–S10.

4 Auerbach JD: HIV/AIDS and aging: interventions for older adults. J Acquir Immune Defic Syndr 2003; 33(suppl 2):S57–S58.

5 Brooks JT, Buchacz K, Gebo KA, Mermin J: HIV infection and older Americans: the public health perspective. Am J Public Health 2012;102:1516–1526.

6 Golub SA, Tomassilli JC, Pantalone DW, Brennan M, Karpiak SE, Parsons JT: Prevalence and correlates of sexual behavior and risk management among HIV-positive adults over 50. Sex Transm Dis 2010; 37:615–620.

7 Golub SA, Botsko M, Gamarel KE, Parsons JT, Brennan M, Karpiak SE: Dimensions of psychological well-being predict consistent condom use among older adults living with HIV. Aging Int 2011;36:346–360.

8 Emlet CA: Experiences of stigma in older adults living with HIV/AIDS: a mixed-methods analysis. AIDS Patient Care STDS 2007;21:740–752.

9 Chambers LA, Wilson MG, Rueda S, Gogolishvili D, Shi MQ, Rourke SB; Positive Aging Review Team: Evidence informing the intersection of HIV, aging and health: a scoping review. AIDS Behav 2014;18: 661–675.

10 Rabkin JG, McElhiney MC, Ferrando SJ: Mood and substance use disorders in older adults with HIV/AIDS: methodological issues and preliminary evidence. AIDS 2004;18(suppl 1):S43–S48.
11 Centers for Disease Control and Prevention: HIV among people aged 50 and over. 2016. CDC.gov/hiv/group/age/olderamericans/index.html (retrieved April 18, 2016).
12 Smith RD, Delpech VC, Brown AE, Rice BD: HIV transmission and high rates of late diagnoses among adults aged 50 years and over. AIDS 2010;24:2109–2115.
13 Swearingen SG, Klausner JD: Sildenafil use, sexual risk behavior, and risk for sexually transmitted diseases, including HIV infection. Am J Med 2005;118:571–577.
14 Jiang J, Yang X, Ye L, Zhou B, Ning C, Huang J, Liang B, Zhong X, Huang A, Tao R, Cao C, Chen H, Liang H: Pre-exposure prophylaxis for the prevention of HIV infection in high risk populations: a meta-analysis of randomized controlled trials. PLoS One 2014;9:e87674.
15 American Psychological Association: Diagnostic and Statistical Manual of Mental Disorders, ed 5. Arlington, American Psychiatric Publishing, Washington, DC.
16 Zanjani F, Saboe K, Oslin D: Age difference in rates of mental health/substance abuse and behavioral care in HIV-positive adults. AIDS Patient Care STDS 2007;21:347–355.
17 Linsk NL: Experience of older gay and bisexual men living with HIV/AIDS. J Gay Lesbian Bisexual Id 1997;2:285–308.
18 White W, Grant JS, Pryor ER, Keltner NL, Vance DE, Raper JL: Do social support, stigma, and social problem-solving skills predict depressive symptoms in people living with HIV? A mediation analysis. Res Theory Nurs Pract 2012;26:182–204.
19 Mavandadi S, et al: Psychological well-being among individuals aging with HIV: the value of social relationships. J Acquir Immune Defic Syndr 2009;51:91–98.
20 Havlik RJ, Brennan M, Karpiak SE: Comorbidities and depression in older adults with HIV. Sex Health 2011;8:551–559.
21 Oursler KK, Goulet JL, Leaf DA, Akingicil A, Katzel LI, Justice A, Crystal S: Association of comorbidity with physical disability in older HIV-infected adults. AIDS Patient Care STDS 2006;20:782–791.
22 Dubé MP, Sattler FR: Inflammation and complications of HIV disease. J Infect Dis 2010;201:1783–1785.
23 Chesney MA, Chambers DB, Taylor JM, Johnson LM: Social support, distress, and well-being in older men living with HIV infection. J Acquir Immune Defic Syndr 2003;33(suppl 2):S185–S193.
24 Löckenhoff CE, Carstensen LL: Socioemotional selectivity theory, aging, and health: the increasingly delicate balance between regulating emotions and making tough choices. J Pers 2004;72:1395–1424.
25 Whitehead NE, Hearn LE, Burrell L: The association between depressive symptoms, anger, and perceived support resources among underserved older HIV positive black/African American adults. AIDS Patient Care STDS 2014;28:507–512.
26 Kalichman SC, Heckman T, Kochman A, Sikkema K, Bergholte J: Depression and thoughts of suicide among middle-aged and older persons living with HIV-AIDS. Psychiatr Serv 2000;51:903–907.
27 Lichtenstein B, Laska MK, Clair JM: Chronic sorrow in the HIV-positive patient: issues of race, gender, and social support. AIDS Patient Care STDS 2002;16:27–38.
28 Grov C, Golub SA, Parsons JT, Brennan M, Karpiak SE: Loneliness and HIV-related stigma explain depression among older HIV-positive adults. AIDS Care 2010;22:630–639.
29 Heckman TG, Heckman BD, Kochman A, Sikkema KJ, Suhr J, Goodkin K: Psychological symptoms among persons 50 years of age and older living with HIV disease. Aging Ment Health 2002;6:121–128.
30 Pence BW, O'Donnell JK, Gaynes BN: Falling through the cracks: the gaps between depression prevalence, diagnosis, treatment, and response in HIV care. AIDS 2012;26:656–658.
31 Han B, Gfroerer JC, Colliver JD, Penne MA: Substance use disorder among older adults in the United States in 2020. Addiction 2009;104:88–96.
32 Wu LT, Blazer DG: Substance use disorders and psychiatric comorbidity in mid and later life: a review. Int J Epidemiol 2014;43:304–317.
33 Green TC, Kershaw T, Lin H, Heimer R, Goulet JL, Kraemer KL, Gordon AJ, Maisto SA, Day NL, Bryant K, Fiellin DA, Justice AC: Patterns of drug use and abuse among aging adults with and without HIV: a latent class analysis of a US veteran cohort. Drug Alcohol Depend 2010;110:208–220.
34 Rabkin JG, McElhiney MC, Ferrando SJ: Mood and substance use disorders in older adults with HIV/AIDS: methodological issues and preliminary evidence. AIDS 2004;18(suppl 1):S43–S48.
35 Schlaerth KR: Older adults and illegal drugs. Geriatrics Aging 2007;10:361–364.
36 Bertholet N, Cheng DM, Samet JH, Quinn E, Saitz R: Alcohol consumption patterns in HIV-infected adults with alcohol problems. Drug Alcohol Depend 2010;112:160–163.
37 Hansen NB, Cavanaugh CE, Vaughan EL, Connell CM, Tate DC, Sikkema KJ: The influence of personality disorder indication, social support, and grief on alcohol and cocaine use among HIV-positive adults coping with AIDS-related bereavement. AIDS Behav 2009;13:375–384.

38 Edelman EJ, Tetrault JM, Fiellin DA: Substance use in older HIV-infected patients. Curr Opin HIV AIDS 2014;9:317–324.
39 Emlet CA: Current knowledge and future directions on aging and HIV research. Behav Med 2014;40: 143–148.
40 Justice AC, Dombrowski E, Conigliaro J, Fultz SL, Gibson D, Madenwald T, et al: Veterans aging cohort study (VACS): overview and description. Med Care 2006;44:S13–S18.
41 Schonfeld L, King-Kallimanis BL, Duchene DM, Etheridge RL, Herrera JR, Barry KL, Lynn N: Screening and brief intervention for substance misuse among older adults: the Florida BRITE project. Am J Public Health 2010;100:108–114.
42 Centers for Disease Control and Prevention (CDC): Health Behaviors of Adults: United States, 2008–2010. USA Department of Health and Human Services. Atlanta, GA, National Center for Health Statistics, 2013.
43 Dawson DA, Grant BF, Stinson FS, Zhou Y: Effectiveness of the derived alcohol use disorders identification test (AUDIT-C) in screening for alcohol use disorders and risk drinking in the US general population. Alcohol Clin Exp Res 2005;29:844–854.
44 Grant BF, Dawson DA, Stinson FS, Chou SP, Dufour MC, Pickering RP: The 12-month prevalence and trends in DSM-IV alcohol abuse and dependence: United States, 1991–1992 and 2001–2002. Drug Alcohol Depend 2004;74:223–234.
45 Williams EC, Bradley KA, Balderson BH, McClure JB, Grothaus L, McCoy K, Rittmueller SE, Catz SL: Alcohol and associated characteristics among older persons living with human immunodeficiency virus on antiretroviral therapy. Subst Abus 2014;35:245–253.
46 Baum MK, Rafie C, Lai S, Sales S, Page JB, Campa A: Alcohol use accelerates HIV disease progression. AIDS Res Hum Retroviruses 2010;26:511–518.
47 Freiberg MS, McGinnis KA, Kraemer K, Samet JH, Conigliaro J, Curtis Ellison R, Bryant K, Kuller LH, Justice AC; VACS Project Team: The association between alcohol consumption and prevalent cardiovascular diseases among HIV-infected and HIV-uninfected men. J Acquir Immune Defic Syndr 2010; 53:247–253.
48 Hahn JA, Samet JH: Alcohol and HIV disease progression: weighing the evidence. Curr HIV/AIDS Rep 2010;7:226–233.
49 Justice A, Sullivan L, Fiellin D: HIV/AIDS, comorbidity, and alcohol: can we make a difference? Alcohol Res Health 2010;33:258–266.
50 Hendershot CS, Stoner SA, Pantalone DW, Simoni JM: Alcohol use and antiretroviral adherence: review and meta-analysis. J Acquir Immune Defic Syndr 2009;52:180–202.
51 Wutoh AK, Elekwachi O, Clarke-Tasker V, Daftary M, Powell NJ, Campusano G: Assessment and predictors of antiretroviral adherence in older HIV-infected patients. J Acquir Immune Defic Syndr 2003; 33(suppl 2):S106–S114.
52 Hinkin CH, Hardy DJ, Mason KI, Castellon SA, Durvasula RS, Lam MN, Stefaniak M: Medication adherence in HIV-infected adults: effect of patient age, cognitive status, and substance abuse. AIDS 2004;18(suppl 1):S19–S25.
53 Lovejoy TI, Heckman TG, Sikkema KJ, Hansen NB, Kochman A, Suhr JA, Garske JP, Johnson CJ: Patterns and correlates of sexual activity and condom use behavior in persons 50-plus years of age living with HIV/AIDS. AIDS Behav 2008;12:943–956.
54 Brennan-Ing M, Porter KE, Seidel L, Karpiak SE: Substance use and sexual risk differences among older bisexual and gay men with HIV. Behav Med 2014; 40:108–115.
55 Siconolfi DE, Halkitis PN, Barton SC, Kingdon MJ, Perez-Figueroa RE, Arias-Martinez V, Karpiak S, Brennan-Ing M: Psychosocial and demographic correlates of drug use in a sample of HIV-positive adults ages 50 and older. Prev Sci 2013;14:618–627.
56 Brennan C: Smoking can have negative impact on immune response to HAART. HIV Clin 2013;25:6–9.
57 Mdodo R, Frazier EL, Dube SR, Mattson CL, Sutton MY, Brooks JT, Skarbinski J: Cigarette smoking prevalence among adults with HIV compared with the general adult population in the United States: cross-sectional surveys. Ann Intern Med 2015;162: 335–344.
58 Fredriksen-Goldsen KI, Kim HJ, Emlet CA, Muraco A, Erosheva EA, Hoy-Ellis CP, Goldsen J, Petry H: The Aging and Health Report: Disparities and Resilience Among Lesbian, Gay, Bisexual, and Transgender Older Adults. Seattle Institute for Multigenerational Health, 2011.
59 Ompad DC, Kingdon M, Kupprat S, Halkitis SN, Storholm ED, Halkitis PN: Smoking and HIV-related health issues among older HIV-positive gay, bisexual, and other men who have sex with men. Behav Med 2014;40:99–107.
60 Parsons JT, Starks TJ, Millar BM, Boonrai K, Marcotte D: Patterns of substance use among HIV-positive adults over 50: implications for treatment and medication adherence. Drug Alcohol Depend 2014; 139:33–40.
61 Skalski LM, Sikkema KJ, Heckman TG, Meade CS: Coping styles and illicit drug use in older adults with HIV/AIDS. Psychol Addict Behav 2013;27:1050–1058.
62 Durvasula R: HIV/AIDS in older women: unique challenges, unmet needs. Behav Med 2014;40:85–98.
63 Barroso J, Sandelowski M: Substance abuse in HIV-positive women. J Assoc Nurses AIDS Care 2004;15: 48–59.

64 Neundorfer MM, Harris PB, Britton PJ, Lynch DA: HIV-risk factors for midlife and older women. Gerontologist 2005;45:617–625.
65 Heckman TG, Barcikowski R, Ogles B, Suhr J, Carlson B, Holroyd K, Garske J: A telephone-delivered coping improvement group intervention for middle-aged and older adults living with HIV/AIDS. Ann Behav Med 2006;32:27–38.
66 Heckman TG, Carlson B: A randomized clinical trial of two telephone-delivered, mental health interventions for HIV-infected persons in rural areas of the United States. AIDS Behav 2007;11:5–14.
67 Heckman TG, Sikkema KJ, Hansen N, Kochman A, Heh V, Neufeld S: A randomized clinical trial of a coping improvement group intervention for HIV-infected older adults. J Behav Med 2011;34:102–111.
68 Orsulic-Jeras S, et al: Counseling older adults with HIV/AIDS: a strength-based model of treatment. J Ment Health Couns 2003;25:233–244.
69 Bartels SJ: Improving system of care for older adults with mental illness in the United States. Findings and recommendations for the president's new freedom commission on mental health. Am J Geriatr Psychiatry 2003;11:486–497.
70 Emlet CA, Poindexter CC: Unserved, unseen, and unheard: integrating programs for HIV-infected and HIV-affected older adults. Health Soc Work 2004; 29:86–96.
71 Cunningham PJ: Beyond parity: primary care physicians' perspectives on access to mental health care. Health Aff (Millwood) 2009;28:w490–w501.
72 Meris D: Responding to the mental health and grief concerns of homeless HIV-infected gay men. Gay Lesbian Soc Serv 2001;13:103–111.
73 Brennan-Ing M, Seidel L, London AS, Cahill S, Karpiak SE: Service utilization among older adults with HIV: the joint association of sexual identity and gender. J Homosex 2014;61:166–196.
74 Emlet CA, Farkas KJ: Correlates of service utilization among midlife and older adults with HIV/AIDS: the role of age in the equation. J Aging Health 2002;14: 315–335.
75 Gongvatana A, Morgan EE, Iudicello JE, Letendre SL, Grant I, Woods SP; the HIV Neurobehavioral Research Program (HNRP) Group: A history of alcohol dependence augments HIV-associated neurocognitive deficits in persons aged 60 and older. J Neurovirol 2014;20:505–513.

David W. Pantalone, PhD
Department of Psychology
University of Massachusetts Boston
100 Morrissey Boulevard, Boston, MA 02125 (USA)
E-Mail david.pantalone@umb.edu

Brennan-Ing M, DeMarco RF (eds): HIV and Aging. Interdiscipl Top Gerontol Geriatr.
Basel, Karger, 2017, vol 42, pp 101–118 (DOI: 10.1159/000448547)

# Disability among Persons Aging with HIV/AIDS

Suzanne G. Leveille · Saurja Thapa

College of Nursing and Health Sciences, University of Massachusetts Boston, Boston, Mass., USA

**Abstract**

Persons surviving to older ages with HIV/AIDS often face an accelerated aging accompanied by increased comorbidity and decline in health and function. In this chapter, we review the process of disablement among persons aging with HIV/AIDS, from chronic conditions to impairments and functional limitations, leading to disability. Chronic immune activation related to chronic HIV infection may contribute to early development of chronic conditions that are common in older adults resulting in premature disablement. Anatomical and physiological changes related to the aging process make people vulnerable to physical and cognitive impairments. In old age, quality of life depends mainly on avoidance and management of age-associated diseases rather than chronological parameters. Interventions to manage chronic conditions associated with aging may have a significant impact on quality of life in older persons with HIV infection. Because of the complexity of physical and cognitive impairments among persons aging with HIV infection, a range of supports and interventions will be needed to effectively address the problem of disablement in this population.



## Introduction

As people age, they confront numerous risks to independent functioning. The presence of comorbid conditions combined with age-related physical changes result in physical impairments and other health problems leading to frail health and disability. Success in treatment and management of HIV infection has added HIV/AIDS to the list of chronic conditions affecting older adults. Accumulating evidence leads to the observation that specific burdens experienced by patients aging with HIV/

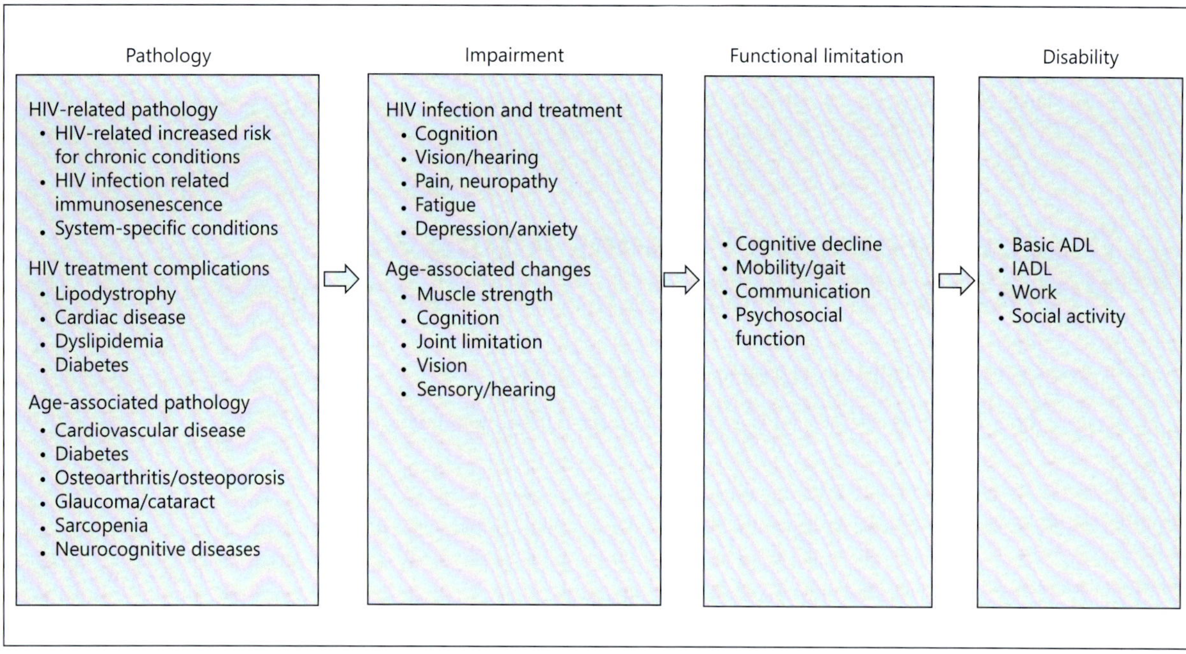


**Fig. 1.** The disablement model adapted for HIV and aging (Nagi [1]).

AIDS include: diminishing physical function, frailty, and risks for disability. Persons surviving to older ages with HIV/AIDS face more rapid aging accompanied by increased comorbidity and accelerated decline in health and function. In this chapter, we will review the pathway to disability in old age among persons living with HIV/AIDS.

## The Disablement Pathway

A long accepted theoretical model, the disablement model, provides a conceptual framework for understanding disability in the context of aging [1]. Developed by Said Nagi in the 1960s, this pathway model describes a process of decline that originates in pathology leading to impairments, then to functional limitations and finally, to disability. The model uses an etiological construct that has been validated by studies examining the causes and progression of disability [2, 3]. An adaptation of this model for conceptualizing the hypothetical disablement pathway among persons aging with HIV is shown in figure 1. HIV is a complex chronic condition in which the pathology, and the treatment, poses risks for health and functioning that may worsen in the face of aging when other non-HIV related chronic conditions emerge. Active pathology, whether from disease or age-related changes that places a person at risk for disability, involves the interruption of normal cellular activity and subsequent interference with homeostatic maintenance of the normal state. According to Nagi [1], active pathology can result from infection, trauma, metabolic imbalance, degenerative disease processes or other causes.

The term 'impairment' refers to the loss or abnormality at the tissue, organ, or body system level. Active pathology usually contributes to impairments, but not all impairments are associated with a definitive active pathology [1]. Also, impairments can occur in areas distinct from the original pathology, for example, pain and weakness in the legs that originate from spinal conditions, or reduced endurance and strength due to deconditioning in part related to aging cardio-respiratory systems.

In the Nagi model, functional limitation refers to restriction in performance of the individual. For example, a common functional limitation that might result from a cerebrovascular accident could include carrying out mobility tasks such as walking or getting in and out of a bed or chair. Functional limitations also include tasks that are considered non-physical, such as communication or reasoning. These functional limitations might or might not be related to specific impairments secondary to, for example, a cerebrovascular accident.

Disability is the limitation in the performance of socially defined roles and tasks within a socio-cultural and physical environment rather than individual functioning. According to Nagi, not all impairments or functional limitations precipitate disability. For instance, a person with severe neuropathy in their feet may have significant limitation in gait and balance and yet may be fully employed in the community. Another person with similar limitations may be homebound and require assistance with daily activities. In this chapter, we will discuss the impact of aging with HIV/AIDS infection, comorbidity, and treatments as it relates to the domains described in the disablement model.

## Pathology

In conceptualizing the domain of pathology on the disablement pathway, we consider multiple systems that are impacted by this chronic complex condition. Using this systems approach, we will describe HIV-associated conditions and their associated symptoms that contribute to impairments and limitations, and subsequent disablement among infected persons. We also will review several of the common age-associated chronic diseases affecting the major systems and physiological functions that contribute to disability.

### *HIV-Associated Pathology*

HIV/AIDS and its treatment increase the risk for chronic diseases such as diabetes mellitus and cardiovascular diseases [4]. Other chronic conditions that occur earlier or more frequently in persons with HIV/AIDs include osteoporosis with bone fractures, neurocognitive diseases, some cancers, and kidney failure [4, 5]. Not only are chronic conditions more common in this population, it is estimated that the overall burden of comorbidity among persons living with HIV/AIDS is comparable to that of persons 10 years older in the general population [5]. Individually, these chronic conditions are often associated with functional difficulty in older adults, but it is the combined burden of multiple chronic conditions that often sets older adults on a course of progressive disability. Notably, the problem of comorbidity may arise not only from chronic HIV/AIDS infection, but also from the effects of treatment such as long-term use of combination antiretroviral therapy (cART), which is the current standard of care in HIV/AIDS management. The well-documented lipodystrophy, or abnormal body fat distribution, associated with cART places HIV-infected adults at high risk for impaired glucose metabolism and diabetes and their sequelae [4]. The causes of these abnormalities are complex, multifactorial, and mostly attributed to HIV/AIDS infection [6].

*HIV Infection-Related Comorbidity*

Life expectancy continues to grow among persons with HIV infection, primarily due to treatment with cART [4, 7]. However, the longer life expectancy is accompanied by the emergence of chronic conditions, especially in the older age groups [4, 7]. HIV infection is a major source of inflammation in both treated and untreated individuals. The disease contributes to a chronic inflammatory condition, unlike what is observed in the aging process, and to the increased incidence of age-associated conditions including cardiovascular, bone, metabolic, and neurocognitive diseases [8, 9]. There is a higher prevalence of cytomegalovirus infection among HIV-infected individuals, similar to that found in older adults, and part of an immune risk phenotype contributing to atherosclerosis [8]. Immune changes in T-cell profiles related to aging may be difficult to distinguish from immune changes in chronic HIV infection [8]. Recent evidence points to the association between this chronic inflammation and elevated cardiovascular risk among HIV patients [10]. Immunosenescence may contribute to age-associated chronic conditions. In persons infected with HIV, elevated IL-6 levels, a general measure of inflammation, and an HIV-specific measure of CD-8 T-cell activation, were each associated with poorer physical function in middle-aged patients with HIV infection [11]. In summary, chronic immune activation related to HIV infection may contribute to the early development of chronic conditions associated with chronic inflammation in older adults, leading to premature disablement [12].

*HIV Treatment Related Problems (cART)*

The emergence of cART treatment in 1996 led to a significant decrease in the overall AIDS mortality and morbidity, and an increase in life expectancy for HIV patients. However, this effective treatment is accompanied by serious adverse effects such as the 'lipodystrophy syndrome' that includes central lipohypertrophy and peripheral subcutaneous lipoatrophy, either of which can become a major problem for HIV patients [13]. Lipohypertrophy and lipoatrophy are independently associated with adverse metabolic consequences including dyslipidemia, insulin resistance, metabolic syndrome, increased level of systemic inflammation, or immune activation. These problems can increase the risk for cardiovascular disease, diabetes, and mortality. For example, the effects of specific antiretroviral drugs on glucose transport and mitochondrial function also leads to the loss of subcutaneous fat and collection of ectopic fat in the liver and muscle in HIV patients leading to diabetes mellitus [6].

*Endocrine System*

Metabolic syndrome is common among people living with HIV and includes accumulation of abdominal fat, elevated triglycerides and cholesterol (dyslipidemia), hypertension, and glucose intolerance. Many aspects of aging with HIV, including long-term treatment with cART can place patients at risk for metabolic syndrome. For example, patients receiving cART often experience lipodystrophy syndrome, as described above, or other metabolic disturbances (dyslipidemia, insulin resistance) [13]. Central obesity that is otherwise referred to as central fat accumulation, or android, abdominal or truncal obesity, is widely observed in patients with HIV infection [14]. Similarly, diabetes mellitus which occurs more often in the general population of aging adults is growing in prevalence among persons aging with HIV who are on long-term cART therapy [15]. Diabetes and its associated chronic conditions including vision problems and neuropathy can have serious consequences for daily functioning in older adults. However, research has shown that regardless of diabetic complications, the disease itself seems to directly contribute to functional decline [16].

Renal problems arising from age-associated diminished renal function may be compounded among older adults living with HIV. The infection increases the risk for renal disease because the kidney serves as an HIV reservoir. Low CD4 cell count and use of cART are commonly associated with higher risk for acute kidney failure. HIV-associated nephropathy rapidly progresses to end-stage renal disease, a situation more common among African-Americans than whites [17]. Due to the renal toxicity caused by antiretroviral agents, adjustment in the dose is required for people with renal insufficiency [18]. It is the most common cause of end-stage renal disease among the HIV-infected patients. Kidney failure is a particularly debilitating condition that contributes to frailty and functional loss [19].

*Cardiovascular System*

There is an increased risk of acute myocardial infarction and advanced subclinical cardiovascular disease among persons who have HIV infection compared to age-matched uninfected persons [20]. The risk for CVD is complex in that it may derive to some extent from other health risks and conditions, specifically diabetes. But even among those without diabetes, there is an increased risk for myocardial infarction in persons with HIV/AIDS [6, 21]. The duration of cART has been linked with an increased risk for cardiovascular disease, especially among those with other risk factors [18]. Accumulating evidence suggests that the presence of HIV virus is associated with increased CVD risk, supporting the idea that there is an inflammatory pathway whereby HIV infection contributes to CVD [7]. Of note, the association between HIV and risk for MI is mainly found among those who have low CD4 counts and evidence of HIV mRNA in their blood [22]. Among older adults with HIV, cardiovascular disease can be addressed by treating hypertension, dyslipidemia, elevated triglycerides, obesity, insulin resistance, and diabetes and altering lifestyle such as quitting smoking, exercising, and healthy eating habits.

Conditions of the cardiovascular system can limit endurance and contribute to other impairments. As the heart gets older, the ability to pump blood is diminished and it has to work harder to pump enough blood throughout the body. Certain medications, emotional stress, physical exertion, illness, injuries, and infection are some of the common risk factors that contribute to problems such as angina, arteriosclerosis, and high blood pressure. The functional abilities of older adults with coronary heart disease (CHD) may become increasingly limited with age depending on the severity of disease. Research suggests that men with CHD are more physically limited due to greater risk for depression [23]. Older adults with diabetes and high blood pressure are also at increased risk of developing CHD [24]. Age-related changes compound the effects of CHD in older adults and contribute to impairments such as limited endurance and strength resulting in further restrictions in physical activity.

*HIV Infection and the Brain*

Among the HIV-infected individuals, central nervous system involvement and changes in neurobehavioral status, particularly occurs in the advanced stages of the illness. The HIV-positive patient with impairments in memory, executive function, and psychomotor functioning can demonstrate significant difficulties with performance on structured tasks of medication management ability and adherence to medication regimens in everyday life [25]. The age-related declines in cognition that have been observed in HIV patients are well documented, but they are not considered to be entirely related to biological aging processes. Chronic disease, particularly cardiovascular disease can have a significant deleterious effect on the brain and on neurocognitive function [26]. Hence, cognitive difficulties in persons aging with HIV can be related to exposure to different diseases and also substance use over the course of a lifetime [27].

*HIV-Associated Neuropathy*

One of the most frequent complications of HIV infection, affecting as many as half of those infected with the virus, is HIV-associated sensory neuropathy (HIV-SN). The disorder may be due to the viral infection or also to toxic effects of specific antiretroviral medications that are becoming less commonly prescribed [28]. These 2 conditions are sometimes difficult to distinguish clinically and lead to a similar constellation of symptoms. As with other neuropathies, HIV-SN can lead to sensory loss, chronic or intermittent pain, and may interfere with sleep and functioning [28]. There are 2 types of HIV-associated distal sensory peripheral neuropathy, HIV-associated polyneuropathy, the more common of the 2, and ART toxic neuropathy. Almost 30–67% of patients infected with HIV are found to have any one of the 2 neuropathies [29]. Other factors associated with HIV-SN include diabetes and use of neurotoxic antiretroviral medications [29]. The problem of HIV-SN is associated with aging, thus, it is likely that the problem will emerge in coming years as a major contributor to disability among aging persons infected with HIV/AIDS.

*Skeletal System*

Individuals infected with HIV are susceptible to a range of musculoskeletal diseases including opportunistic bone infections, osteonecrosis, osteopenia, and osteoporosis. Both HIV infection and cART place patients at increased risk for bone loss [30]. New evidence points to a substantial increase in fracture risk among older adults with HIV infection compared to other older persons [30]. Immune activation, HAART use, abnormal vitamin D metabolism, and premature menopause are some of the factors contributing to accelerated bone loss in people with HIV. In the general population, hip fracture is a sentinel event contributing to functional decline, institutionalization, and death [31]. Very little research has examined the risk of osteoporosis or other age-associated chronic musculoskeletal disease among patients with HIV infection. A recent study reported that body fat changes among HIV-infected adults using chronic cART therapy resulted in lower cartilage volume, possibly placing them at increased risk for osteoarthritis, compared to controls without HIV [14]. Of note, arthritis is the leading cause of disability in the US [32]. More research is needed to determine the possible role of HIV in the development of debilitating musculoskeletal diseases of old age.

*Non-HIV Pathology Associated with Aging*

A number of age-associated conditions place older people at risk for progressive functional losses and disability. In recent years, a number of studies have examined the occurrence and correlates of age-associated loss of skeletal muscle, frequently referred to as sarcopenia. The model in figure 2 shows not only the overall complexity but the many mechanisms that influence development of sarcopenia [33]. Notably, many of the conditions contributing to sarcopenia, shown in the model, are the very conditions that are commonly seen among adults with HIV/AIDS. As described above, body composition changes are a hallmark of long-term cART, and may contribute to sarcopenia in this population.

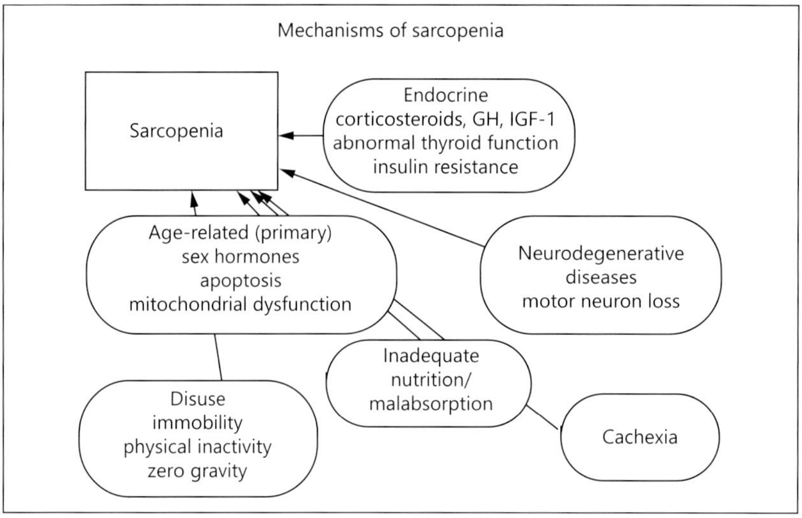


**Fig. 2.** Mechanisms of sarcopenia (Cruz-Jentoft et al. [33]).

*Summary*
In general, age-related quality of life depends mainly on age-associated diseases rather than chronological parameters, and includes pathological changes in the immune, cardiovascular, musculoskeletal, endocrine, and central nervous systems. Musculoskeletal conditions, such as arthritis and spine diseases, can lead to chronic pain and changes in the joint structure [34]. Limiting movement to prevent discomfort exacerbates the effects of many chronic conditions in aging adults, leading to further loss of function. Interventions to manage chronic conditions associated with aging may have a significant impact on the quality of life in the aging population of persons with HIV.

## Impairments

Chronic diseases associated with aging lead to impairments across many body systems. In addition, anatomical and physiological changes related to the aging process make people vulnerable to physical and cognitive impairments. Sensory losses are among the most common age-associated impairments. In the US, more than 25% of adults aged 70 years and older have hearing impairment and 15% have impaired vision [35]. Other common impairments include balance problems, which increase the fall risk, and sensory loss related to neuropathies particularly affect feeling in the feet. Losses of muscle strength and endurance pose challenges to mobility, placing elderly at increased risk for falls and fall injuries. Cognitive changes associated with aging affect many cognitive domains and are not restricted to memory loss. Here we will review some of the most common and debilitating impairments in the population of persons infected with HIV.

*HIV-Associated Impaired Cognition*

HIV has the ability to infect the brain and cause cognitive impairment in HIV seropositive individuals, thus, impaired cognition is one of the major complications associated with the infection. Although cART has been successful in decreasing the incidence of HIV dementia and some severe forms of HIV-associated cognitive problems, subtle forms of HIV-associated neurocognitive disorder are still prevalent [36]. Among the HIV-positive patients with advanced infection, HIV-associated cognitive impairment still continues to be a huge clinical problem [36]. Interventions to manage the chronic neurocognitive impairments of HIV infection are key to preventing a cascade of problems, in part related to the poor adherence to treatment and poor decision-making regarding self-care and disability prevention.

*HIV-Associated Impaired Vision*

Persons who are HIV seropositive may develop ocular manifestations of HIV infection that may lead to visual impairment or even blindness [9]. Although the incidence of opportunistic infections affecting the eye, such as *Cytomegalovirus retinitis*, has declined by 80% since the introduction of cART, this opportunistic infection continues to be the most frequent reason for vision loss, in part due to cART treatment failure [37]. HIV damage to the eye is extremely common in HIV-infected individuals, frequently related to vascular abnormalities affecting the conjunctiva and retina. Some of the current causes of vision loss among the HIV-infected patients are cataract, immune reconstitution uveitis with secondary macular edema, epiretinal membranes, and HIV retinopathy [37]. In addition, the higher prevalence of diabetes among persons with HIV places them at risk for vision loss related to diabetic eye diseases. Vision loss not only contributes to disability, but also places older adults at risk for depression, falls, and fall injuries [38, 39].

*HIV-Associated Hearing Impairment*

While conflicting evidence has been reported about the relation between HIV/AIDs and age-related hearing loss, more consistent results show a low-tone hearing loss among middle-aged adults with HIV/AIDS that is not typically associated with aging [40, 41]. Low-tone hearing loss is associated with the duration of illness and low CD4 counts, but not with other disease-related factors including viral load. Another hazard to hearing is related to ototoxicity from drugs used to treat HIV/AIDS and associated conditions, the most common iatrogenic source of auditory disorders.

*HIV-Associated Fatigue*

Fatigue being one of the earliest symptoms of HIV infection often continues as an everyday complaint and bothersome symptom among patients at all stages of HIV disease, impairing quality of life due to decreased functional capacity [42–44]. In a study of over 13,000 HIV patients in the US, 37% were found to have fatigue reported during medical visits, and it was most commonly associated with diagnosis of AIDS, presence of depression, or anemia [43]. Measures such as CD4 count and viral load were not associated with fatigue. Others have reported that socioeconomic factors are among the strongest predictors of fatigue, specifically, unemployment and low income [44]. Use of cART was also associated with fatigue. Surprisingly, results of laboratory tests did not predict level of fatigue in general [44]. In a longitudinal study of HIV-related fatigue, psychological factors were most strongly associated with fatigue, including number of stressful events and presence of depression and anxiety [42]. Physiological measures also had little bearing on fatigue levels in that study. Most studies on HIV-related fatigue have not addressed the role of chronic conditions such as kidney or heart diseases that are more common in patients aging with HIV, but those who live with these chronic conditions may have an increased risk for problems with debilitating fatigue.

*HIV-Associated Depression and Psychological Conditions*

Persons infected with HIV face a host of psychological challenges emanating from within and often triggered by their external environment. Depression is very common in this population, though the prevalence of depression in persons with HIV infection varies depending upon the regions and populations [45]. Proper treatment of this chronic condition is crucial because it not only impacts the quality of life but, if not treated effectively, it can place patients at risk for other problems related to the complex demands of chronic HIV infection. In her extensive review on the topic of depression and HIV infection, Rabkin [46] concluded that while depression prevalence may decline with age in the population without HIV infection, there does not seem to be a similar age-associated decline in depression rates among persons with HIV. Depression rates vary widely between studies, but this condition is second only to substance abuse among psychiatric disorders in persons with HIV, and is as treatable as in other populations. Depression assessment and treatment should be a routine aspect of HIV care [46].

Multiple factors have been attributed to the association between HIV and depression, the latter of which is often associated with poor cognitive and physical function [47, 48]. Grov et al. [49] found that depression was significantly related to increased HIV-associated stigma, increased loneliness, and decreased cognitive functioning in older adults with HIV infection. Therefore, efforts should be made toward diminishing HIV-related stigma and loneliness which will help in reducing the overall rate of depression, thereby improving the overall health [49]. Among many other barriers, stigma is considered as one of the important barriers to access healthcare, which negatively impacts physical, mental, and overall well-being [50].

*Chronic Pain in HIV and Aging*

Chronic pain can be related to a number of diseases and conditions, and it is often difficult to attribute it to a specific pathology in older adults. There is very little pain research specifically in older patients with HIV to date. A new study of primary care patients receiving treatment for HIV/AIDS reported that 40% had at least one diagnosis of a chronic pain condition, and 69% reported pain during at least one visit in the 1-year study [51]. However, patients in this study were aged 18–65 years. Similar to the general population, musculoskeletal pain was the most common pain condition reported [51]. In the US, it is estimated that over 40% of adults experience a chronic pain condition in a given year [52]. Among older adults, the prevalence is nearly 60% [31]. Common pain conditions include arthritis, low back pain, neuropathy, headaches, and muscle pain. Chronic pain can lead to many other problems such as muscle tension, limited mobility, poor sleep and eating habits, depression and anxiety, thereby affecting a person's overall quality of life [53]. Careful assessment for the presence of impairments is key to early intervention as much impairment is treatable, and treatment can prevent or delay disabling consequences.

*Balance and Gait Impairments*
HIV infection and treatments are associated with balance and gait dysfunction [54]. These balance problems and sensorimotor deficits in middle-aged HIV patients may lead to more serious mobility difficulties with the aging of the HIV population. This is an area that requires much more research as the preservation of mobility is key to preventing physical disability in old age. Development of effective strategies to prevent the progression of mobility losses could have a substantial impact on the population aging with HIV.

## Functional Limitations

Functional limitations are limitations in the performance of the whole organism or person. These include limitations in physical, emotional, and cognitive performance [55]. Extensive epidemiologic literature has demonstrated a decline in functional performance in older populations [3, 56, 57]. Very few studies have examined the impact of HIV infection and treatment on functional limitations and physical performance in aging persons. In a study of persons aged 45–65 living with HIV infection, limitations in physical performance were associated with biomarkers of disease including low CD4 and CD8 proportions [11]. Functional limitations in this study were based on a variety of assessment measures including the short physical performance battery (SPPB) that has become a standard measure of lower body mobility performance in research and clinical care [58]. This measure is a composite of 3 tests, a 4-meter usual-paced walk, a timed test of standing up and down from a chair 5 times without using arms, and 3 tests of standing balance. Using validated cut-points, the 3 tests are scored from 0 to 4, and summed for a maximal score of 12 [58]. Low scores on the SPPB are predictive of disability, hospitalization, and mortality in general populations of older adults [2, 3]. Few studies of HIV patients have reported SPPB or other functional measures. Bauer compared effects of obesity on SPPB sub-scores in HIV seropositive and seronegative persons, and found that persons with HIV performed worse than their seronegative counterparts, and also that these effects were compounded by obesity

[59]. The average age of participants in this study was below age 40, thus these results do not address the possible effects of age on performance among persons with HIV.

There is a good deal of heterogeneity in reports regarding effects of aging on the brain. In the general population, declines in processing speed, memory, and spatial ability are fairly common with age [60]. Cognitive difficulties related to pathology versus aging are sometimes challenging to sort out clinically, but the focus of clinical care becomes one of maintaining optimal cognitive function through healthy behaviors and ongoing monitoring for changes requiring intervention. With emerging evidence demonstrating the close link between cognitive function and mobility [61], it is critically important to address this issue in persons aging with HIV who may have longstanding neurocognitive deficits along with sensorimotor impairments as they approach old age.

## Disability

In general, disability in older populations refers to the ability of maintaining daily activities without help from others. These daily activities are often referred to as basic activities of daily living (ADL: bathing, dressing, eating, transferring from a bed or chair, and using the toilet) and instrumental ADL (IADL: shopping, preparing meals, doing housework, and managing money). Rates of ADL and IADL disabilities increase with age, and in general, persons who have chronic conditions are much more at risk for disability as they age. Socioeconomic status is a strong predictor of both functional limitations and disability in the aging population [62]. Older women have higher incidence and prevalence of disability than men as they age [63]. Race is also an important risk factor for disability. In the general population of older adults in the US, recent estimates show that 25% of blacks versus 17% of whites have difficulty with IADL, and 15% blacks versus 10% of whites have difficulty with ADL [64].

Very few studies have examined the impact of HIV on disability in persons aging with HIV compared to those without HIV. Oursler studied 6,500 veterans aged 50 and older and found only modest differences in disability according to HIV status [65]. However, when the groups were stratified by age, HIV was found to predict a 3-fold faster decline in disability scores among those aged 55 and older with HIV compared to their age peers who were uninfected. Of note, the terminology for disability often varies between studies. The outcome measure used in the veterans study was described as 'physical function' and 'limitation' yet the description of the measure included ADL and IADL, which we refer to as measures of disability consistent with the Nagi model [66].

A recent national study found that nearly half of people aged 65 and older in the US report having difficulty or needing help with daily activities [67]. Nearly 30% receive help from others with one or more daily activities, and this percentage increased markedly with age to 59% of persons aged 85–89 years, and 76% of those aged 90 and older. Nearly all from this group reported having one or more close family members or friends in their network, and on average, older adults reported having 4 people in their close network. More than half of those receiving help obtained help from their close relatives and friends, or their informal care network [67]. These findings have important implications for the population aging with HIV. The lack of resources and isolation that is very common in this population will result in greater needs for formal care networks to address disability needs as persons with HIV reach older ages. These changes will come at a time when demographically, the US population is aging rapidly as the baby boom generation moves over 65. The number of older adults requiring personal assistance is likely to surge with this expansion of the older population. Competition for resources is likely to result in more and more unmet needs. Community-level solutions to these impending challenges will be necessary in the coming decades. Greater efforts in the area of disability prevention must be considered in anticipation of the convergence of the demographic shift in both aging populations, those with and without HIV infection.

## The Psychosocial and Environmental Context

Since Nagi's original work, Verbrugge and Jette [66] and others have expanded the disablement model to encompass a psychosocial and environmental context for the disablement process. In describing the context, Verbrugge and Jette [66] asserted that there are 3 additional domains to be considered: predisposing factors, intra-individual, and extra-individual factors. These are particularly relevant for the population aging with HIV/AIDS, where social and psychological factors often place individuals at increased risk for functional limitations and disability.

### *Predisposing Factors*

These include sociodemographic, behavioral, and lifestyle factors that may have long preceded development of HIV/AIDS. Persons with HIV/AIDS are often from disadvantaged and vulnerable populations, those with low incomes, and from racial, ethnic, and sexual minority communities. Behavioral risks, including intravenous drug use and having unprotected sex with multiple partners, are not only risk factors for contracting HIV infection but are also associated with a number of other infections and health problems that can compound the impact of HIV infection on general health. For example, hepatitis B and C are more associated with these behaviors, and can be very debilitating chronic conditions exacerbating health problems related to HIV infection. Problems with substance use can contribute to poor adherence to medical management of primary and secondary conditions associated with HIV infection. Long term homelessness, associated with the risk for onset of HIV infection, also places people at high risk for many chronic conditions and their consequences. Management of HIV/AIDS and HIV comorbidity is particularly challenging in the context of homelessness for patients and providers alike.

*Intra-Individual Factors*
Psychological factors including mood and coping skills are critically important for the management and self-management of HIV infection and associated morbidity. Depression and anxiety are common in the aging population, and those who have chronic conditions, requiring a good deal of management and adaptation to sustain healthy living, often struggle with mood disorders. Living into old age with HIV and the burden of the associated stigma can lead to chronic depression and social isolation [49]. Every step of the disablement pathway can be mediated or exacerbated by psychosocial issues, which are common among persons with HIV/AIDS.

*Extra-Individual Factors*
The social environment of people aging with HIV/AIDS infection can have a tremendous impact on their health and function into their later years. Those who have strong informal and formal supports are in a much better position to weather disabling chronic conditions associated with aging, such as arthritis and heart disease. Access to healthcare is key to aging successfully with HIV infection. Health insurance may or may not cover all of the healthcare needs for persons aging with HIV infection, and this may vary widely depending on where people are living. Proximity to and availability of medical and rehabilitative services are often factors influencing whether people obtain the necessary treatment and medications to manage their health and recover from health event. Inadequate rehabilitation can lead to a spiral of declining function in the face of aging with comorbidity. For example, lack of rehabilitation following cardiac hospitalizations or surgical events such as fractures, can contribute to further losses of function and mobility, and deteriorating self-care. Interventions to keep persons with HIV/AIDS infection engaged in their self-healthcare can reduce the risk of permanent hospitalizations and worsening disability. Social support can foster self-management and adherence to healthcare recommendations [68]. Where people who experience isolation may have limited informal supports, the formal social support system including case management can help in filling the gap of daily help and encouragement that family and friends can provide.

## Prevention and Management of Disability

The key to disability prevention is optimal health and self-management with aging. Because of the complexity of physical and cognitive impairments among persons aging with HIV infection, a range of support and interventions will be needed to effectively address the needs of this population. An individualized targeted risk-reduction approach may be needed for some, while others may benefit from interventions available to the general community of older persons. Physical activity, for example, is key for preventing mobility loss as people age. Engagement in exercise programs for older adults in the community is one strategy that can successfully reduce mobility limitations

[69]. Others with more severe impairment may benefit from rehabilitative care before engaging in community-based exercise and other health programs. Other types of impairments, including sensory losses may require adaptive equipment, including canes, glasses or hearing aids. Prioritizing rehabilitative impairments and modifiable conditions may yield the most benefit in disability prevention. Addressing cognitive deficits may improve coping and self-management skills, and could improve the quality of life. Research is needed to determine the best strategies for disability prevention among persons aging with HIV, though initially evaluating the benefits of established approaches for disability prevention will be an important first step.

## Conclusion

In the coming decades, the problem of disablement in the population of persons with HIV will continue to grow. For now, it is important to note that the shift from a condition characterized by opportunistic infections to where HIV/AIDS has become a chronic disease is mainly evident in a subset of patients, primarily in developed countries. Even in the US only about 1 in 4 persons infected with HIV is receiving cART and are virally suppressed [70]. In resource poor countries, it is a limited population of patients that have ongoing access to cART, and thus are living longer as a result of reductions in opportunistic infections. A number of efforts are underway to increase access and engagement in healthcare, which will ultimately increase life expectancy and the concomitant risk for developing chronic conditions both HIV-related and age-associated. Although we are learning more and more about prevention and management of disability in older adults in general, the growing population of persons aging with and without HIV will create a significant challenge for health and social support systems that serve aging persons living with disability. A public health approach that anticipates the needs of the aging population with and without HIV will be best suited to prevent and manage the challenges of disability.

## References


1 Nagi SZ: Some conceptual issues in disability and rehabilitation; in Sussman MB (ed): Sociology and Rehabilitation. Washington, American Sociological Association, 1965.

2 Guralnik JM, Ferrucci L, Pieper CF, Leveille SG, Markides KS, Ostir GV, Studenski S, Berkman LF, Wallace RB: Lower extremity function and subsequent disability: consistency across studies, predictive models, and value of gait speed alone compared with the short physical performance battery. J Gerontol A Biol Sci Med Sci 2000;55:M221–M231.

3 Guralnik JM, Ferrucci L, Simonsick EM, Salive ME, Wallace RB: Lower-extremity function in persons over the age of 70 years as a predictor of subsequent disability. N Engl J Med 1995;332:556–561.

4 Meir-Shafrir K, Pollack S: Accelerated aging in HIV patients. Rambam Maimonides Med J 2012; 3:e0025.

5 Guaraldi G, Orlando G, Zona S, Menozzi M, Carli F, Garlassi E, Berti A, Rossi E, Roverato A, Palella F: Premature age-related comorbidities among HIV-infected persons compared with the general population. Clin Infect Dis 2011;53:1120–1126.

6 Grinspoon S: Diabetes mellitus, cardiovascular risk, and HIV disease. Circulation 2009;119:770–772.
7 Barrett L, Fowke KR, Grant MD: Cytomegalovirus, aging, and HIV: a perfect storm. AIDS Rev 2012;14:159–167.
8 Tsoukas C: Immunosenescence and aging in HIV. Curr Opin HIV AIDS 2014;9:398–404.
9 Pathai S, Bajillan H, Landay AL, High KP: Is HIV a model of accelerated or accentuated aging? J Gerontol A Biol Sci Med Sci 2014;69:833–842.
10 Mooney S, Tracy R, Osler T, Grace C: Elevated biomarkers of inflammation and coagulation in patients with HIV are associated with higher Framingham and VACS risk index scores. PLoS One 2015;10:e0144312.
11 Erlandson KM, Allshouse AA, Jankowski CM, Lee EJ, Rufner KM, Palmer BE, Wilson CC, MaWhinney S, Kohrt WM, Campbell TB: Association of functional impairment with inflammation and immune activation in HIV type 1-infected adults receiving effective antiretroviral therapy. J Infect Dis 2013;208:249–259.
12 Brinkley TE, Leng X, Miller ME, Kitzman DW, Pahor M, Berry MJ, Marsh AP, Kritchevsky SB, Nicklas BJ: Chronic inflammation is associated with low physical function in older adults across multiple comorbidities. J Gerontol A Biol Sci Med Sci 2009;64:455–461.
13 Cofrancesco J Jr, Freedland E, McComsey G: Treatment options for HIV-associated central fat accumulation. AIDS Patient Care STDS 2009;23:5–18.
14 Fillipas S, Tanamas SK, Davies-Tuck ML, Wluka AE, Wang Y, Holland AE, Cherry CL, Cicuttini F: The relationship between body composition and knee structure in patients with human immunodeficiency virus. Int J STD AIDS 2015;26:133–138.
15 Polsky S, Floris-Moore M, Schoenbaum EE, Klein RS, Arnsten JH, Howard AA: Incident hyperglycaemia among older adults with or at-risk for HIV infection. Antivir Ther 2011;16:181–188.
16 Maty SC, Fried LP, Volpato S, Williamson J, Brancati FL, Blaum CS: Patterns of disability related to diabetes mellitus in older women. J Gerontol A Biol Sci Med Sci 2004;59:148–153.
17 Wei A, Burns GC, Williams BA, Mohammed NB, Visintainer P, Sivak SL: Long-term renal survival in HIV-associated nephropathy with angiotensin-converting enzyme inhibition. Kidney Int 2003;64:1462–1471.
18 Panel on Antiretroviral Guidelines for Adults and Adolescents: Guidelines for the use of antiretroviral agents in HIV-1-infected adults and adolescents. Department of Health and Human Services 2009, pp 1–161.
19 Delgado C, Shieh S, Grimes B, Chertow GM, Dalrymple LS, Kaysen GA, Kornak J, Johansen KL: Association of self-reported frailty with falls and fractures among patients new to dialysis. Am J Nephrol 2015;42:134–140.
20 Triant VA, Lee H, Hadigan C, Grinspoon SK: Increased acute myocardial infarction rates and cardiovascular risk factors among patients with human immunodeficiency virus disease. J Clin Endocrinol Metab 2007;92:2506–2512.
21 Triant VA: Epidemiology of coronary heart disease in patients with human immunodeficiency virus. Rev Cardiovasc Med 2014;15(suppl 1):S1–S8.
22 Freiberg MS, Chang CC, Kuller LH, Skanderson M, Lowy E, Kraemer KL, Butt AA, Bidwell Goetz M, Leaf D, Oursler KA, Rimland D, Rodriguez Barradas M, Brown S, Gibert C, McGinnis K, Crothers K, Sico J, Crane H, Warner A, Gottlieb S, Gottdiener J, Tracy RP, Budoff M, Watson C, Armah KA, Doebler D, Bryant K, Justice AC: HIV infection and the risk of acute myocardial infarction. JAMA Intern Med 2013;173:614–622.
23 Ahto M, Isoaho R, Puolijoki H, Laippala P, Romo M, Kivela SL: Functional abilities of elderly coronary heart disease patients. Aging (Milano) 1998;10:127–136.
24 Halter JB, Musi N, McFarland Horne F, Crandall JP, Goldberg A, Harkless L, Hazzard WR, Huang ES, Kirkman MS, Plutzky J, Schmader KE, Zieman S, High KP: Diabetes and cardiovascular disease in older adults: current status and future directions. Diabetes 2014;63:2578–2589.
25 Hinkin CH, Castellon SA, Durvasula RS, Hardy DJ, Lam MN, Mason KI, Thrasher D, Goetz MB, Stefaniak M: Medication adherence among HIV+ adults: effects of cognitive dysfunction and regimen complexity. Neurology 2002;59:1944–1950.
26 Waldstein SR, Wendell CR: Neurocognitive function and cardiovascular disease. J Alzheimers Dis 2010;20:833–842.
27 Foley J, Ettenhofer M, Wright MJ, Siddiqi I, Choi M, Thames AD, Mason K, Castellon S, Hinkin CH: Neurocognitive functioning in HIV-1 infection: effects of cerebrovascular risk factors and age. Clin Neuropsychol 2010;24:265–285.
28 Ellis RJ, Rosario D, Clifford DB, McArthur JC, Simpson D, Alexander T, Gelman BB, Vaida F, Collier A, Marra CM, Ances B, Atkinson JH, Dworkin RH, Morgello S, Grant I; CHARTER Study Group: Continued high prevalence and adverse clinical impact of human immunodeficiency virus-associated sensory neuropathy in the era of combination antiretroviral therapy: the CHARTER study. Arch Neurol 2010;67:552–558.

29 Evans SR, Ellis RJ, Chen H, Yeh TM, Lee AJ, Schifitto G, Wu K, Bosch RJ, McArthur JC, Simpson DM, Clifford DB: Peripheral neuropathy in HIV: prevalence and risk factors. AIDS 2011;25:919–928.
30 Ofotokun I, Weitzmann MN: HIV-1 infection and antiretroviral therapies: risk factors for osteoporosis and bone fracture. Curr Opin Endocrinol Diabetes Obes 2010;17:523–529.
31 Leveille SG: Musculoskeletal aging. Curr Opin Rheumatol 2004;16:114–118.
32 Centers for Disease Control and Prevention (CDC): Prevalence and most common causes of disability among adults – United States 2005. MMWR Morb Mortal Wkly Rep 2009;58:421–426.
33 Cruz-Jentoft AJ, Baeyens JP, Bauer JM, Boirie Y, Cederholm T, Landi F, Martin FC, Michel JP, Rolland Y, Schneider SM, Topinkova E, Vandewoude M, Zamboni M; European Working Group on Sarcopenia in Older People: Sarcopenia: European consensus on definition and diagnosis: report of the European working group on sarcopenia in older people. Age Ageing 2010;39:412–423.
34 Woolf AD, Pfleger B: Burden of major musculoskeletal conditions. Bull World Health Organ 2003;81: 646–656.
35 Dillon CF, Gu Q, Hoffman H, Ko CW: Vision, hearing, balance, and sensory impairment in Americans aged 70 years and over: United States, 1999–2006. Hyattsville, National Center for Health Statistics, 2010.
36 Sacktor N, McDermott MP, Marder K, Schifitto G, Selnes OA, McArthur JC, Stern Y, Albert S, Palumbo D, Kieburtz K, De Marcaida JA, Cohen B, Epstein L: HIV-associated cognitive impairment before and after the advent of combination therapy. J Neurovirol 2002;8:136–142.
37 Stewart MW: Human immunodeficiency virus and its effects on the visual system. Infect Dis Rep 2012; 4:e25.
38 Gates S, Fisher JD, Cooke MW, Carter YH, Lamb SE: Multifactorial assessment and targeted intervention for preventing falls and injuries among older people in community and emergency care settings: systematic review and meta-analysis. BMJ 2008;336:130–133.
39 Horowitz A, Reinhardt JP, Kennedy GJ: Major and subthreshold depression among older adults seeking vision rehabilitation services. Am J Geriatr Psychiatry 2005;13:180–187.
40 Luque AE, Orlando MS, Leong UC, Allen PD, Guido JJ, Yang H, Wu H: Hearing function in patients living with HIV/AIDS. Ear Hear 2014;35:e282–e290.
41 Torre P 3rd, Hoffman HJ, Springer G, Cox C, Young MA, Margolick JB, Plankey M: Hearing loss among HIV-seropositive and HIV-seronegative men and women. JAMA Otolaryngol Head Neck Surg 2015; 141:202–210.
42 Barroso J, Leserman J, Harmon JL, Hammill B, Pence BW: Fatigue in HIV-infected people: a three-year observational study. J Pain Symptom Manage 2015;50:69–79.
43 Sullivan PS, Dworkin MS: Prevalence and correlates of fatigue among persons with HIV infection. J Pain Symptom Manage 2003;25:329–333.
44 Jong E, Oudhoff LA, Epskamp C, Wagener MN, van Duijn M, Fischer S, van Gorp EC: Predictors and treatment strategies of HIV-related fatigue in the combined antiretroviral therapy era. AIDS 2010;24: 1387–1405.
45 Nyirenda M, Chatterji S, Rochat T, Mutevedzi P, Newell ML: Prevalence and correlates of depression among HIV-infected and -affected older people in rural South Africa. J Affect Disord 2013;151:31–38.
46 Rabkin JG: HIV and depression: 2008 review and update. Curr HIV/AIDS Rep 2008;5:163–171.
47 Clifford DB: HIV-associated neurocognitive disease continues in the antiretroviral era. Top HIV Med 2008;16:94–98.
48 Vance DE, Farr KF, Struzick T: Assessing the clinical value of cognitive appraisal in adults aging with HIV. J Gerontol Nurs 2008;34:36–41.
49 Grov C, Golub SA, Parsons JT, Brennan M, Karpiak SE: Loneliness and HIV-related stigma explain depression among older HIV-positive adults. AIDS Care 2010;22:630–639.
50 Mahajan AP, Sayles JN, Patel VA, Remien RH, Sawires SR, Ortiz DJ, Szekeres G, Coates TJ: Stigma in the HIV/AIDS epidemic: a review of the literature and recommendations for the way forward. AIDS 2008;22(suppl 2):S67–S79.
51 Jiao JM, So E, Jebakumar J, George MC, Simpson DM, Robinson-Papp J: Chronic pain disorders in HIV primary care: clinical characteristics and association with healthcare utilization. Pain 2016;157: 931–937.
52 Tsang A, Von Korff M, Lee S, Alonso J, Karam E, Angermeyer MC, Borges GL, Bromet EJ, Demytteneare K, de Girolamo G, de Graaf R, Gureje O, Lepine JP, Haro JM, Levinson D, Oakley Browne MA, Posada-Villa J, Seedat S, Watanabe M: Common chronic pain conditions in developed and developing countries: gender and age differences and comorbidity with depression-anxiety disorders. J Pain 2008;9:883–891.
53 Makris UE, Abrams RC, Gurland B, Reid MC: Management of persistent pain in the older patient: a clinical review. JAMA 2014;312:825–837.
54 Bauer LO, Ceballos NA, Shanley JD, Wolfson LI: Sensorimotor dysfunction in HIV/AIDS: effects of antiretroviral treatment and comorbid psychiatric disorders. AIDS 2005;19:495–502.
55 Nagi SZ: An epidemiology of disability among adults in the United States. Milbank Mem Fund Q Health Soc 1976;54:439–467.

56 Abellan van Kan G, Rolland Y, Andrieu S, Bauer J, Beauchet O, Bonnefoy M, Cesari M, Donini LM, Gillette Guyonnet S, Inzitari M, Nourhashemi F, Onder G, Ritz P, Salva A, Visser M, Vellas B: Gait speed at usual pace as a predictor of adverse outcomes in community-dwelling older people an international academy on nutrition and aging (IANA) task force. J Nutr Health Aging 2009;13:881–889.
57 Jette AM: Toward a common language for function, disability, and health. Phys Ther 2006;86:726–734.
58 Guralnik JM, Simonsick EM, Ferrucci L, Glynn RJ, Berkman LF, Blazer DG, Scherr PA, Wallace RB: A short physical performance battery assessing lower extremity function: association with self-reported disability and prediction of mortality and nursing home admission. J Gerontol 1994;49:M85–M94.
59 Bauer LO, Wu Z, Wolfson LI: An obese body mass increases the adverse effects of HIV/AIDS on balance and gait. Phys Ther 2011;91:1063–1071.
60 Hedden T, Gabrieli JD: Insights into the ageing mind: a view from cognitive neuroscience. Nat Rev Neurosci 2004;5:87–96.
61 Montero-Odasso M, Verghese J, Beauchet O, Hausdorff JM: Gait and cognition: a complementary approach to understanding brain function and the risk of falling. J Am Geriatr Soc 2012;60:2127–2136.
62 Minkler M, Fuller-Thomson E, Guralnik JM: Gradient of disability across the socioeconomic spectrum in the United States. N Engl J Med 2006;355:695–703.
63 Leveille SG, Penninx BW, Melzer D, Izmirlian G, Guralnik JM: Sex differences in the prevalence of mobility disability in old age: the dynamics of incidence, recovery, and mortality. J Gerontol B Psychol Sci Soc Sci 2000;55:S41–S50.
64 Siordia C: Precision in estimates of disability prevalence for the population aged 65 and over in the United States by race and ethnicity. J Frailty Aging 2014;3:187–192.
65 Oursler KK, Goulet JL, Crystal S, Justice AC, Crothers K, Butt AA, Rodriguez-Barradas MC, Favors K, Leaf D, Katzel LI, Sorkin JD: Association of age and comorbidity with physical function in HIV-infected and uninfected patients: results from the veterans aging cohort study. AIDS Patient Care STDS 2011;25:13–20.
66 Verbrugge LM, Jette AM: The disablement process. Soc Sci Med 1994;38:1–14.
67 Freedman VA, Spillman BC: Disability and care needs among older Americans. Milbank Q 2014;92:509–541.
68 Landi F, Onder G, Cesari M, Russo A, Barillaro C, Bernabei R: Pain and its relation to depressive symptoms in frail older people living in the community: an observational study. J Pain Symptom Manage 2005;29:255–262.
69 Chou CH, Hwang CL, Wu YT: Effect of exercise on physical function, daily living activities, and quality of life in the frail older adults: a meta-analysis. Arch Phys Med Rehabil 2012;93:237–244.
70 Skarbinski J, Rosenberg E, Paz-Bailey G, Hall HI, Rose CE, Viall AH, Fagan JL, Lansky A, Mermin JH: Human immunodeficiency virus transmission at each step of the care continuum in the United States. JAMA Intern Med 2015;175:588–596.

Suzanne G. Leveille, PhD, RN
College of Nursing and Health Sciences
University Massachusetts Boston
100 Morrissey Blvd., Boston, MA 02125 (USA)
E-Mail Suzanne.Leveille@umb.edu

Brennan-Ing M, DeMarco RF (eds): HIV and Aging. Interdiscipl Top Gerontol Geriatr.
Basel, Karger, 2017, vol 42, pp 119–133 (DOI: 10.1159/000448549)

# Application of Geriatric Principles and Care Models in HIV and Aging

Aroonsiri Sangarlangkarn[a, b] · Anchalee Avihingsanon[b, c] · Jonathan S. Appelbaum[d]

[a]Department of Geriatrics and Palliative Care, Mount Sinai Medical Center, New York, N.Y., USA; [b]HIV Netherlands Australia Thailand Research Collaboration, Thai Red Cross AIDS Research Centre, and, [c]Department of Medicine, Faculty of Medicine, Chulalongkorn University, Bangkok, Thailand; [d]Department of Clinical Sciences, Florida State University College of Medicine, Tallahassee, Fla., USA

**Abstract**

People aging with HIV present a unique challenge for providers. HIV-infected patients experience accentuated aging and multimorbidity, but are typically disconnected from geriatric care, which is limited by a shortage of geriatric providers worldwide. Consequently, HIV providers are tasked with managing multiple age-related illnesses, within service networks that are historically not designed to care for aging patients. While comfortable with the management of antiretroviral therapy, HIV providers may have limited training on how to recognize or manage geriatric syndromes, especially in the context of multimorbidity. The result is an emerging, vulnerable population, and the question is how to best care for them.

As part of the answer, we offer examples of how providers can use geriatric principles to improve the care of aging HIV-infected patients. We begin by describing basic geriatric concepts and examples of care models, and subsequently use a patient case to illustrate their applications at the patient level. At the system level, we discuss how HIV service networks can use components of geriatric care models to meet the needs of aging HIV-infected patients. Lastly, we identify aging-specific guidelines and service integration as important areas for future endeavors. 

## Introduction

As of 2015, more than 50% of HIV-infected patients in the United States were 50 years and older [1]. They may experience accentuated aging [2, 3] and increased multimorbidity [4], but are not usually connected to geriatric care, possibly due to a shortage of geriatric providers in multiple disciplines and inadequate integration between HIV and geriatric service networks. As a result, HIV providers currently bear the responsibility of managing multiple age-related diseases, within service networks that were not designed for aging patients. While comfortable with HIV-related issues, HIV providers may have limited training on how to recognize or treat age-related illnesses in the setting of multimorbidity. This has resulted in an emerging, vulnerable population, and we are faced with the question of how to best care for them.

To help answer this question, we offer examples of how geriatric principles and care models may be applied to the aging HIV-infected population. Since globally validated research in this area is limited, these strategies should be tailored based on local needs assessment, available resources, and cultural nuances. We first begin with basic geriatrics concepts and examples of geriatric care models. For application at the patient level, we present a patient case to describe the complex socioeconomic conditions surrounding the aging HIV-infected patient, then offer a case-based example of how multidisciplinary teams may use geriatric principles to improve the patient's condition. At the system level, we discuss how HIV service networks can draw from components of geriatric care models to prepare for the needs of aging HIV-infected patients. Lastly, we identify areas of critical need for future research.

## Basic Concepts in Geriatrics

Although aging HIV-infected patients may face unique stigma and discrimination, they experience many health-related issues that are similar to those in the uninfected. As a result, basic concepts in geriatrics [5] may be relevant to this unique population.

Diseases in aging HIV-infected patients, much like those in the uninfected patients, are often multiple and multifactorial [4]. Termed *multimorbidity*, these diseases do not simply coexist with one another, but often have synergistic interactions that together increase morbidity and mortality. With increased multimorbidity, HIV-infected patients are at risk of iatrogenic illnesses and care fragmentation due to involvement of various clinicians in multiple settings. Specialists may focus on a single disease within their field and prescribe treatments that unintentionally worsen a patient's other conditions. Treatment guidelines for one disease may clash with another, and multiple concurrent treatments may increase care burdens without benefits on mortality or quality of life [6]. As a result, disease-centric guidelines should be grounded in *patient-centered outcomes*, such as care preferences, function, symptom burden, and quality of life. *Coordination of care* is also crucial, since aging HIV-infected patients may use medical and social services from both HIV and geriatric service networks. Care should be provided through integrated, multilevel systems that follow patients through various care settings and coordinate between transitions to avoid conflicting interventions, duplications, and errors.

Additionally, multimorbidity creates multifaceted needs, and effective care cannot be delivered by one person alone. Care is best delivered by *multidisciplinary teams*, which may include nurses, social workers, pharmacists, and other disciplines. Team effectiveness will depend on the psychosocial environment surrounding the patient, and providers should consider how *psychosocial determinants* may affect care plans, such as living situations, family relationships, caregiver availability, religion/spirituality, and local availability of services.

Despite increased multimorbidity in some patients, providers should avoid *ageism* and keep in mind that aging occurs at different rates between individuals, and within the same individual in different organs. Aging is not a disease, and chronological age should be viewed in conjunction with aging phenotypes. For example, many HIV-infected patients age well with minimal symptoms, while others experience increased prevalence of age-related illnesses. These patients with accentuated aging phenotype may have *typical presentations of diseases*, symptoms of which are often dismissed as part of aging. Systematic screenings for age-related illnesses can help prevent under-diagnoses of reversible and treatable conditions.

## Examples of Care Models Utilizing Geriatric Concepts

Due to limited space, we choose the Geriatrics Resources for Assessment and Care of Elders (GRACE) model as an example due to its comprehensive home-based components, then apply it to a patient case to illustrate how multidisciplinary teams may use the GRACE model to care for aging HIV-infected patients. Other examples are listed in table 1, with links to external resources that provide greater detail. Since the evidence on globally validated geriatric care models is limited, these models will likely require tailoring in resource-limited settings.

### *Geriatrics Resources for Assessment and Care of Elders (GRACE)*

GRACE was developed to improve care quality for community-dwelling adults 65 years and older with low income [12]. As part of a geriatrician-led multidisciplinary intervention, the GRACE support team, consisting of a nurse practitioner and a social worker with special training in GRACE, visits patients at home to perform a baseline comprehensive geriatric assessment. This assessment aims to provide comprehensive information on the patient, and to proactively assess for 12 target domains: advance care planning, health maintenance, medication management, difficulty walking/falls, chronic pain, visual impairment, hearing loss, urinary incontinence, depression, malnutrition/weight loss, dementia, and caregiver burden. The assessment includes medical and psychosocial history, medication review, functional assessment, home safety evaluation, review of social support, and advance directives.

After in-home assessments, the GRACE support team meets with the larger GRACE interdisciplinary team consisting of a geriatrician, pharmacist, physical therapist, mental health social worker, and community-based service liaison from the same health system as the primary care physician (PCP). All members work together to develop a prioritized care plan based on patient's care goals. If any of the 12 target

**Table 1.** Examples of geriatric care models

| Program information | Description | Populations served | External resources |
|---|---|---|---|
| Geriatric Resources for Assessment and Care of Elders (GRACE)<br>Country: United States | As part of a geriatrician-led multidisciplinary team, GRACE nurse practitioners and/or social workers visit patients at home to perform baseline assessments and explore psychosocial determinants. They work with primary care physicians to develop and coordinate care plans that provide comprehensive health/social services | Community-dwelling adults 65 years and older with low income | graceteamcare.indiana.edu |
| The United States Department of Veterans Affairs (VA)<br>Country: United States | The VA provides coordinated, comprehensive services consolidated by geographic areas using multidisciplinary teamwork and nationwide integrated medical records [7]. It also runs home-based primary care (VA HBPC) program [8] for veterans with limited mobility | US veterans of all ages | www.va.gov/health |
| Program for All-Inclusive Care of the Elderly (PACE)<br>Country: United States | PACE multidisciplinary team acts as care managers and coordinates care across settings, including acute, long-term, and primary care [9]. They provide comprehensive medical and supportive services at home, in the community, and at PACE centers which serve as adult day care that patients visit several times per week | Nursing-home eligible, community-dwelling patients 55 years and older who have Medicare and Medicaid | www.npaonline.org |
| System of Integrated Care for Older Persons (SIPA)<br>Country: Canada | A multidisciplinary team based in local community centers works with, but does not replace, primary care physicians to provide comprehensive, coordinated health/social services. They reduce institutional service utilization with 24-hour availability, rapid team mobilization, and home support services [10] | Moderately impaired community-dwelling adults 64 years and older | – |
| Program of Research to Integrate Services for the Maintenance of Autonomy (PRISMA)<br>Country: Canada | A multidisciplinary team performs standardized assessment and coordinates individualized care with primary care physicians through a single entry point. Care is integrated using computerized clinical chart that communicates between institutions for client monitoring purposes [11] | Moderately to severely impaired community-dwelling adults who are 65 years or older | www.prisma-qc.ca |

domains is deficient, corresponding GRACE protocols are activated to provide recommendations based on published guidelines.

Once the care plan is finalized, the GRACE support team meets with the PCP in person to review a computer-generated summary of the assessment and suggestions to obtain PCP approval. Collaborating with the PCP, the GRACE support team implements and coordinates the care plan across multiple diseases, providers, and sites of care using face-to-face and telephone contacts with patients, family members/

caregivers, and providers. Team reviews occur at regular intervals to track success in care implementations, and patients receive a minimum of one contact/month and one reassessment/year to check for new problems.

### Application at the Patient Level: Applying GRACE to the Case of Mr. Elder

*Baseline In-Home Comprehensive Assessment*

Mr. Elder has a change in the ability for self care, which may be an atypical presentation of various medical conditions in the setting of multimorbidity. As the first step, an in-home comprehensive assessment should be performed to avoid attributing these changes incorrectly to age and prevent underdiagnoses of treatable conditions. Detecting abnormalities early can prevent future complications, while a normal result provides a baseline for future comparisons. In-home visits are an important component, since they have been shown to delay the onset of disability and reduce nursing home placement in the uninfected elderly [13–15].

Members of the multidisciplinary team, with the most flexible availability and mobility, can be trained to perform in-home comprehensive assessment. Since a standardized comprehensive geriatric assessment has not been validated in the aging HIV-infected population, providers may assemble a set of assessment tools that fit

| Case example |
|---|
| Mr. Elder is a 61-year-old African-American gay man with well-controlled HIV, diabetes, chronic kidney disease, hypertension, knee osteoarthritis, and stroke 3 years prior with residual right-hand weakness. He follows up in a clinic with you, his PCP. |
| Past medical history: Mr. Elder contracted HIV through sex. He was diagnosed in 1990 when he presented with meningoencephalitis due to toxoplasmosis. His last CD4 was 550 cells/mm$^3$, viral load was undetectable. His diabetes and blood pressure were well-controlled. |
| Social history: Mr. Elder dropped out of high school at 16 years. He used to work as a postman but became disabled when he had a stroke. He lives alone in a low-income housing project. His lifelong partner died a year prior from AIDS-related complications, and he has not been sexually active since. He has no children and has been estranged from his sister, the only remaining family member, due to his sexual orientation. She has not seen him in 30 years and does not know that he has HIV. He has been reclusive most of his life, since he worries that others would discover his HIV status. He does everything himself and has no help at home. |
| The problem: Mr. Elder says he has not been feeling well and has lost 8 lbs. since last visit. He was admitted to the hospital twice in the past few months for uncontrolled diabetes and blood pressure, so you have not seen him for a while. He also feels weak and fell multiple times at home after discharge. His sugar level and blood pressure are high today, unlike prior visits. His CD4 is now 200 cells/mm$^3$, viral load is 200,000 copies/ml. It seems that Mr. Elder has not been adherent to his medications for HIV or other chronic conditions. |

into their workflow, cover the same domains as the GRACE model, and have prior use in the HIV-infected population when possible. For example, although the Mini-Mental Status Exam is a popular cognitive screening tool in the traditional comprehensive geriatric assessment, it is proprietary and does not thoroughly test for executive function which may be impaired by HIV-associated neurocognitive disorders [16]. As a result, screening tools that test both cortical and subcortical functions, such as the Montreal Cognitive Assessment, may be more suitable [16].

*Summary of Mr. Elder's Health Status*

Mr. Elder has a subacute change in health status in the context of multimorbidity, suffering from multiple illnesses that interact to exacerbate one another [4]. Using the social ecological model (fig. 1) [22], we describe dynamic interactions between per-

| **Case example continued** |
|---|
| Assessments and findings: The multidisciplinary team, consisting of a nurse practitioner and a social worker, performs baseline assessments in Mr. Elder's home. |
| Other than the medical and psychosocial history known prior to the PCP, the team finds that Mr. Elder suffers from severe depressive symptoms (45/60 on Center for Epidemiologic Studies Depression Scale [17]), coexisting with mild cognitive impairment (21/30 on Montreal Cognitive Assessment). Despite these impairments, safety assessments corroborated with Mr. Elder's landlord did not reveal wandering, unattended stove tops, or firearms in the home. |
| Assessing for functional ability using the Basic and Instrumental Activities of Daily Living [18], we find that Mr. Elder has problems with medication management and gait instability, with frailty (4/5 on Fried Frailty Index [19]), limited mobility due to knee pain (20 seconds on get-up and go test [20]), and multiple falls outside the home. As a result, Mr. Elder has been skipping meals since he is afraid he will fall if he goes grocery shopping. He has also stopped cleaning the bathroom since he fears he may slip on wet surfaces. As part of home safety evaluation, the team finds that the bathroom indeed presents safety hazards as reported by Mr. Elder. He does not have non-slip mats in the bathroom, and there are no grab bars to help with balance. The bathtub also has a tall edge that requires Mr. Elder to clear a height of 0.5 meters to get in for a shower. Luckily, he has no problems with hearing, or incontinence. |
| On review of medications, you find that Mr. Elder had problems sleeping in the hospital due to beeping monitors on his wards, and was started on zolpidem 10 mg nightly that continued on discharge, even though he sleeps well at home. He was instructed to inject short-acting insulin 10 units at breakfast, 15 units at lunch and dinner. However, Mr. Elder got confused and has been injecting 40 units of insulin every morning instead, although he is unsure since he could not read the small syringe very well. The residual weakness in his right hand from prior stroke also makes insulin injection difficult. |
| Using the HIV primary care guidelines from the Infectious Diseases Society of America [21], the team finds that although Mr. Elder is up-to-date on all his vaccines and most healthcare maintenance, he has not had a bone densitometry screen, and his last gonorrhea/chlamydia screens were performed 3 years ago. He has not chosen a proxy for healthcare or financial decisions, and has not thought about care preferences earlier. When asked, he mentions that the most important goals are pain control and functional independence. |

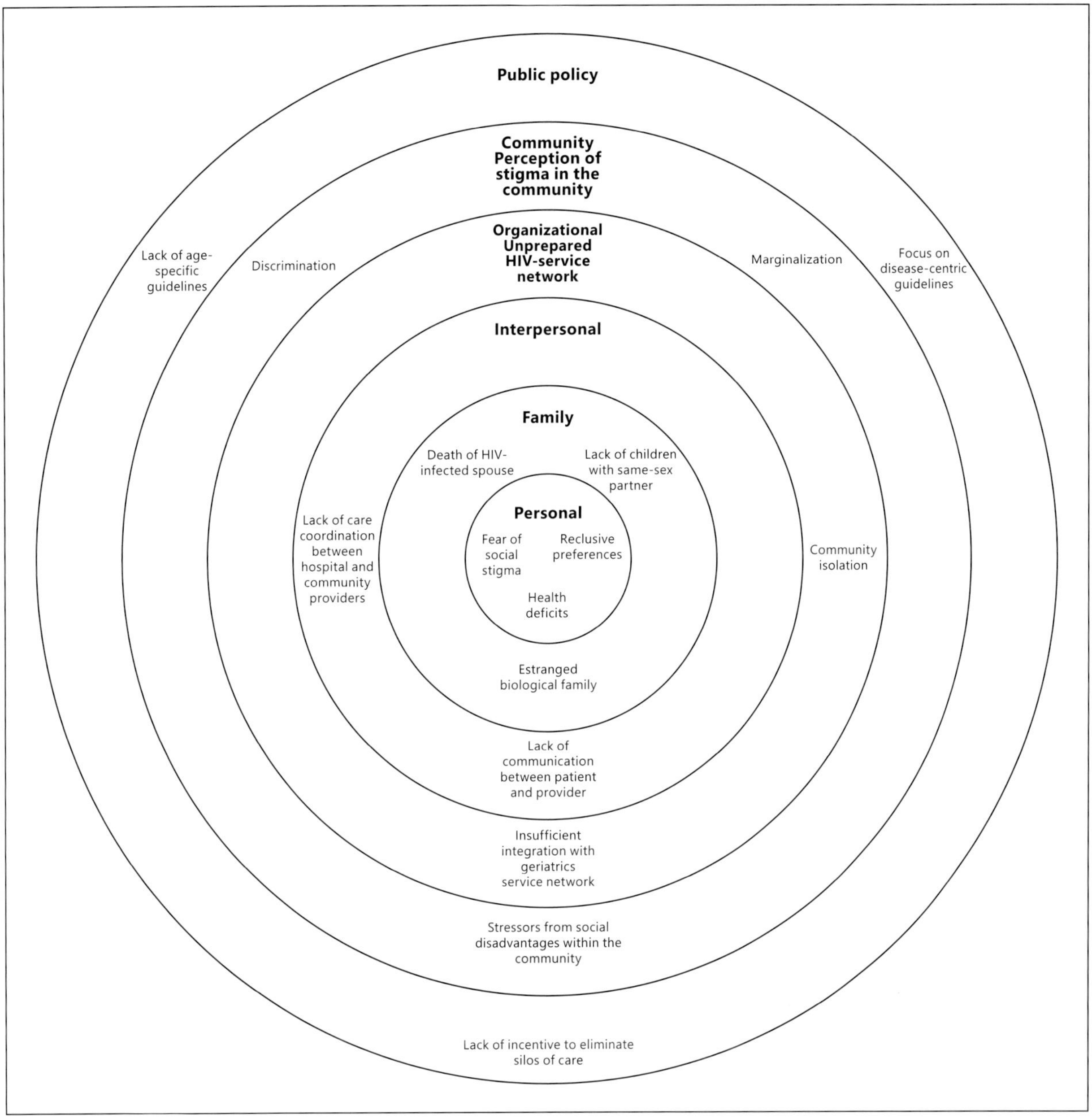


**Fig. 1.** Social ecological model depicting factors that affected Mr. Elder's health.

sonal, family, interpersonal, organizational, community, and public policy factors that affect Mr. Elder [23].

At the *personal* level, Mr. Elder's reclusive preferences and fear of social stigma may influence him to self-isolate instead of seeking help when difficulties arise. For example, Mr. Elder prefers to skip meals instead of asking others for help with grocery shopping, likely contributing to his weight loss. His health deficits also impede on his ability to care for self. For example, the residual weakness from prior stroke creates difficulties with frequent insulin injections, while his cognitive impairment, depression, and limited education may affect adherence to all types of medications, leading to uncontrolled diabetes, blood pressure, and HIV. His falls and functional impairment may result from frailty, chronic knee pain from osteoarthritis, low glucose level from incorrect insulin injections causing dizziness, and sedating side effects of zolpidem.

*Family* factors contribute to Mr. Elder's lack of social support, including a lack of children with same-sex partners, and estrangement from biological family members who are uninvolved and unaware of his HIV status and healthcare preferences. It is also likely that Mr. Elder used to receive help only from his HIV-infected partner, and his partner's death severely compromised his support structure [24].

At the *interpersonal* level, Mr. Elder's complications may have worsened due to poor coordination between hospital and community providers. The lack of communication between Mr. Elder and his providers about difficulties with the insulin regimen also *contribute* to the problem.

At the *organizational* level, HIV service networks may need further adjustments to fully prepare for the care of aging HIV-infected patients. Currently, the assessment and modification of home environment are not consistently part of routine care for functionally impaired HIV-infected patients, and may contribute to safety hazards in Mr. Elder's environment. The failure to reconcile medication lists and assess for changes in medication needs during care transitions led Mr. Elder to continue to take zolpidem at home [25], although it is no longer necessary now that Mr. Elder is back home with less noise interruption. Insufficient integration with geriatric service network also limits Mr. Elder's ability to benefit from traditional geriatric services that can help patients with functional and cognitive impairments during care transitions.

At the *community* level, social isolation, marginalization, discrimination, and stigma may prevent Mr. Elder from fully integrating into his community and benefiting from its support structure. Mr. Elder may also be distressed by social disadvantages within his community, including poverty, unemployment, housing issues, or lack of recreational opportunities.

At the *policy* level, lack of evidence-based guidelines specific to aging HIV-infected patients presents a challenge to HIV providers. The current focus on disease-centric guidelines fails to accommodate multimorbidity, and distracts from patient-centered outcomes. Lack of directives and incentives to eliminate silos of care also *contribute* to Mr. Elder's health status.

*Overall Management Strategy in the Setting of Multimorbidity*

Each aging HIV-infected individual is unique and complex. They cannot be defined simply by one-dimensional characteristic, such as chronological age which subscribes to ageism, or single disease entities that dismiss the effect of multimorbidity and the multifactorial nature of their illnesses. More importantly, different patients have different goals and preferences. As a result, applying disease-centric guidelines homogeneously to every patient without consideration of individual preferences, aging phenotypes, or multimorbidity disregards each person's unique health needs and likely will not provide patient-centered care.

Recognizing that not all aging HIV-infected patients should be approached the same way, clinicians may utilize prognostic tools such as the Veterans Aging Cohort Study (VACS) index [26] to prioritize care plans. Using prognosis to establish timeframes, providers can elicit care goals, identify diseases and risk factors that affect these goals, calculate the likely effects and lag time to benefit [27] of various care guidelines on these goals, and use this information to prioritize interventions and guide shared decision making with patients and caregivers [6].

*Initial Interventions*

Initial efforts should focus on immediate needs and maintenance of function [28]. After in-home assessments, the GRACE support team should elicit preferences from Mr. Elder before meeting with the full multidisciplinary team to help prioritize interventions in the context of multimorbidity. Subsequently, the plan should be discussed with Mr. Elder and his PCP, and modified as necessary to arrive at a care plan supported by all involved parties.

To achieve functional independence, the team recommended non-slip mats, grab bars, and shower chairs to help Mr. Elder shower safely, as well as a bedside commode and nightlight to help minimize nighttime bathroom trips in dark environments that may cause falls. To prevent fractures, the team recommended bone density scan to screen for osteoporosis as Mr. Elder is at risk [21], and fall prevention/maintenance of function are important to Mr. Elder.

Before discussing useful services, the community-based services liaison has a long discussion with Mr. Elder to assure him that his HIV status will not be revealed to non-health care workers. Despite this, Mr. Elder refuses home attendants, housekeeping services, help with errands by local volunteers, and referral to HIV-related support group in the local community, as he is uncomfortable with prolonged interactions with strangers at this time. However, he accepts a medical alert system wristband, arranged transportations to appointments, home delivery of pre-sorted medications, and meal delivery based on the menu that Mr. Elder and the team nutritionist work on together.

As part of the falls evaluation, the pharmacist may review medication list to ensure that falls caused by medication side effects are not misdiagnosed as symptoms of another condition, lest more medications be prescribed to treat side effects, initiating what is known as the prescribing cascade [29]. With sedating side effects of zolpidem suspected as the culprit, the team discusses fall risks with Mr. Elder, weighed against likely little benefit of sleep aid now that he is no longer in a noisy hospital environment. The team makes a shared decision with Mr. Elder to taper zolpidem and monitor for improvement. Without orthostatic hypotension, the PCP feels comfortable increasing Mr. Elder's blood pressure medication to achieve better control of his hypertension. However, without proof of reliable food intake, the team suggests a more lenient diabetic goal to prevent hypoglycemia that may precipitate falls, using once/day, pre-filled syringes for ease of use. Mr. Elder gets new eyeglasses so that he can read small print on the syringes, but the team warns him about possible increased falls while getting used to new eyewear [30]. The nurse works with Mr. Elder to make sure that he feels comfortable with the new syringes. All medication changes were discussed with the PCP to avoid errors.

The team tackles depression in conjunction with pain, since they can exacerbate one another. They suggest collaborative care programs that offer a choice of medications and/or psychotherapy in clinic [31] or at home [32], combined with patient education by the team's mental health social worker. The physical therapist visits Mr. Elder at home to discuss exercise routines, while the team consults a pain specialist to provide a safe regimen for his knee pain.

*Mid-Range Interventions*

After dealing with acute issues, mid-range interventions may include regular check-ups to monitor progress on care plans and management of non-urgent issues. For example, interval check-ups on Mr. Elder may involve assessments of food intake, weight changes, glucose or blood pressure level to adjust medications, or pill counts to monitor adherence.

Non-urgent issues may include chronic disease management, healthcare maintenance, advance care planning, and integration into the community or the family unit. They should be guided by lag time to benefit [27] and prognosis based on the VACS index [26]. For example, if Mr. Elder has a VACS index of 70 (predicted 5-year mortality of 47%), the team may advise Mr. Elder to prioritize advance care planning over gonorrhea/chlamydia screening or tertiary prevention for stroke. Initial efforts should focus on identifying a proxy for finance and healthcare decisions, who preferably knows the patient's HIV status. The team may consult with Mr. Elder on whether his sister should be recruited as his advocate or proxy, and the pros and cons of sharing HIV diagnosis with her and her family. If family is not available, integration into the local community may help expand social support and foster a sense of empowerment.

*Long-Term Interventions*

Long-term interventions address care plans that may be implemented at the time of eventual decline. Providers should avoid discussing specific treatments, such as intubation or feeding tubes, since it is difficult to make decisions that encompass all future scenarios in which these treatments may be necessary. On the contrary, providers should focus on 'living' instead of 'dying', and ask about activities that bring meaning, as well as desired levels of function and quality of life. Using these preferences, the team can recommend treatments that accomplish these goals at the time of eventual decline, regardless of the types of illness that may occur. Mr. Elder should also discuss the types and amount of leeway in decision making with his proxy [33].

### Application at the System Level

A successful application of geriatric principles at the patient level requires concurrent changes at the system level. Drawing from examples of care models in table 1, we provide a generalized action plan that helps prepare systems for the care of aging HIV-infected patients.

*Build a Multidisciplinary Team That Follows Patients across the Continuum of Care*
To facilitate care coordination, multidisciplinary teams should not be divided by syndromes (e.g., pain control or hepatitis C co-management), but by cohorts of patients to be followed longitudinally, so the whole patient is cared for (e.g., Programs for All Inclusive Care of the Elderly (PACE), GRACE, System of Integrated Care for Older Persons (SIPA), Program of Research to Integrate Services for the Maintenance of Autonomy (PRISMA); table 1). Team members should be trained to provide a comprehensive set of common services across the continuum of HIV. They may include initial screenings (e.g., GRACE, PRISMA), ongoing HIV care, management of common comorbidities, and end-of-life care. The responsibility for each provider should be determined by the team to ensure safety and comfort for all involved.

*Provide Comprehensive Healthcare Services*
Comprehensive services are needed to address multimorbidity and psychosocial factors among aging HIV-infected patients (e.g., Veterans Affairs (VA), PACE, GRACE, SIPA). This requires the capacity to comprehensively assess for psychological, cognitive, functional, financial, nutritional, and medication needs (e.g., GRACE, PRISMA). Services can be provided accordingly to ensure that basic needs are met so patients can effectively participate in care [34]. Linkages to community agencies that serve older adults may help expand options and availability of services.

For example, since HIV-infected patients are at risk of mental health issues and substance use disorders, treatment adherence may be dictated by access to mental health and substance abuse services. Access should include both pharmacologic and behavioral therapy to maximize success and prevent relapses. HIV neuropathy and chronic pain also affect compliance, and providing pain services through anesthesiologists, neurologists, or palliative care providers can improve the quality of life. With higher risk of metabolic and cardiovascular disease, nutritionist consultations and services to provide healthy meals in community centers or delivered to home can help patients maintain a healthy weight and a healthy life. HIV-infected patients with severe cognitive impairment and high caregiver burden may benefit from adult day programs (e.g., PACE centers), respite services, and consultations with geriatricians, who can also help with advance care planning. Care coordinators, social workers or volunteers can be trained to lead support groups as a confidential forum to discuss disease burden and share effective resources. Using these examples as guidance, providers should determine the types and extent of appropriate services for their population based on patient/caregiver needs and resource assessment. Certain services may need to be created depending on local disease patterns, what existing staff can take on, and what can be outsourced.

*Focus on Patient-Centered Outcomes*

Much of current literature offers single-disease guidelines based on ideal patients without addressing multimorbidity in aging HIV-infected patients. Consequently, policy makers should advocate for multimorbidity protocols (e.g., GRACE) that help prioritize interventions and encourage patient/public engagement [35]. Patient/caregiver representatives should be involved in deciding which cross-disease, universal, patient-centered outcomes should be used to measure quality. These may include function, symptom burden, or quality of life [6].

*Integrate Geriatric and HIV Networks of Services*

Service network integration can improve quality, efficiency, and cost-effectiveness. Literature on integrated care [36, 37] may provide applicable strategies for policy makers.

Financial strategies include pooling of funds, as form follows financing. For a US-based example, pooling Medicare/Medicaid funds for dual-eligible HIV-infected patients into per capita payments to replace fee-for-service models may increase cost-effectiveness (e.g., PACE). Administrative strategies include inter-agency planning to streamline eligibility and access (e.g., VA, PRISMA), decentralization/consolidation of functions to reduce complexities (e.g., VA, PACE), or joint purchasing/commissioning to improve resource management. Organizational strategies include co-location of services or affiliations of care networks (e.g., VA, PACE), joint ownership/merger, or joint contracting/program management. Service delivery strategies include integrated information systems (e.g., VA, PRISMA), centralized referral/intake structure (e.g., VA, PRISMA), and joint training to update HIV providers with skills in geriatrics and help geriatricians provide effective consultations for complicated HIV cases. Clinical strategies include shared clinical records (e.g., VA, PRISMA), joint decision support tools and practice guidelines, joint care planning, shared assessment procedures, and joint diagnostic codes.

Integration with geriatric service networks should take into account the unique care needs of HIV-infected patients, who may be reluctant due to concerns of confidentiality or discrimination [38], fear of being judged as old/disabled [39], or disruptions to long-standing relationships with their HIV providers [40]. The system should address potential barriers and provide appropriate reassurance to help patients engage in beneficial services.

*Provide Coordination and Monitoring across Care Settings*

To provide seamless transitions, a single multidisciplinary team should be designated as the care manager (e.g., PACE, GRACE, SIPA, PRISMA). They should monitor patients across care settings, take responsibility for coordinating care among clinicians (e.g., PACE, GRACE, SIPA, PRISMA), provide rapid support during medical crises to prevent hospitalization or emergency room visits (e.g., SIPA), and help patients process treatment options based on goals of care [6]. A multi-tiered strategy might be necessary, starting with simple programs that coordinate care for independent patients and advancing to highly integrated programs as their needs increase.

For mobile patients, the HIV service networks should simplify care coordination by co-locating services in one location (e.g., VA, PACE). Geographic consolidation can increase patient engagement by strengthening long-term relationships with providers, and reducing concerns regarding HIV status disclosure to multiple care systems. Consolidation also limits the number of handoffs, minimizes errors, encourages collaborations, and decreases travel time.

With increased disability and cognitive impairment as more HIV-infected patients age [2–4], building capacity for home-bound patients is also essential. Home-based programs (e.g., VA HBPC, GRACE, SIPA) should provide close monitoring, timely interventions, adaptations to create a therapeutic home environment, coordination with other providers, support to relieve caregiver burden, and comprehensive services that optimize function, cognition, and quality of life. Benefits include maximizing functional independence, promoting patient autonomy, reducing the need for hospitalization or institutionalization, avoiding emergency department or outpatient clinic visits, assisting during transitions of care, and providing continuity of care throughout the disease continuum, from diagnosis to the end of life [13].

## Future Directions

Future efforts should create changes at both the patient and system levels. At the patient level, research should explore age-specific treatment and screening guidelines for aging HIV-infected patients at both ends of the spectrum: when interventions should occur earlier, and when interventions are no longer appropriate due to poor prognosis and multimorbidity. Dedicated efforts for patients in resource-limited settings may be needed, since they may develop different pathology from those in developed countries due to different ART regimens and socioeconomic factors. At the system level, we should create and validate care models for aging HIV-infected patients that provide patient-centered protocols and descriptions of appropriate roles and timing of care involvement by various disciplines. Emphasis on developing countries is crucial, since validated care models in high-burden, resource-limited settings such as Asia or Africa are currently absent. Policy makers should also focus on capacity building and integration of HIV and geriatric service networks. Aging HIV-infected patients are a unique and vulnerable population. Building HIV and aging care models of the future will require persistence, creativity, collaboration, and a flexible system within which to exercise them.

## References


1 Brooks J, Buchacz K, Gebo KA, Mermin J: HIV infection and older Americans. the public health perspective. Am J Public Health 2012;102:1516–1526.

2 Althoff KN, McGinnis KA, Wyatt CM, Freiberg MS, Gilbert C, Oursler KK, Rimland D, Rodriguez-Barradas MC, Dubrow R, Park LS, Skanderson M, Shiels MS, Gange SJ, Gebo KA, Justice AC: Comparison of risk and age at diagnosis of myocardial infarction, end-stage renal disease, and non-AIDS-defining cancer in HIV-infected versus uninfected adults. Clin Infect Dis 2015;60:627–638.

3 Pathai S, Bajillan H, Landay AL, High KP: Is HIV a model of accelerated or accentuated aging? J Gerontol A Biol Sci Med Sci 2014;69:833–842.

4 Schouten J, Wit FW, Stolte IG, Kootstra NA, van der Valk M, Geerlings SE, Prins M, Reiss P: Cross-sectional comparison of the prevalence of age-associated comorbidities and their risk factors between HIV-infected and uninfected individuals: the AGEhIV cohort study. Clin Infect Dis 2014;59:1787–1797.

5 Emory University, Division of Geriatric Medicine and Gerontology: The Emory 'BIG 10' Basics in Geriatrics. http://medicine.emory.edu/documents/geriatrics-big10.pdf (accessed July 7, 2015).

6 Tinetti M, Fried TR, Boyd CM: Designing health care for the most common chronic condition – multimorbidity. JAMA 2012;307:2493–2494.

7 Kizer KW, Dudley RA: Extreme makeover: transformation of the veterans health care system. Annu Rev Public Health 2009;30:313–339.

8 Beales JL, Edes T: Veteran's affairs home based primary care. Clin Geriatr Med 2009;25:149–154.

9 Eng C, Pedulla J, Eleazer GP, McCann R, Fox N: Program of all-inclusive care for the elderly (PACE): an innovative model of integrated geriatric care and financing. J Am Geriatr Soc 1997;45:223–232.

10 Béland F, Bergman H, Lebel P, Dallaire L, Fletcher J, Contandriopoulos AP, Tousignant P: Integrated services for frail elders (SIPA): a trial of a model for Canada. Can J Aging 2006;25:5–42.

11 MacAdam M: PRISMA: program of research to integrate the services for the maintenance of autonomy. A system-level Integration model in Quebec. Int J Integr Care 2015;15:e018.

12 Counsell SR, Callahan CM, Buttar AB, Clark DO, Frank KI: Geriatric resources for assessment and care of elders (GRACE): a new model of primary care for low-income seniors. J Am Geriatr Soc 2006;54:1136–1141.

13 Stuck AE, Aronow HU, Steiner A, Alessi CA, Büla CJ, Gold MN, Yuhas KE, Nisenbaum R, Rubenstein LZ, Beck JC: A trial of annual in-home comprehensive geriatric assessments for elderly people living in the community. N Engl J Med 1995;333:1184–1189.

14 Stuck AE, Egger M, Hammer A, Minder CE, Beck JC: Home visits to prevent nursing home admission and functional decline in elderly people: systematic review and meta-regression analysis. JAMA 2002;287:1022–1028.

15 Bernabei R, Landi F, Gambassi G, Sgadari A, Zuccala G, Mor V, Rubenstein LZ, Carbonin P: Randomised trial of impact of model of integrated care and case management for older people living in the community. BMJ 1998;316:1348–1351.

16 Valcour V, Paul R, Chiao S, Wendelken LA, Miller B: Screening for cognitive impairment in human immunodeficiency virus. Clin Infect Dis 2011;53:836–842.

17 Grov C, Golub SA, Parsons JT, Brennan M, Karpiak SE: Loneliness and HIV-related stigma explain depression among older HIV-positive adults. AIDS Care 2010;22:630–639.

18 Noelker LS, Browdie R: Sidney Katz, MD: a new paradigm for chronic illness and long-term care. Gerontologist 2014;54:13–20.

19 Fried LP, Tangen CM, Walston J, Newman AB, Hirsch C, Gottdiener J, Seeman T, Tracy R, Kop WJ, Burke G, McBurnie MA: Frailty in older adults: evidence for a phenotype. J Gerontol A Biol Sci Med Sci 2001;56:M146–M156.

20 Mathias S, Nayak US, Isaacs B: Balance in elderly patients: the 'get-up and go' test. Arch Phys Med Rehabil 1986;67:387–389.
21 Aberg JA, Gallant JE, Ghanem KG, Emmanuel P, Zingman BS, Horberg MA: Primary care guidelines for the management of persons infected with HIV: 2013 update by the HIV medicine association of the infectious diseases society of America. Clin Infect Dis 2014;58:1–10.
22 Emmons K: Health behaviours in a social context; in Berkman L, Kawachi I (eds): Social Epidemiology. New York, Oxford University Press, 2000.
23 Stokols D: Translating social ecological theory into guidelines for community health promotion. Am J Health Promot 1996;10:282–298.
24 Poindexter C, Shippy RA: Networks of older New Yorkers with HIV: fragility, resilience, and transformation. AIDS Patient Care STDS 2008;22:723–733.
25 By the American Geriatrics Society 2015 Beers Criteria Update Expert Panel: American geriatrics society 2015 updated beers criteria for potentially inappropriate medication use in older adults. J Am Geriatr Soc 2015;63:2227–2246.
26 Justice AC, Modur SP, Tate JP, Althoff KN, Jacobson LP, Gebo KA, Kitahata MM, Horberg MA, Brooks JT, Buchacz K, Rourke SB, Rachlis A, Napravnik S, Eron J, Willig JH, Moore R, Kirk GD, Bosch R, Rodriguez B, Hogg RS, Thorne J, Goedert JJ, Klein M, Gill J, Deeks S, Sterling TR, Anastos K, Gange SJ: Predictive accuracy of the veterans aging cohort study index for mortality with HIV infection: a North American cross cohort analysis. J Acquir Immune Defic Syndr 2013;62:149–163.
27 Lee SJ, Leipzig RM, Walter LC: Incorporating lag time to benefit into prevention decisions for older adults. JAMA 2013;310:2609–2610.
28 Reuben DB: Medical care for the final years of life 'when you're 83, it's not going to be 20 years'. JAMA 2009;302:2686–2694.
29 Kalisch L, Caughey G, Roughead E, Gilbert A: The prescribing cascade. Aust Prescr 2011;24:162–166.
30 Cumming RG, Ivers R, Clemson L, Cullen J, Hayes MF, Tanzer M, Mitchell P: Improving vision to prevent falls in frail older people: a randomized trial. J Am Geriatr Soc 2007;55:175–181.
31 Unützer J, Katon W, Callahan CM, Williams JW Jr, Hunkeler E, Harpole L, Hoffing M, Della Penna RD, Noël PH, Lin EH, Areán PA, Hegel MT, Tang L, Belin TR, Oishi S, Langston C; IMPACT Investigators: Collaborative care management of late-life depression in the primary care setting: a randomized controlled trial. JAMA 2002;288:2836–2845.
32 Bruce ML, Raue PJ, Reilly CF, Greenberg RL, Meyers BS, Banerjee S, Pickett YR, Sheeran TF, Ghesquiere A, Zukowski DM, Rosas VH, McLaughlin J, Pledger L, Doyle J, Joachim P, Leon AC: Clinical effectiveness of integrating depression care management into Medicare home health: the depression CAREPATH randomized trial. JAMA Intern Med 2015;175:55–64.
33 Sudore RL, Knight SJ, McMahan RD, Feuz M, Farrell D, Miao Y, Barnes DE: A novel website to prepare diverse older adults for decision making and advance care planning: a pilot study. J Pain Symptom Manage 2014;47:674–686.
34 Meyer JP, Chen NE, Springer SA: HIV treatment in the criminal justice system: critical knowledge and intervention gaps. AIDS Res Treat 2011;2011:680617.
35 Lorenc A, Robinson N: A tool to improve patient and public engagement in commissioning sexual and reproductive health and HIV services. J Fam Plann Reprod Health Care 2015;41:8–12.
36 Kodner DL, Spreeuwenberg C: Integrated care: meaning, logic, applications, and implications – a discussion paper. Int J Integr Care 2002;2:e12.
37 Leutz WN: Five laws for integrating medical and social services: lessons from the United States and the United Kingdom. Milbank Q 1999;77:77–110, iv–v.
38 Turton M, Naidoo S: Stigma and disclosure as barriers to regular dental care for people living with HIV/AIDS in Kwazulu-Natal and Western Cape, South Africa. Ethn Inequal Health Soc Care 2014;7:49–59.
39 Emlet CA: 'You're awfully old to have this disease': experiences of stigma and ageism in adults 50 years and older living with HIV/AIDS. Gerontologist 2006;46:781–790.
40 Cervia JS: Easing the transition of HIV-infected adolescents to adult care. AIDS Patient Care STDS 2013; 27:692–696.

Aroonsiri Sangarlangkarn
Department of Geriatrics and Palliative Care
24928 Gov. Stockley Rd
Georgetown, DE 19947 (USA)
E-Mail junes@post.harvard.edu

Brennan-Ing M, DeMarco RF (eds): HIV and Aging. Interdiscipl Top Gerontol Geriatr.
Basel, Karger, 2017, vol 42, pp 134–143 (DOI: 10.1159/000448559)

# Sexual Health, Risk and Prevention

Teri Aronowitz

Department of Nursing, University of Massachusetts Boston, Boston, Mass., USA

**Abstract**

Sexuality is an important aspect of health across the lifespan and includes sex, gender identities, sexual orientation, intimacy, pleasure, reproduction, and free from coercion and discrimination. In 2010, individuals 50 years and older living with HIV in the US made up 8.5 per 100,000 persons affected by the virus, with African Americans accounting for 46% of seroconversion in the same year, which was 10.7 times greater than Whites. African American women are particularly at-risk. Although there are many promising HIV prevention interventions to date, there are few that focus specifically on older adults. This chapter raises methodological concerns in research that focuses on sexual health of older adults living with HIV infection and special concerns regarding the older adult population's sexual health risk and suggested clinical interventions.



There are more than 40.3 million individuals 65 years and older in the US [1], accounting for over 13% of the population [2]. Sexuality is an important aspect of health across the lifespan and includes sex, gender identities, sexual orientation, intimacy, pleasure, reproduction, and free from coercion and discrimination [3]. There is very little written about sexuality and aging [4], and there are no federally funded programs for HIV prevention among older adults [5]. This chapter will present methodological concerns regarding the current research on sexual behaviors among older adults, discuss the increase in HIV seroconversion among older adults, and the population at most risk in the US, present some of the possible HIV prevention interventions strategies and review specific concerns regarding HIV risk in older adults.

### Methodological Concerns Regarding Sexual Research of Older Adults

In understanding the needs for sexual health in those that are aging, we need accurate data on which to build knowledge and prevention interventions. However, there are numerous methodological issues that are complicating the advancement of sexual health in those that are aging and those living with HIV infection. There are conflicting findings regarding sexual activity among older adults, a lack of consistent definitions, and the stigmatization of aging.

Research findings from a national probability sample of 3,005 US adults 57–85 years found that the majority of the participants reported being sexually active but had noted a decline in sexual activity with age [6]. Of those that were sexually active, 50% of both men and women complained of at least one sexual problem. Women experienced low desire and difficulty with vaginal lubrication and men expressed erectile difficulties. Less than a third of them reported these difficulties to their healthcare provider. Healthcare providers do not assess sexual health concerns among their patients, particularly older adults. In one study, general practitioners reported they felt sex was a private concern for an older person and did not want to risk causing offense by assessing sexual health [7].

In another study, older adults reported that they maintain their usual sexual activity throughout their life; however, this was dependent on one's overall health and the health of a partner [2]. In a study of older adults living in subsidized independent living facilities, most of the 166 participants experienced intimate physical contact such as kissing and hugging from daily to once a month. Most of these individuals did not partake in masturbation or sexual contact [8]. Questions about relationships need to be included in the studies, for the decline in sexual activity may be due to lack of a partner or the partner's health. Additionally, most research examining sexual function with aging are not longitudinal thereby not allowing for an understanding of prior levels of sexual function to assess the current function [9].

Another methodological concern is how sexual dysfunction is defined. Historically, sexual decline was thought to be a universal consequence of growing old. In fact, there is an overwhelming belief that older adults are not sexually active [10]. On the one hand there is the stereotype that older adults are asexual and on the other hand our culture is extending middle age into later life, with an obsession on self-improvement. There are images of older adults seeming eternally youthful and sexy, and also the unattractive or ill asexual individual who is shamed for any sexual expression [11].

So older adults must grow old without aging, and it is their responsibility to accomplish this through physical fitness and sexual function. The redefinition of aging in popular terms, such as 'boomers', ignores the realities of poverty and health disparities in old age [12]. Boomers are represented in the media as physically fit and attractive. They are not represented as impoverished, which represents ageist attitudes. At times, ageist attitudes are expressed as humorous with some degree of fact, increasing the negative effects on older adults. In addition, sexual expression in assisted living and long-term care facilities is viewed in many facilities as problematic and may be restricted by means that may include involuntary pharmaceutical measures [11], which are against the Declaration of Sexual Health statement [13], which states that sexual activity should be free of coercion and discrimination. The World Health Organization statement suggests the need to address sexual health needs across the lifespan.

An additional methodological concern in population-based studies on sexual health of older adults is that the researchers have not asked the participants about sexual orientation and there is an assumption that all older adults are heterosexual [6, 14]. Certainly researchers are studying specific populations such as lesbian women [15] and MSM [16, 17], but there is a lack of representation of older LGBT sexuality [4]. This lack of population-based data on LGBT elders emphasizes the heteronormative bias regarding older adults [18].

One population-based study includes information about sexual orientation. The inclusion criteria were individuals over 50 years of age and 5,045 (82% of population) individuals who participated in the survey. The majority of the population of both sexes engaged in solo masturbation and partnered sexual activities (including oral sex and intercourse). Overall condom usage rates were low (2/3 of the men and women stated they did not use a condom on last sexual encounter). The majority of the sample was identified as heterosexual (91.2% for men and 95.1% for women) [19]. These findings contradict some of the other studies in regard to sexual activity, and although the participants were asked about their sexual orientation there was no attempt to oversample the LGBT community. It is clear from the findings that there is a need to advance sexual health promotion and include condom use.

### Healthcare-Related Clinical Issues

As of the 1960s, gerontologist and sexologist were writing that sexual activity, particularly sexual intercourse, was a healthy and necessary part of aging. Urological research around the same time redefined male erectility as a physiological response and erectile dysfunction as a treatable problem [12]. More recently, Female Sexual Arousal Disorder is stated to be very prevalent and age-related [12], but there is no diagnostic criteria for this disorder. Sexual dysfunction is now seen as technical fixes and there are broad marketing campaigns for sexual function products. Meanwhile, research studies have not captured the new definitions of sexual dysfunction, excluding from sampling exclusion criteria older adults with sexual problems that are secondary to medication use or a medical condition [9]. Considering the number of older adults with comorbidities who are on medications, excluding them from studies that have as the primary purpose of the investigations the understanding of sexual health and behaviors of older adults seriously biases the sample.

Stigma related to HIV affects the general public's beliefs of the factual information about HIV transmission. In one study, people believed that sexual HIV transmission could occur in 2 male partners who are both HIV negative [20]. An example of discrimination was a published report by AARP, where the eviction of a former university provost from an assisted living facility occurred because of his HIV diagnosis [21]. There is a reluctance of healthcare providers to inquire about sexual health, particularly in older adults. This is accentuated when the older adult engages in the same sex sexual behavior. For example, many providers consider lesbian women at low risk because they have not comprehensively assessed the women's sexual history, for many lesbian women has had male partners [15]. The LGBT population over 65 is the first generation to be able to openly live as LGBT individuals. Nevertheless, they face health disparities secondary to the denial of their civil and human rights [22]. Using non-judgmental, open-ended questions regarding relationship status and sexual orientation is the first step in correcting these health disparities.

A systematic review discovered 4 themes that affect the diagnosis and treatment of sexually transmitted infections (STIs) and HIV in older adults [23]. These themes were: (1) health literacy, (2) social and demographic changes in aging, (3) hidden diagnoses of STIs, and (4) barriers to dialogue. Health literacy included lack of sexual health information targeted toward older adults and the biases of healthcare providers related to assumptions that older adults are asexual. Social and demographic changes included new relationships after the death of a long-term partner, divorce, increased longevity, and multiple partners. Hidden diagnoses of STIs were due to the lack of perceived vulnerability on the part of the adults and the misconceptions about older adult sexuality among healthcare providers. And finally barriers to dialogue included heterosexism among healthcare providers, providers' anxiety about discussing sexual health concerns, and inconsistent condom use among older adults.

In 2013, there were 446,253 new STI diagnoses among older adults, which is more than double the rates in this population 10 years previously [23]. With the prediction of over 50% of HIV-positive individuals to be over 50 in 2015 and the increase rates of STIs there is an overbearing need to implement interventions. These should be focused on increasing knowledge and positive attitudes about condom use in older adults. Additionally, interventions should be geared toward healthcare providers to train them on performing sexual health histories. One strategy would be to work with professional organizations to mandate curricular changes to include sexual health concerns in all areas of healthcare. Programs are presently not addressing sexual health concerns.

### HIV/AIDS in Older Adults in United States

Although gerontologists usually use 65 and above in referring to older adults, the literature on the aging HIV population uses age 50 and above to discuss the phenomenon because of the Center for Disease Control's (CDC) age stratification of HIV/AIDS [24]. In 2010, individuals 50 years and older living with HIV in the US made up 12–22% of all new infections and these rates are rising [25]. Despite these growing rates of seroconversion, the CDC presently mandates HIV testing only for individuals aged 64 and younger [26], and no nationally supported HIV primary prevention interventions are available for older adults [27]. The lack of attention to these health concerns may be secondary to the recent increase in STI and HIV rate increases in the older adult population.

HIV affects certain communities at a higher rate. African Americans accounted for 46% of seroconversions in 2010, which was 10.7 times greater than Whites [28]. AIDS is the fifth leading cause of death among African American women aged 45–54 years [29]. The mechanism of transmission among African American women of all ages is heterosexual activity [30]. By the age of 65 years or older, African Americans are 6 times more likely to have HIV as compared to the overall older adult population [25]. Hispanic individuals are also more likely to be represented among the older adults with new HIV diagnoses, and by the age of 60 years they are 2 times more likely to have HIV as compared with the overall older adult population [25].

Inconsistent condom use among all older adults is considered a major contributing factor to these HIV rates [31]. There is a low perceived susceptibility of STIs among older adults [32] and misconceptions about HIV and STIs are common [11]. Researchers have questioned the role that men who have sex with men and women may play on the rates of HIV among African American women [33, 34]. However, one study found that African American HIV-positive heterosexually identifying men who have sex with men are less likely to engage in sex with female partners than HIV-positive bisexually identified African American men [35].

Religiosity has played a significant role in HIV and homosexuality stigma within the African American community. Black Sexual Politics is a critical framework used to understand sexual communication between African American women and men. Black Sexual Politics is defined as 'a set of ideas and social practices that are shaped by gender, race, and sexuality that frame black men and women's treatment of one another, as well as how African Americans are perceived and treated by others' [36]. One focus group study found that even though African American women were placed at risk of exposure to HIV infection due to risk behaviors of some African American men, the shared experiences of racial discrimination among men and women contributed to the women's empathetic attitudes toward men [37]. The women were more understanding about men's extramarital relationships with men than with another women. Interventions that emphasize condom use rather than sexual orientation would provide a chance for these women to have open communication with male partners and increase safe sex practices.

## HIV Prevention Interventions

There are 3 levels of prevention: primary, secondary, and tertiary. Primary prevention focuses on preventing disease before it occurs. Secondary prevention aims at reducing the impact of the disease once it has been contracted. And tertiary prevention focuses on decreasing the impact of the disease. In HIV prevention, an example of primary prevention intervention would be those that focus on increasing condom use.

Considering the lack of knowledge regarding HIV and STIs, low perceived risk, inconsistent condom use, and increases in HIV prevalence, there is an urgent need for health education directed toward older adults. Despite the fact that risk reduction interventions that focus on specific at-risk populations and individuals living with HIV/AIDS have shown effective results in increased safe sex practices, none thus far have focused on older adults [38]. Brief educational sessions conducted by nurses in primary care settings and STI clinics have shown an increase in condom use among adults [39, 40]. Group sex education in public housing and community settings has also shown a decrease in risky sexual behaviors [41]. Although these studies are encouraging and important, the population they focused on were middle-aged individuals. One recent study showed promise as to the feasibility and acceptability of a community health promotion intervention with older adults [32].

In addition to primary health clinics and community settings for interventional venues, increasing religious social capital has been shown to be effective, especially for African American women [42]. Approximately 80% of African Americans state that religion is very important in their lives and African American women make up over 60% of the congregants in historically Black churches [43]. African American faith-based organizations have been committed to HIV prevention interventions [44]. Since African American women are currently disproportionately affected by HIV, developing a community participatory action project with the church leaders to increase religious social capital is a powerful means of reaching this population for health promotion. A randomized clinical trial in Atlanta, Georgia recruited younger women (aged 18–34 years) and successfully enhanced abstinence and safe sex practices, and religious social capital [42]. This same intervention should also be adapted for older women.

### Intervention for HIV-Positive Adults

Sexuality of older adults with HIV is highly stigmatized, and any health promotion intervention related to HIV has rarely focused on older adults [27]. This does not allow for meeting the basic human rights and social justice of older adults. The Declaration on Sexual Health [13] stated that HIV-positive adults have a right to enjoy their sexuality, therefore, interventions to advance sexual health promotion in this population is needed. Secondary HIV prevention interventions focus on decreasing transmission between seroconcordant partners. For example, a study that focused on reducing sexual risk behaviors among HIV-positive adults 45 years and older was based on the information-motivation-behavioral skills model for HIV risk behavior change [38]. It consisted of 3 two-hour sessions with a 12-month follow-up. Because studies have reported high rates of unprotected intercourse among people living with HIV [45], the main goal was to increase safe sex practices, specifically condom use. This group intervention showed an increase in condom use, and could possibly be adapted to older adults. Both older adults that are HIV negative and HIV positive need more health promotion education.

Another secondary HIV prevention study was conducted with low income Black women living with HIV infection in Boston, Massachusetts. The intervention was a peer-led, structured writing exercise using the film 'Women's Voices Women's Lives' as a prompt to small group writing. The film included prevention messages that included what experiences women have after testing positive for HIV, stigma, negotiating safe sex, and survivorship [46]. The study design was a randomized controlled feasibility trial to effect change in safe sex behavior (negotiating for safe sex) and condom use. The sample included 110 women (intervention, $n = 56$; comparison, $n = 54$). Retention was 85.5%. Repeated-measures analysis indicated that intervention group condom use ($n = 69$, $F = 8.02$, d.f. = 1, $p < 0.01$) and safe sex ($n = 71$, $F = 13.02$, d.f. = 1, $p < 0.01$) was higher than that of comparison group. This study demonstrates the feasibility of a tailored, peer-led, and culturally relevant intervention and tentative efficacy in populations affected by health disparities.

## Specific Concerns of HIV Risk among Older Adults

Because of the lack of open sexual communication between healthcare providers and older adults, we have seen an increase in individuals with STIs and HIV. Older adults desire active, satisfying sex lives [38]. As healthcare providers, we need to make sure that older adults are aware of the risk of STI and HIV and how to protect themselves, and at the same time know how to instruct them on how to adapt to the normal physiological changes of the reproductive organs with aging so they can enjoy their sexual experiences. Men experience a decrease in testosterone and estrogen levels at the same time that women experience menopause with decreases in androgens and estrogen. These hormonal changes can cause erectile dysfunction in men and urogenital atrophy in women [47].

Older adults are at greater risk of HIV transmission and the progression from HIV to AIDS. One study showed that among HIV-positive older adults, approximately half were diagnosed with HIV and AIDS at the same time or were diagnosed with AIDS within a year of their initial HIV diagnosis [48]. This might be due to the older adult not seeking testing because they did not believe they were at risk, or that the clinician underestimated the risk of HIV and mistook a nonspecific symptom such as fatigue as related to aging [48]. Additionally, due to decreases in estrogen levels and the friability of the vaginal mucosa postmenopausal women are at increased risk of HIV infection during heterosexual contact [49]. Furthermore, many older adults do not consider sex without a condom as risky sexual behavior because they are no longer concerned about contraception. Health promotion education is needed in regard to HIV and STI.

Depression has been reported as prevalent among HIV-positive adults [50]. HIV/AIDS-related stigma is believed to contribute to its occurrence [51]. Depression and stigma can then affect HIV treatment adherence and further decrease the person's reliance on social support because of rejection concerns [52]. In a study of HIV-positive individuals 50 years and older who lived in the community, investigators examined the role of depression, stigma, and loneliness on the quality of life [52]. Higher levels of HIV stigma and loneliness increased the risk of a major depression. It will be important to assess older adults for depression and provide social support to prevent or treat depression. Depression will affect the older adult's ability to develop intimate relationships. Depressed feelings could also make older adults feel that it is not worth protecting themselves and actually increase their risky behaviors.

## Summary

Despite prevailing societal stereotypes that older adults lack interest in sexual activity, many older adults continue to be sexually active with long-term or new partners. Older adults are at increasing risk of HIV, due to their lack of knowledge about condom use, and their lack of perceived risk of HIV. Several normal physical changes of aging make women at particular risk and interfere with enjoyment of sexual activity in both sexes. Regular sexual activity actually decreases the vaginal atrophy that occurs with aging, and individuals should be instructed that simulation helps increase lubrication. Preventing vaginal atrophy would help women to lubricate and prevent friability of the vagina. This in turn would decrease the HIV risk. Men can be instructed on the use of a penile ring to help maintain erections. There is a great need for the development and testing of interventions to address the lack of knowledge, to assess attitudes about condom use, and to increase behavioral skills needed to practice safe sexual activities. It would be best to apply Hillman's holistic model to guide intervention development and the assessment of sexual health in older adults, for sexuality is shaped by biological, psychological, social, cultural, environmental, and institutional factors [53].

## References


1 US Census Bureau: 65 + in the United States: 2010. Current Population Reports. 2014. http://www.census.gov/content/dam/Census/library/publications/2014/demo/p23-212.pdf (retrieved June 2014).

2 Roney L, Kazer MW: Geriatric sexual experiences: the seniors tell all. Appl Nurs Res 2015;28:254–256.

3 World Health Organization: Defining sexual health: report of a technical consultation on sexual health 28–31. January 2002. Geneva, WHO, 2006. http://www.who.int/reproductivehealth/topics/gender_rights/defining_sexual_health.

4 de Vries B: Introduction to special issue: sexuality and aging: a late-blooming relationship. Sex Res Soc Policy 2009;6:1–4.

5 Hillman J: A call for an integrated biopsychosocial model to address fundamental disconnects in an emergent field: an introduction to the special issue on 'sexuality and aging'. Ageing Int 2011;36:303–312.

6 Lindau ST, Schumm LP, Laumann EO, Levinson W, O'Muircheartaigh CA, Waite LJ: A study of sexuality and health among older adults in the United States. N Engl J Med 2007;357:762–774.

7 Gott M, Hinchliff S, Galena E: General practitioner attitudes to discussing sexual health issues with older people. Soc Sci Med 2004;58:2093–2103.
8 Ginsberg TB, Pomerantz SC, Kramer-Feeley V: Sexuality in older adults: behaviours and preferences. Age Ageing 2005;34:475–480.
9 Hayes R, Dennerstein L: The impact of aging on sexual function and sexual dysfunction in women: a review of population-based studies. J Sex Med 2005;2: 317–330.
10 Kazer MW: Sexuality in older adults changing misconceptions. J Gerontol Nurs 2013;39:2–3.
11 Hillman J: Knowledge, attitudes, and experience regarding HIV/AIDS among older adult inner-city latinos. Int J Aging Hum Dev 2008;66:243–257.
12 Katz S, Marshall B: New sex for old: lifestyle, consumerism, and the ethics of aging well. J Aging Stud 2003;17:3–16.
13 WHO Defining Sexual Health: Report of a Technical Consultation on Sexual Health 28–31. Geneva, World Health Organization, 2002.
14 Gott M, Hinchliff S: How important is sex in later life? The views of older people. Soc Sci Med 2003;56: 1617–1628.
15 Matebeni Z, Reddy V, Sandfort T, Southey-Swartz I: 'I thought we are safe': southren African lesbians' experiences of living with HIV. Cult Health Sex 2013; 15(suppl):34–47.
16 Owen G, Catalan J: 'We never expected this to happen': narratives of ageing with HIV among gay men living in London, UK. Cult Health Sex 2012;14:59–72.
17 Rojas Castro D, Coquelin V, Sempé S, Jablonski O, Le Gall JM, Andreo C, Spire B: Barebacking and sexual health in the French setting: 'noKondom zone' workshop. AIDS Care 2012;24:1046–1051.
18 Thompson EH: Expressions of manhood: reconciling sexualities, masculinities, and aging. Gerontologist 2004;44:714–719.
19 Schick V, Herbenick D, Reece M, Sanders SA, Dodge B, Middlestadt S, Fortenberry JD: Sexual behaviors, condom use, and sexual health of Americans over 50: implications for sexual health promotion for older adults. J Sex Med 2010;7(suppl 5):315–329.
20 Herek GM, Widaman KF, Capitanio JP: When sex equals AIDS: symbolic stigma and heterosexual adults' inaccurate beliefs about sexual transmission of AIDS. Soc Probl 2005;52:15–37.
21 Walker BS: AARP Bulletin. 2010. http://www.aarp.org/relationships/caregiving/info-12-2010living_with_HIV.html.
22 Zelle A, Arms T: Psychosocial effects of health disparities of lesbian, gay, bisexual, and transgender older adults. J Psychosoc Nurs Ment Health Serv 2015;53:25–30.
23 Nash P, Willis P, Tales A, Cryer T: Sexual health and sexual activity in later life. Rev Clin Gerontol 2015; 25:22–30.
24 Poindexter C, Emlet C: HIV-infected and HIV affected older adults; in Beckman B (ed): Handbook of Social Work in Health and Aging. New York, Oxford University Press, 2006, pp 91–99.
25 CDC Basic Information about AIDS. 2010. http://www.cdc.gov/hiv/topics/basic/index.htm#spread.
26 Branson BM, Handsfield HH, Lampe MA, Janssen RS, Taylor AW, Lyss SB, Clark JE: Revised recommendations for HIV testing of adults, adolescents, and pregnant women in health-care settings. MMWR Recomm Rep 2006;55:1–17; quiz CE1–CE4.
27 Orel NA, Wright JM, Wagner J: Scarcity of HIV/AIDS risk-reduction materials targeting the needs of older adults among state department of public health. Gerontologists 2004;44:693–696.
28 Centers for Disease Control and Prevention: Diagnoses of HIV infection among adults aged 50 years and older in the United States and dependent areas 2007–2010. HIV Surveill Suppl Rep 2013;18:6.
29 Heron M: Deaths: leading causes for 2007. Natl Vital Stat Rep 2011;59:1–95.
30 CDC HIV/AIDS Fact Sheet: HIV among African Americans. Atlanta, US Department of Health and Human Services, CDC, 2007.
31 Ward E, Disch W, Schensul J, Levy J: Understanding low-income, minority older adult self-perceptions of HIV risk. J Assoc Nurses AIDS Care 2011;22:26–37.
32 Gedin TC, Resnick B: Increasing risk awareness and facilitating safe sexual activity among older adults in senior housing. J Community Health Nurs 2014;31: 187–197.
33 Lauby JL, Millett GA, LaPollo AB, Bond L, Murrill CS, Marks G: Sexual risk behaviors of HIV-positive, HIV-negative, and serostatus-unknown black men who have sex with men and women. Arch Sex Behav 2008;37:708–719.
34 Prabhu R, Owen CL, Folger K, McFarland W: The bisexual bridge revisited: sexual risk behavior among men who have sex with men and women, San Francisco, 1998–2003. AIDS 2004;18:1604–1606.
35 Millett G, Malebranche D, Mason B, Spikes P: Focusing 'down low': bisexual black men, HIV risk and heterosexual transmission. J Nati Med Assoc 2005; 97(7 suppl):52S–59S.
36 Collins PH: Black Sexual Politics: African Americans, Gender and the New Racism. New York and London, Routledge, 2004, p 7.
37 Goparaju L, Warren-Jeanpiere L: African American women's perspectives on 'down low/DL' men: implications for HIV prevention. Cult Health Sex 2012;14: 879–893.

38 Illa L, Echenique M, Jean GS, Bustamante-Avellaneda V, Metsch L, Mendez-Mulet L, Eisdorfer C, Sanchez-Martinez M: Project roadmap: reeducing older adults in maintaining AIDS prevention: a secondary intervention for older HIV-positive adults. AIDS Educ Prev 2010;22:138–147.
39 Jemmott LS, Jemmott JB, Hutchinson MK, Cederbaum JA, O'Leary A: Sexually transmitted infection/HIV risk reduction interventions in clinical practice settings. J Obstet Gynecol Neonatal Nurs 2008;37:137–145.
40 Jemmott LS, Jemmott JB, O'Leary A: Effects on sexual risk behavior and STD rate of brief HIV/STD prevention interventions for African American women in primary care settings. Am J Public Health 2007;97:1034–1040.
41 Carey MP, Senn TE, Vanable PA, Coury-Doniger P, Urban MA: Brief and intensive behavioral interventions to promote sexual risk reduction among STD clinic patients: results from a randomized controlled trial. AIDS Behav 2010;14:504–517.
42 Wingood GM, Robinson LR, Braxton ND, Er DL, Conner AC, Renfro TL, Rubtsova AA, Hardin JW, DiClemente RJ: Comparative effectiveness of a faith-based HIV intervention for African American women: importance of enhancing religious social capital. Am J Public Health 2013;103:2226–2233.
43 Pew Forum on Religion and Public Like: US Religious Landscape Survey. 2008. http://religions.pewforum.org/pdf/report-religious-landscape-study-full.pdf.
44 Adedoyin C: A systematic review of the roles of congregations and faith-based organizations in the care and support of African Americans living with HIV/AIDS in the United States. Soc Work Christ 2013;40:184–205.
45 Kalichman SC, Rompa D, Cage M: Group Intervention to reduce HIV transmission risk behavior among persons living with HIV/AIDS. Behav Modif 2005;29:256–285.
46 DeMarco RF, Chan K: The sistah powah structured writing intervention: a feasibility study for aging, low-income, HIV-positive black women. Am J Health Promot 2013;28:108–118.
47 Horstman AM, Dillon EL, Urban RJ, Sheffiled-Moore M: The role of androgens and estrogens on healthy aging and longevity. J Gerontol A Biol Sci Med Sci 2012;67:1140–1152.
48 Linley L, et al: HIV/AIDS Diagnoses among Persons Fifty Years and Older in 33 States, 2001–2005. Atlanta, National HIV Prevention Conference, December 2007.
49 Shaw JK: HIV and the older adult: a hidden epidemic. HIV Medical Alert 2001;5:1–4.
50 Rabkin JG: HIV and depression: 2008 review and update. Curr HIV/AIDS Rep 2008;5:163–171.
51 Vanable PA, Carey MP, Blair DC, Littlewood RA: Impact of HIV-related stigma on health behaviors and psychological adjustment among HIV-positive men and women. AIDS Behav 2006;10:473–482.
52 Grov C, Golub SA, Parsons JT, Brennan M, Karpiak SE: Loneliness and HIV-related stigma explain depression among older HIV-positive adults. AIDS Care 2010;22:630–639.
53 Hillman J: Sexual issues and aging within the context of work with older adult patients. Prof Psychol Res Pr 2008;39:290–297.

Teri Aronowitz, PhD, APRN, FNP-BC
Department of Nursing
University of Massachusetts Boston
100 Morrissey Blvd., Boston, MA 02125 (USA)
E-Mail Teri.aronowitz@umb.edu

Brennan-Ing M, DeMarco RF (eds): HIV and Aging. Interdiscipl Top Gerontol Geriatr.
Basel, Karger, 2017, vol 42, pp 144–158 (DOI: 10.1159/000448560)

# Stigma in an Aging Context

Charles A. Emlet

University of Washington, Tacoma, Wash., USA

**Abstract**

Both the Joint United Nations Program on HIV/AIDS and the US National HIV/AIDS Strategy identify HIV stigma as a barrier to care, a barrier to service access, and deleterious to personal and social well-being. This chapter discusses the topic of HIV stigma from a conceptual basis, including the mechanisms of prejudice and discrimination, and defining anticipated, enacted, and internalized stigma. Stigma is then placed in a historical context of HIV and AIDS, and events exacerbating HIV stigma are discussed. The components of HIV stigma are then applied to the population of older adults (age 50 years and older) who are at-risk of or living with HIV infection. The importance of intersectionality is discussed with regard to race, ethnicity, gender, sexual orientation, gender identity, and in particular, age. Drawing upon the HIV and gerontological literature, the chapter outlines characteristics found to be protective against stigma and placing older adults at greater risk for HIV stigma. Stigma management strategies are outlined and finally, implications of working with older adults related to HIV stigma are provided.


## Introduction

The updated National HIV/AIDS Strategy for the US [1] identified HIV stigma as a major concern, and articulates the need to eliminate HIV stigma in its vision statement. The national strategy identifies the goal of reducing stigma and discrimination as part of lessening HIV-related health disparities to improve health outcomes for individuals living with HIV. The strategy clearly recognizes the interaction of HIV stigma and other forms of stigma and discrimination in what Reidpath and Chan [2] have called layering. This is the recognition that many individuals who face HIV stigma also experience, the compounding effects of stigma from substance use, homophobia, racism and/or other factors, including age. Recently, HIV research has begun to explore the phenomenon of intersectionality, acknowledging that multiple social categories intersect and reflect interlocking systems of oppression [3]. The intersectionality of stigma, therefore, is quite relevant to the intersection of one's experiences of HIV status, gender, race, sexuality orientation, and other components of identity [4]. While the topic of HIV stigma is prominent in the updated National HIV/AIDS Strategy, there are few references to older adults overall, and the document does not address, in any way, ageism as a compounding or complicating factor in living with HIV. By the very omission of this issue, the National Strategy marginalizes the impact HIV stigma has on older people living with or at risk for HIV. This chapter will provide a fundamental and conceptual understanding of stigma in general, across conditions, and focus specifically on HIV-related stigma as it impacts older adults with regard to prevention, care, treatment (including retention in care), and compounding psychosocial factors.

## Stigma as a Construct

The concept of stigma, or devaluing an individual or group due to particular characteristics they possess, is ancient in origin. The Greeks, according to Goffman [5], coined the term 'stigma' and tied it to exposing something bad about the moral character of an individual. McGough provides an historical account of how individuals who were identified as having sexually transmitted diseases in Europe during the 1700s were stigmatized and given inferior care, or no care at all; and how personal characteristics such as gender, for example, could positively or negatively influence care based on the power and status held by an individual [6].

While the concept of stigma has existed for centuries, the seminal modern work on the phenomenon is most often linked to Goffman, who suggested that the term stigma is used to describe an attribute of an individual that is 'deeply discrediting' [5, p 3]. As important as discrediting, Goffman highlights the significance of relationships in the stigmatizing process. The work of Link and Phelan [7] in the conceptualization of stigma helps to further elucidate the importance of various types of relationships in the stigma process. They identify 4 key components of stigma, including: (1) creating a distinction between an attribute and a label; (2) understanding human differences and the creation of negative attributes; (3) the creation of separation using an 'us and them' mentality; and (4) how these components create status loss and discrimination.

In the first component of stigma, Link and Phelan [7] draw an important distinction from Goffman's work by reframing the stigmatizing characteristic as a label as opposed to an attribute. Throughout the literature, stigma is commonly acknowledged to be a socially constructed phenomenon that may differ by time and place

[7]. It is associated with power and social inequity [8], whereby the individual or group enacts stigma through social prejudice to reduce their perception of personal risk [9]. Because of the subjectivity of social phenomena specific to human differences, Link and Phelan use the term label in place of Goffman's attribute. They suggest that a label is something that is affixed – in this case by society – and thus, the validity of that label can be left in question. The concept of an attribute or mark, they suggest, not only lacks validity, but it is also something that cannot be removed.

The second component of stigma is that labeled differences are tied to stereotypes, an idea which emanates directly from Goffman. Stereotyping is described as a cognitive process in which group-based beliefs link a person to a set of undesirable characteristics [7, 10]. In the case of HIV-related stigma, an individual may be tied to group-based beliefs about populations commonly associated with HIV, such as those who inject drugs or engage in same-sex activity. Because many people view sexuality through a heteronormative lens; they may view relationships outside of heterosexuality as different and thus stigmatizing.

The third component of stigma, according to Link and Phelan, is creating a difference between 'us and them' based on the social label. By projecting a negative value onto the other [11], there is a psychological payoff for the stigmatizing individual who, in essence, creates a sense of self-protection from the label. Link and Phelan [7] suggest that this linking of labels to undesirable attributes 'becomes a rationale for believing that negatively labeled persons are fundamentally different from those who do not share the label' [p 370].

The idea of creating an 'us and them' dichotomy sets the stage for the fourth component of stigma; status loss and discrimination. Labeling and stereotyping may lead to the cognitive creation of an 'us and them' mentality, which in turn may result in devaluation of the person or group (status loss), which then opens the door to discrimination. UNAIDS refers to HIV discrimination as 'the unfair and unjust treatment (act or omission) of an individual based on his or her real or perceived (HIV) status' [12, p 2]. Link and Phelan [7] conclude that the inclusion of this component of status loss and discrimination is necessary and that the term stigma 'cannot hold the meaning we commonly assign it when this aspect is left out' [p 370]. The act of discrimination is behavioral, and in some frameworks, it is referred to as enacted stigma or the extent to which an individual experiences prejudice and/or discrimination emanating from others [10, 13].

While Link and Phelan's conceptualization of stigma does not specifically identify the internalization of negative labels and status loss, it is important to consider. Deacon suggests that, even in the absence of direct discrimination, stigma can and often has a negative impact on the self-concept and actions of stigmatized people [9]. Earnshaw and Chaudoir [10] refer to internalized stigma as the degree to which a stigmatized person endorses the negative beliefs and feelings associated with their label. Through status loss and a power differential, individuals may change their behavior, withdraw socially, and thus place themselves at further disadvantage [9, 11]. Another form of internalized stigma manifests as internalized homophobia, or the negative self attributes toward oneself, often experienced by gay men [14]. Internalized homophobia has also been linked to depression and other complications of adjustment [15].

## Defining Stigma

While Goffman [5] defined stigma as 'an attribute that is deeply discrediting' [p 3], Link and Phelan [7] suggest a more specific definition, offering greater utility that embodies their 4 major components. Therefore, they define stigma as existing when 'elements of labeling, stereotyping, separation, status loss, and discrimination occur together in a power situation that allows them' [p 377]. An important element in this definition is that of power loss in the stigmatized group and accompanying loss of social status, thereby enabling discrimination to occur. Building on this understanding of stigma conceptually, we can turn to HIV-related stigma specifically and how that construct impacts older adults living with HIV infection.

### *HIV Stigma*

HIV stigma has been defined as prejudice, discounting, discrediting, and discrimination directed at people perceived to have HIV or AIDS [16], and has been conceptualized as encompassing enacted, anticipated, and internalized components. While enacted stigma has previously been defined, anticipated stigma signifies how much a person living with HIV expects to experience enacted stigma; while internalized stigma is the degree to which negative attributes and beliefs about people with HIV infection are endorsed and accepted [10].

### *HIV Stigma in Historical Context*

HIV stigma has existed since early in the epidemic. HIV stigma has been described as one of the largest barriers to coping with HIV/AIDS [17] and has been characterized as the third epidemic – the epidemic of social, economic, political, and cultural responses to AIDS [8].

In the early days of the epidemic, HIV was associated with sexual and drug-using behaviors provoking intense, value-laden reactions [18]. Such reactions were based on the assumptions that HIV could have been avoided if one had taken better care of oneself or was more careful [19]. Also, HIV/AIDS was seen as a 'gay disease', suggesting immoral behavior resulting in infection and illness [9]. Thus, segments of society engaged in blaming the victim. People living with HIV were stigmatized, as some believed individuals deserved their illness because of their behavior [20]. Even individuals seen as 'innocent', such as Ryan White, faced considerable stigma and discrimination after contracting HIV through a blood transfusion. After being diagnosed with AIDS, White was refused re-entry into his school of 360 students, with 117 parents and 50 teachers signing a petition encouraging school leaders to ban White from attending the school [21].

While there is evidence that HIV-related stigma has been reduced over the years, it persists [22]. Gorman [23] reminds us that cases of discrimination related to HIV status still find their way into the US court system regularly. She references a case in which a Pennsylvania man, in 2012, was denied a job as a nursing assistant after revealing his HIV status to his employer. Up until 2009, HIV-positive individuals were not allowed to enter the US. The lifting of the travel ban allowed the 2012 International AIDS Conference to be held in the US for the first time in over 20 years [23]. Discrimination associated with HIV continues to exist even when there is no clear evidence of risk. For example, the FDA's position on not accepting blood donations from men who have sex with men was finally relaxed in December of 2015, after being in existence for more than 30 years [24]. While this change in policy is welcomed, the amount of time it took to revisit the antiquated policy reflects a discriminatory stance based on a homophobic position. The criminalization of HIV is another example of HIV stigma manifesting in law and policy. The Positive Justice Project has documented that 34 states have criminal statutes based on perceived exposure to HIV [25]. Many of these statutes are out of date with current clinical knowledge about HIV, including the ability to maintain an undetectable viral load, which makes the possibility of HIV transmission very unlikely.

Unfortunately, the enduring impact of HIV-related stigma continues to have significant interpersonal and social consequences. It negatively impacts mental, psychological and emotional health, quality of life; can be a barrier to safe sex practices [18]; can lead to delayed diagnosis and treatment due to fear of a positive diagnosis [17] and poorer retention in care [26]. Thus, HIV stigma can negatively impact individuals ranging from those at risk for HIV all the way to negatively affecting retention in HIV care and treatment. While stigma has maintained its virulence since the advent of the HIV epidemic, we have learned considerably about its components and mechanisms.

*Understanding Types and Components of Stigma*

Stigma research has grown in complexity over the past decade, significantly adding to our understanding of this complex and multidimensional phenomenon. Stigma and its components have not been consistently defined or understood in research [9], and the literature is inconsistent in the labeling of various types of stigma [8–10, 17, 27, 28]. In this chapter, we will focus the discussion on the stigma framework of Earnshaw and Chaudoir [10], as this framework is comprehensive, distinguishes between mechanisms of stigma based on HIV status (persons living with HIV and those who are not), and includes the impacts of stigma as negative health outcomes.

Earnshaw and Chaudoir [10] stigma framework 'disentangles parallel, yet distinct, individual processes that occur for HIV-uninfected and HIV-infected people in

**Table 1.** Elements of the HIV stigma framework by Earnshaw and Chaudoir [10]

| | Mechanism | Psychological component |
|---|---|---|
| HIV uninfected person | Prejudice<br>Stereotyping<br>Discrimination | Negative emotion<br>Group-based belief of HIV<br>Behavioral expression |
| Person living with HIV | Enacted<br>Anticipated<br>Internalized | Experience of prejudice and discrimination<br>Expect they will experience prejudice and discrimination<br>Endorsement of negative beliefs of others |

Adapted from Earnshaw and Chaudoir [10].

response to the stigmatized nature of HIV' [p 1160]. The framework recognizes that different stigma mechanisms exist based on whether you are an infected or uninfected individual. These mechanisms are psychological responses to the knowledge that: (1) the devalued characteristic may threaten one's health and imply moral blemishes; or (2) that one is in possession of that characteristic and is subject to the negative treatment of others (table 1).

These components of stigma may impact older people differently depending on their gender, sexual orientation, social networks, and other characteristics. It is critical that we understand the multifaceted elements of stigma, including intersectionality and their differential impact on the lives of HIV-infected older persons so that social and individual interventions can be conceptualized, implemented, and evaluated [30].

## The Impact of HIV Stigma on Older Adults

### *Prevention and Testing*

Older people are very diverse and heterogeneous, and older adults living with or at-risk of HIV are no exception. Differences in gender, sexual orientation and/or gender identity, ethnicity and race, HIV cohort or HIV transmission route will all influence one's knowledge of HIV, and its impact on one's life [31, 32]. While the body of knowledge concerning HIV stigma in general is quite substantial [17, 33], our knowledge about how HIV impacts older persons specifically is less developed.

There is empirical evidence that HIV stigma negatively impacts HIV testing [34]. but there is less age-specific evidence related to stigma and HIV testing. A recent study by Ford et al. [35] found that HIV testing among older adults is low (<5%). Additionally, stereotyping of older adults, including ageist beliefs about HIV risk and sexuality, serve as barriers to knowledge of HIV information and testing rates. We can argue that the routine testing recommendations by the CDC reinforce this belief as the CDC recommends screening for HIV infection routinely for all patients aged 13–64 years [36], tacitly suggesting that adults over 64 are asexual and/or without substance use risk behavior. Thus, anticipated stigma and the lack of HIV knowledge and information, coupled with institutional ageism, can all serve to create barriers to older adults obtaining timely HIV testing. The urgency to change HIV stigmatizing and ageist beliefs is reinforced when we examine the proportion of older adults who receive a late diagnosis of HIV. The CDC tracks individuals found to have an AIDS-defining illness at the time of their HIV diagnosis; these cases point to long-term undiagnosed HIV infection, and thus, more advanced disease, poorer prognosis, and poorer clinical outcomes. The rates of late diagnosis rise continuously with age, from 41% for those in their early 50s; to 53% of those in their early 70s; to even higher rates for those in their late 70s and 80s [37]. Thus, age increases the likelihood of delayed HIV diagnosis, reinforcing the need for improved testing in this population and the removal of stigmatizing practices and attitudes among healthcare providers, the general public, and older adults themselves.

*Components of Stigma among Older Adults Living with HIV*

HIV-related stigma has been shown to create barriers to HIV prevention, testing and care [1], and has been well documented among older populations living with HIV [38–41]. The various components of stigma discussed previously (anticipated, enacted, and internalized) have been associated with negative health and psychosocial outcomes among older adults. Research has noted specific ways in which the components of stigma manifest among older adults and negatively impact their lives. For example, with regard to enacted stigma, Foster and Gaskins [40] report, in their study of older HIV-positive African Americans, that participants frequently heard disparaging remarks from others about people living with HIV, which in turn had negative impacts on their self-worth and self-image. Emlet [39] found that among older adults living with HIV/AIDS in the Pacific Northwest, one-third believed that people avoided them due to their HIV disease; and 50% believed people were uncomfortable being around them because of their HIV-positive serostatus. Haile et al. [41] interviewed 10 poor, older gay and bisexual African American men in New York. The men discussed how dehumanizing societal views and attitudes are towards HIV, including those in the healthcare system, robbed them of their personhood, relegating them to an HIV ghetto.

The judgments of others through enacted stigma may have serious impacts on the psychological health of older adults living with HIV. Internalized stigma negatively impacts self-esteem and psychological well-being. Psaros et al. [42] studied HIV-positive older women and found that the profound experiences of internalized stigma led these women to believe that no one would enter into an intimate relationship with them; describing themselves as 'dirty'. Similarly, Emlet's [39] study of stigma among older adults found that 48% felt ashamed of their illness at least some of the time.

Older adults also experience anticipated stigma. Wallach and Brotman [44] studied older adults living with HIV in Quebec, Canada. They found that older adults hid their HIV-seropositive status from their family members, including adult children, to reduce anticipated stigma, while Poindexter and Shippy [45] explored diagnosis disclosure among 34 older adults living with HIV in New York City. Approximately half hid their HIV diagnosis to 'protect themselves from rejection, harsh judgment or difficult practical ramifications from family, church members or employment' [p 371]. Unfortunately, by limiting disclosure due to anticipated stigma, one limits the potential for greater social support. More recently, Brennan et al. [47] examined the topic of HIV disclosure within religious congregations. They found that although 47% of subjects had not disclosed their status, disclosure of HIV status was not related to any change in participation within the congregation, and that relationships remained viable for both those who did and those who did not disclose their HIV status. The interplay between stigma, disclosure, and social support is quite complex and requires additional research.

The negative physical and mental health outcomes associated with stigma may be exacerbated by the phenomenon of multi-stigmatizing labels or 'layering' which occurs when one experiences stigma from HIV and other identities, such as age, sexual orientation, race, or ethnicity [2]. The phenomenon of intersectionality often refers to HIV and race, gender or social orientation but can also exist with age. For example, in a qualitative study of HIV-related stigma and ageism, Emlet [38] found that nearly 70% of older adults living with HIV had experiences of both HIV-related stigma and ageism and felt the negative impact of both experiences. Additionally, other stigmatized characteristics such as sexual orientation can further contribute to negative consequences through homophobia or transphobia. Recently, Emlet et al. [48] studied risk and protective factors associated with quality of life among 226 older gay and bisexual men living with HIV disease. They found that lifetime victimization (enacted stigma due to sexual orientation) was a significant risk factor for lowered physical and mental health quality of life in this sample.

HIV stigma among older adults, therefore, is not only a multidimensional issue within itself, but also needs to be viewed in the context of other compounding factors, including ageism, homophobia, transphobia or stigmatization due to other factors such as substance use histories, or racism. Layering, therefore, can compound the impacts of stigma on an older person living with HIV and complicate the development of interventions designed to address a stigmatizing condition when, in fact, multiple stigmas may co-exist.

*Stigma Management*

In the early days of AIDS epidemic, individuals often found it difficult to hide their diagnosis due to severe weight loss (wasting syndrome) or other physical marks such as Kaposi's sarcoma in what Goffman [5] would have called abominations of the body. Currently, in the majority of cases of HIV, particularly in the developed world, such physical symptoms are rarely obvious, and individuals living with HIV can decide to whom they want to disclose their diagnosis. Stigma management is a key issue for those experiencing anticipated or enacted stigma and plays an important role in their HIV care, and in their social and personal lives. In a meta-analysis of studies on HIV disclosure, Smith et al. [49] found a negative association between HIV stigma and disclosure, and between stigma and social support. In their final analysis, Smith et al. [49] suggested that, 'when people living with HIV felt that HIV carried a greater stigma, they reported less social support' [p 1272]. In their study of older African Americans living with HIV, Foster and Gaskins [40] found that these older adults commonly used non-disclosure as a means to manage stigma. This included not seeking care in the area in which they lived to avoid disclosure and potential stigma.

### Risk and Protective Factors for Stigma in HIV-Positive Older Adults

While our understanding of HIV-related stigma among older adults living with HIV is still developing, we are gaining important insights into the mechanisms of stigma in this population and learning more about protective and risk factors. We know from existing research that personal (demographic), psychological, and interpersonal (social) aspects of life can work to lessen or exacerbate HIV stigma in this population.

Recent research on HIV-related stigma among older adults has yielded some important information on factors that are associated with greater or lesser stigma. Often referred to in the health literature as risk and protective factors, these are aspects of an individual that make it more likely (risk) or less likely (protective) that an individual will experience a particular problem – in this case, HIV stigma. These factors may be sociodemographic, such as gender or sexual orientation; interpersonal, such as the amounts and types of social support available or community identity; psychological, such as feelings of mastery, self-efficacy and coping; or intrapersonal, including areas of spirituality. It is important to consider risk and protective factors not only for their identification of overall risk of negative outcomes, but also to closely examine protective factors that may be malleable and therefore amenable to improvement through intervention development.

*Risk Factors*

Various demographic, intrapersonal and psychological factors have been found to be associated with HIV-related stigma among older adults. As an example, Emlet et al. [46] found that women and heterosexual men had increased HIV stigma scores compared to gay and bisexual men in a sample of 378 older adults enrolled in the Ontario HIV Treatment Network Cohort Study, suggesting that one's personal characteristics can potentially influence stigma. Time since HIV diagnosis also influenced stigma in the same study with more newly diagnosed older adults experiencing increased stigma. From a psychological perspective, maladaptive coping and lower levels of mastery were also associated with increased stigma. Grov et al. [43] studied the impact of stigma on 914 older adults in New York City living with HIV and found that HIV stigma was significantly associated with depression and loneliness, suggesting the importance of interplay between interpersonal and psychological factors.

Interpersonal factors, including social support, have been found to have an important and significant influence on HIV stigma among older adults. The previously mentioned study by Emlet et al. [46] in Ontario, Canada, found that lower levels of emotional and informational social support were associated with increased stigma, while Grov et al. [43], in a multivariate analysis, found an association between loneliness, stigma, and depression, suggesting that social isolation is a risk factor for depression and stigma. Slater et al. [50], in their study of 60 gay men between the ages of 50 and 65 found both satisfaction and availability of support to be associated with increased quality of life, while social stigma from HIV, detracted from the quality of life.

*Protective Factors*

A variety of sociodemographic, interpersonal, and psychological factors have also been found to be protective against HIV stigma in this population, that is, associated with lower levels of stigma. In some instances, it is the presence of a characteristic as opposed to the absence of it (for example, social support), while in others researchers have found specific identifiable components that are associated with lower HIV stigma. In contrast to risks of female gender and heterosexual orientation as reported above, Emlet et al. [46], in 2 different studies, found men having sex with men, identified primarily as gay, to have lower stigma scores overall, compared to their female or heterosexual counterparts [51]. The second study, which included 960 individuals in the age group 22–86, also found older age to be a protective factor whereby those over 55 experienced lower levels of stigma than their younger counterparts [51].

Numerous psychological factors have also been found to be protective. Recently, Porter et al. [52] found greater psychological well-being (including mastery) and spirituality to be protective against HIV stigma in a study of 914 older adults from New York City [42]. These findings are consistent with Emlet et al. [46, 51] who found mastery to be protective against stigma. From an interpersonal perspective, social support consistently emerges as an important protective factor with both emotional and informational support associated with lower levels of stigma and increased mental health-related quality of life [29, 48, 50, 51]. In their examination of stigma and psychological well-being in older adults living with HIV, Porter et al. [52] found that interconnectedness (part of spirituality) which includes connections to significant others was an important factor in reduced levels of stigma in their structural equation model.

## Stigma Reduction and Interventions

While the updated National HIV/AIDS Strategy for the US refers to stigma throughout the document, there is no mention of this phenomenon in older adults and no specific aims that address how to reduce stigma. We have evidence that HIV-related stigma exists among older adults [38–40, 50, 52], and there has been a call for the development of more rigorous research that positively impacts the biopsychosocial aspects of aging with HIV [53]. Researchers have successfully implemented rigorous intervention studies focusing on older adults living with HIV, including randomized control trials that sought to improve coping mechanisms [54], decrease depressive symptoms [55], and reduce sexual risk behavior [56].

Although we need to be cautious about the delivery of interventions to older adults that were designed primarily for younger people (potentially limiting their efficacy) [53], we are gaining important information about factors that may lessen or exacerbate stigma in this population, and factors that can enhance quality of life and foster resilience. The number of studies examining resilience among older adults living with HIV is growing [52, 57–59] and the potential exists that attributes found to accompany resilience, such as mastery [57, 59], self-acceptance, and spirituality [52] can be incorporated into stigma interventions.

Development of interventions for HIV-related stigma among older adults, similar to those of any age, need to be multifaceted and include interventions at the community, structural, interpersonal, and intrapersonal levels [33]. Still, as Heckman and Halkitis [53] point out, interventions need to be specific to older adults and should take into account the layering of HIV-related stigma and ageism, and the uneven access to available services. For example, a report on aging with HIV from GMHC, formally known as The Gay Men's Health Crisis, calls on the US Department of Health and Human Services and the Administration on Aging to fund educational and marketing campaigns to challenge HIV stigma and stigma related to homosexuality [60]. We know from research and needs assessments that older adults are much more likely to use services from AIDS Service Organizations than from the aging network [60], and that many agencies on aging still feel unequipped to serve older adults living with HIV, further creating barriers for the delivery of services [61]. There is growing concern about HIV stigma emerging from the long-term care workforce as older adults living with HIV continue to age and need long-term care services such as assisted living and skilled nursing [60]. Thus, stigma-related interventions and provider education continue to be needed at macro levels of care delivery systems, including advocacy and policy change. A recent example of improving providers' knowledge about HIV and aging, and potentially decreasing HIV-related stigma, is the National Older Adults with HIV Initiative (NOAH) [62]. This initiative, which began in New York City, has expanded nationally to dispel myths concerning HIV, aging and sexuality and to increase the competence of service providers to serve older adults. NOAH is an example of a sound and sustained effort to work towards lowering HIV stigma and increasing knowledge in both HIV and aging network providers.

## Conclusion and Implications

Continued new HIV infections among older adults and dramatic increase in the numbers of individuals 'aging in' with HIV will result in an unprecedented need for researchers, clinicians, service providers, and policy makers to focus on this emerging population. While acceptance and improvement in societal views of HIV may have lessened the HIV stigma, it continues to negatively impact people living with HIV at all ages. Older adults will continue to face a layering of HIV stigma and to confront the intersectionality of ageism along with stereotyping about what age means for sexuality and sexual risk behavior.

The improved understanding of how age and HIV stigma intersect has important implications for researchers, policy makers, and providers of care. The body of literature on HIV stigma has grown significantly and there is a need for continued focus on older adults. Stigma researchers should deliberately include older adults in samples from a more general population and pay particular attention to how age impacts various elements of stigma. (Older) Age needs to be more than a sociodemographic variable that is scarcely examined. The significant attention to HIV stigma in the recent National HIV/AIDS strategy is critical to our understanding. Considering the demographic trends discussed in this volume and elsewhere; however, policy makers including those at federal, state, and local levels should consider the impact of this phenomenon on the growing population of older adults. Finally, this topic is highly relevant to clinicians and social service providers. Assessment of HIV stigma and its impact on an individual should be part of any comprehensive assessment of an older adult living with HIV to better identify personal risk and protective factors and help the individual develop and engage social and other support systems.

As we continue to learn more about the impact of aging and HIV in the coming years, it will be critical to carefully and rigorously examine the impact of stigma on intrapersonal well-being, social relations, and care and treatment, including retention in care. Additionally, the projected need for long-term care among older adults living with HIV and LGBT older adults will present the potential for a new and different but no less devastating form of stigma to take hold [53, 54]. HIV and aging service providers, researchers, and policy makers will need to continue working together to combat HIV stigma, as it has plagued the lives of people living with HIV, including older adults, since the beginning of the epidemic.

## Acknowledgements

The author wishes to thank Michele Costa, MSW for her extensive help and editorial work in preparing this chapter.

## References


1 White House Office of National AIDS Policy: National HIV/AIDS strategy for the United States: Updated to 2020. https://www.aids.gov/federal-resources/national-hiv-aids-strategy/nhas-update.pdf.

2 Reidpath DD, Chan KY: A method for the quantitative analysis of the layering of HIV-related stigma. AIDS Care 2005;17:425–432.

3 Ontario HIV Treatment Network: Intersectionality in HIV and other health-related research. Rapid Review #68. 2013. http://www.ohtn.on.ca/Pages/Knowledge-Exchange/Rapid-Responses/Documents/RR68-2013-Intersectionality.pdf.

4 Logie CH, James L, Tharao W, Loutfy MR: HIV, Gender, Race, Sexual Orientation, and Sex Work: A Qualitative Study of Intersectional Stigma Experienced by HIV-Positive Women in Ontario, Canada. PLoS Med 2011;8:e1001124.

5 Goffman E: Stigma: Notes on the Management of Spoiled Identity. New York, Simon and Schuster Inc., 1963.

6 McGough LJ: HIV/AIDS stigma: historical perspectives on sexually transmitted diseases. AMA J Ethics 2005;7:10.

7 Link BG, Phelan JC: Conceptualizing stigma. Annu Rev Soc 2001;27:363–385.

8 Parker R, Aggleton P: HIV and AIDS-related stigma and discrimination: a conceptual framework and implications for action. Soc Sci Med 2003;57:13–24.

9 Deacon H: Towards a sustainable theory of health-related stigma: lessons from the HIV/AIDS literature. J Community Appl Soc 2006;16:418–425.

10 Earnshaw VA, Chaudoir SR: From conceptualizing to measuring HIV stigma: a review of HIV stigma mechanism measures. AIDS Behavior 2009;13:1160–1177.

11 Duffy L: Suffering, shame, and silence: the stigma of HIV/AIDS. J Assoc Nurses AIDS Care 2005;16:13–20.

12 UNAIDS: Reduction of HIV-related stigma and discrimination, 2014. http://www.unaids.org/en/targetsandcommitments/eliminatingstigmaanddiscrimination.

13 USAID: Can we measure HIV/AIDS-related stigma and discrimination?: current knowledge about quantifying stigma in developing countries. 2006. http://www.icrw.org/publications/can-we-measure-hivaids-related-stigma-and-discrimination.

14 Frost DM, Meyer IH: Internalized homophobia and relationship quality among lesbians, gay men, and bisexuals. J Couns Psychol 2009;56:97–109.

15 McLaren S: The interrelations between internalized homophobia, depressive symptoms, and suicidal ideation among Australian gay men, lesbians, and bisexual women. J Homosex 2016;63:156–168.

16 Herek GM, Mitnick L, Burris S, et al: Workshop report: AIDS and stigma: a conceptual framework and research agenda. AIDS Public Policy J 1998;13:36–47.

17 Logie C, Gadalla TM: Meta-analysis of health and demographic correlates of stigma towards people living with HIV. AIDS Care 2009;21:742–753.

18 Valdiserri RO: HIV/AIDS stigma: An impediment to public health. Am J Public Health 2002;92:341–342.

19 Nelson G: The Origin of HIV/AIDS Stigma and How to End it. Huffpost Gay Voices. 2013. http://www.huffingtonpost.com/gary-nelson/hivaids-stigma_b_3982247.html.

20 Rana S, Parikh C: The game of fear, blame and shame: stigma of HIV, a major public health debacle. J Pediatr Neonatal Care 2014;1:00003.

21 American Library Association: Cruel shunning of AIDS victim Ryan White led to greater understanding of disease. 2012. http://dev.atyourlibrary.org/culture/cruel-shunning-aids-victim-ryan-white-led-greater-understanding-disease.

22 UNAIDS: How AIDS changed everything – MDG6: 15 years, 15 lessons of hope from the AIDS response. 2015. http://www.unaids.org/en/resources/documents/2015/MDG6_15years-15lessonsfromtheAIDSresponse.

23 Gorman S: 'What can we learn from disease stigma's long history?' PLOS Speaking Med. 2012. http://blogs.plos.org/speakingofmedicine/2012/11/27/what-can-we-learn-from-disease-stigmas-long-history/.

24 U.S. Food and Drug Administration: Revised recommendations for reducing the risk of human immunodeficiency virus transmission by blood and blood products – questions and answers. 2015. http://www.fda.gov/BiologicsBloodVaccines/BloodBloodProducts/QuestionsaboutBlood/ucm108186.htm

25 Positive Justice Project: Consensus statement on the criminalization of HIV in the United States. 2012. http://www.hivlawandpolicy.org/resources/positive-justice-project-consensus-statement-criminalization-hiv-united-states-positive.

26 Yehia BR, Stewart L, Momplaisir F, Mody A, Holtzman CW, Jacobs LM, Hines J, Mounzer K, Glanz K, Metlay JP, Shea JA: Barriers and facilitators to patient retention in HIV care. BMC Infect Dis 2015;15:246.

27 Emlet CA: Measuring stigma in older and younger adults with HIV/AIDS: an analysis of an HIV stigma scale and initial exploration of subscales. Res Social Work Prac 2005;15:291–300.

28 Berger BE, Ferrans CE, Lashley FR: Measuring stigma in people with HIV: psychometric assessment of the HIV stigma scale. Res Nurs Health 2001;24:518–529.

29 Rueda S, Gibson K, Rourke SB, Bekele T, Gardner S, Cairney J: Mastery moderates the negative effect of stigma on depressive symptoms in people living with HIV. AIDS Behav 2012;16:690–699.
30 Emlet CA: Understanding the impact of stigma on older adults with HIV. APA: Psychology and AIDS Exchange. 2014. http://apa.org/pi/aids/resources/exchange/2014/01/stigma-living.aspx.
31 Brennan DJ, Emlet, CA, Eady A: HIV, sexual health, and psychosocial issues among older adults living with HIV in North America. Ageing Int 2011;36: 313–333.
32 Rosenfeld D, Bartlam B, Smith RD: Out of the closet and into the trenches: gay male baby boomers, aging, and HIV/AIDS. Gerontologist 2012;52:255–264.
33 Mahajan AP, Sayles JN, Patel VA, Remien RH, Sawires SR, Ortiz DJ, Szekeres G, Coates TJ: Stigma in the HIV/AIDS epidemic: a review of the literature and recommendations for the way forward. AIDS 2008;22(suppl 2):S67–S79.
34 Smolak A, El-Bassel N: Multilevel stigma as a barrier to HIV testing in Central Asia: a context quantified. AIDS Behav 2013;17:2742–2755.
35 Ford CL, Mulatu MS, Godette DC, Gaines TL: Trends in HIV testing among U.S. older adults prior to and since release of CDC's routine HIV testing recommendations: national findings from the BRFSS. Public Health Rep 2015;130:514–525.
36 Center for Disease Control and Prevention (CDC): Revised recommendations for HIV testing of adults, adolescents, and pregnant women in health-care settings. MMWR Recomm Rep 2006;55(RR-14). http://www.cdc.gov/mmwr/preview/mmwrhtml/rr5514a1.htm.
37 CDC: Diagnoses of HIV infection among adults aged 50 years and older in the United States and dependent areas, 2007–2010. HIV Surveillance Supplemental Report 2013;18. http://www.cdc.gov/hiv/topics/surveillance/resources/reports/#supplemental.
38 Emlet CA: 'You're awfully old to have this disease': experiences of stigma and ageism in adults 50 years and older living with HIV/AIDS. Gerontologist 2006;46:781–790.
39 Emlet CA: Experiences of stigma in older adults living with HIV/AIDS: a mixed-methods analysis. AIDS Patient Care STDS 2007;21:740–752.
40 Foster PP, Gaskins SW: Older African Americans' management of HIV/AIDS stigma. AIDS Care 2009; 21:1306–1312.
41 Haile R, Padilla MB, Parker EA: 'Stuck in the quagmire of an HIV ghetto': the meaning of stigma in the lives of older black gay and bisexual men living with HIV in New York City. Cult Health Sex 2011;13: 429–442.
42 Psaros C, Barinas J, Robbins GK, Bedoya CA, Safren SA, Park ER: Intimacy and sexual decision making: exploring the perspective of HIV positive women over 50. AIDS Patient Care STDS 2012;26:755–760.
43 Grov C, Golub SA, Parsons JT, Brennan M, Karpiak SE: Loneliness and HIV-related stigma explain depression among older HIV-positive adults. AIDS Care 2010;22:630–639.
44 Wallach I, Brotman S: Ageing with HIV/AIDS: a scoping study among people aged 50 and over living in Quebec. Ageing Soc 2013;33:1212–1242.
45 Poindexter CC, Shippy RA: HIV diagnosis disclosure: stigma management and stigma resistance. J Gerontol Soc Work 2010;53:366–381.
46 Emlet CA, Brennan DJ, Brennenstuhl S, Rueda S, Hart TA, Rourke SB; OHTN Cohort Study Team: Protective and risk factors associated with stigma in a population of older adults living with HIV in Ontario, Canada. AIDS Care 2013;25:1330–1339.
47 Brennan M, Strauss SM, Karpiak SE: Religious congregations and the growing needs of older adults with HIV. J Relig Spiritual Aging 2010;22:307–328.
48 Emlet CA, Fredriksen-Goldsen KI, Kim HJ: Risk and protective factors associated with health-related quality of life among older gay and bisexual men living with HIV disease. Gerontologist 2013;53:963–972.
49 Smith R, Rossetto K, Peterson BL: A meta-analysis of disclosure of one's HIV-positive status, stigma and social support. AIDS Care 2008;20:1266–1275.
50 Slater LZ, Moneyham L, Vance DE, Raper JL, Mugavero MJ, Childs G: Support, stigma, health, coping, and quality of life in older gay men with HIV. J Assoc Nurses AIDS Care 2013;24:38–49.
51 Emlet CA, Brennan DJ, Brennenstuhl S, Rueda S, Hart TA, Rourke SB: The impact of HIV-related stigma on older and younger adults living with HIV disease: does age matter? AIDS Care 2015;27:520–528.
52 Porter KE, Brennan-Ing M, Burr JA, Dugan E, Karpiak SE: Stigma and psychological well-being among older adults with HIV: the impact of spirituality and integrative health approaches. Gerontologist 2015;pii:gnv128.
53 Heckman TG, Halkitis PN: Biopsychosocial aspects of HIV and aging. Behav Med 2014;40:81–84.
54 Heckman TG, Barcikowski R, Ogles B, Suhr J, Carlson B, Holroyd K, Garske J: A telephone-delivered coping improvement group intervention for middle-aged and older adults living with HIV/AIDS. Ann Behav Med 2006;32:27–38.
55 Heckman TG, Sikkema KJ, Hansen N, Kochman A, Heh V, Neufeld S: A randomized clinical trial of a coping improvement group intervention for HIV-infected older adults. J Behav Med 2011;34:102–111.
56 Lovejoy TI, Heckman TG: Depression moderates treatment efficacy of an HIV secondary-prevention intervention for HIV-positive late middle-age and older adults. Behav Med 2014;40:124–133.

57 Fang X, Vincent W, Calabrese SK, Heckman TG, Sikkema KJ, Humphries DL, Hansen NB: Resilience, stress, and life quality in older adults living with HIV/AIDS. Aging Ment Health 2015;19:1015–1021.
58 Emlet CA, Tozay S, Raveis VH: 'I'm not going to die from the AIDS': resilience in aging with HIV disease. Gerontologist 2011;51:101–111.
59 Emlet CA, Furlotte C, Brennan DJ, Pierpaoli C: Understanding the lived experiences of older adults living with HIV in Ontario: an examination of strengths and resilience in a vulnerable population. Poster presented at the 23rd Annual Canadian Conference on HIV/AIDS Research, St. Johns Newfoundland, Canada, May 1–4, 2014.
60 Brennan-Ing M, Seidel L, London AS, Cahill S, Karpiak SE: Service utilization among older adults with HIV: the joint association of sexual identity and gender. J Homosex 2014;61:166–196.
61 Emlet CA, Gerkin A, Orel N: The graying of HIV/AIDS: preparedness and needs of the aging network in a changing epidemic. J Gerontol Soc Work 2009; 52:803–814.
62 Seidel L, Karpiak SE, Brennan-Ing M: Training senior service providers about HIV and aging: evaluation of a multi-year, multi-city initiative. Gerontol Geriatr Educ 2015, Epub ahead of print.
63 National Women's Law Center: Health care refusals harm patients: the threat to LGBT people and individuals living with HIV/AIDS. 2014. http://www.nwlc.org/resource/health-care-refusals-harm-patients-threat-lgbt-people-and-individuals-living-hivaids.
64 National Senior Citizens Law Center: LGBT older adults in long-term care facilities. 2011. http://www.lgbtagingcenter.org/resources/pdfs/NSCLC_LGBT_report.pdf.

Charles A. Emlet, PhD, ACSW
University of Washington, Tacoma
1900 Commerce Street, Campus Box 358425
Tacoma, WA 98402-5825 (USA)
E-Mail caemlet@u.washington.edu

Brennan-Ing M, DeMarco RF (eds): HIV and Aging. Interdiscipl Top Gerontol Geriatr.
Basel, Karger, 2017, vol 42, pp 159–172 (DOI: 10.1159/000448561)

# Social Support Systems and Social Network Characteristics of Older Adults with HIV

Mark Brennan-Ing[a, b] • Liz Seidel[a, c] • Stephen E. Karpiak[a, b]

[a]ACRIA, ACRIA Center on HIV and Aging, [b]New York University College of Nursing and [c]Fordham University Graduate School of Social Service, New York, N.Y., USA

**Abstract**

Social networks of older adults with HIV have been characterized as fragile, with a greater reliance on friends as compared to family. However, we know little about the subgroup differences in the social network constellations of this population, how such characteristics are related to social support resources, and their relationship with psychosocial well-being. We developed a typology of social networks of older HIV-positive adults and examined if they would be related to receipt of informal assistance, perceptions of support sufficiency, and psychosocial well-being. Data were obtained from Research on Older Adults with HIV (n = 914). Participants were 50 years and older, HIV positive, and diverse in terms of race/ethnicity, gender, and sexual orientation. Cluster analysis identified *Isolated, Friend-centered*, and *Integrated* social network types. The *Isolated* reported significantly lower levels of assistance, lower perceptions of support availability and adequacy, greater stigma and psychological distress, and lower well-being compared to their peers. While friends dominate many social networks in this population, a more nuanced interpretation is needed; many have no friends and a substantial proportion receive significant family support. Those with *Isolated* network types will likely need to access a high volume of community-based services as they age as they lack informal support resources.


The introduction of highly active anti-retroviral therapy has had a profound impact on the course of HIV disease, transforming it into a manageable chronic disorder with greatly improved life expectancies [1]. It has been estimated that at the time of this writing in 2015, 50% of those living with HIV in the US were 50 years or older, a proportion that may rise to 71% by 2020 [2–4]. But the long-term consequences of living with this illness are sobering. Adults aging with HIV are encountering the challenges of the onset of illnesses typically associated with those who are decades older [5, 6]. Research finds that older HIV-positive adults report 3 comorbid conditions on average in addition to HIV [6], suggesting high levels of multimorbidity and a considerable burden of disease in this group. Depression is one of the most common comorbidities in this population, and is linked to specific diseases and overall multimorbidity. High rates of depression are of concern, given their relationship to poor adherence to HIV treatment, resulting in poorer clinical outcomes and potential viral mutation and the development of treatment-resistant strains of HIV [6]. Major covariates of depression in this population include perceptions of social isolation (i.e., loneliness) and lack of support [7]. Multimorbidity along with mental health concerns suggest that older adults with HIV will need increasing levels of assistance from their informal social networks. This chapter examines the social network characteristics of older adults with HIV, how these characteristics are related to social support resources they will need as they age, and psychosocial factors related to the quality of life and well-being.

## Social Supports in Later Life

Older adults are increasingly susceptible to shrinking social networks as they experience the loss of partners and friends, deteriorating health, and other life transitions intrinsic to aging [8]. Social support systems are a critical resource in later life as these networks are the source of caregivers who provide both instrumental and emotional support in managing illness and other challenges of old age [9]. Limited social support resources may be exacerbated in the presence of a chronic or serious illness, such as HIV. When people need support, they first turn to close family (spouses and children), then to other relatives, friends and neighbors and when those are not available turn to formal community-based support systems [10]. Additionally, those with chronic illness may perceive themselves as different from their healthy peers, leading to social withdrawal [11]. Being disconnected socially is associated with poorer self-rated health among older adults [12]. Family and friends may also withdraw to avoid the harsh realities of a sick loved-one [13]. These reactions may become intensified when confronting a highly stigmatized illness such as HIV.

## Social Supports and Aging with HIV

Stigma itself is a major catalyst of decreased social resources among people with HIV, by promoting ostracism, rejection, and self-protective withdrawal on the part of the stigmatized individual [14, 15]. Social isolation attributed to HIV stigma is greater among certain subgroups, such as African Americans and heterosexual women [15]. Factors that are related to, but independent of, HIV infection such as, incarceration, homosexuality, and intravenous drug use are other operative sources of stigma [16, 17] and may exacerbate social isolation for those with HIV infection. Although HIV disproportionally affects gay and bisexual men, research finds HIV-positive gay and bisexual men feeling stigmatized by their HIV-negative peers, which may further inhibit HIV disclosure [8, 18]. If people are reluctant to disclose their HIV serostatus, and hence their need for support, the supports may not be forthcoming [19].

*Social Supports and Related Psychosocial Factors*

Social support resources are related to mental health and psychological well-being. In studies of chronic illness in middle-aged and older adults, perceptions of support adequacy and availability were related to greater levels of psychosocial well-being and better adaptation to illness [20]. Among older adults with HIV, Chesney et al. [5] found that when social supports were available for older men with HIV, levels of psychological distress were lower and well-being was enhanced. Others found that among older gay and bisexual men with HIV, perceptions of support were related to better health-related quality of life [21].

*Social Network Types and Social Resources*

Older adults with HIV often have been described as having truncated and dysfunctional social networks, lacking adequate social support resources [22–24]. Friends are frequently the primary source of support, yet research shows that many of their friends are also HIV positive. Those friends may need their own supports as they age and may not be in a position to offer instrumental and emotional support to others [23, 24]. Thus, it is not surprising that social isolation is more prevalent among older adults with HIV compared to their younger counterparts. Emlet [25] reported that 39% of adults over 50 with HIV were socially isolated as compared with 25% of younger adults. Their social isolation is reinforced by the loss of partners, family and friends to HIV/AIDS. Regardless of etiology, social isolation among older adults with HIV most likely contributes to their low levels of perceived social support [24, 26]. Past research has failed to find a significant relationship between social network size and the perceptions of availability and adequacy of social support [24]. However, the qualitative aspects of social networks of older people with HIV with regard to the constellation of available resources (i.e., a description of social network types) remain unexplored.

*How Can We Characterize the Social Networks of Older Adults with HIV?*

Given our current state of knowledge of the social networks of HIV-positive older adults, we were interested in examining potential constellations of support networks in this population and to see if a typology of social networks could be developed that was related to both tangible and perceived social support resources. We were also interested whether such a typology would relate to perceived stigma and psychosocial factors such as loneliness, depression, and psychological well-being. We hypothesized that those having social networks offering greater resources would report lower stigma, loneliness, and depression, and higher levels of psychological well-being compared to their peers.

## The Social Network Typology of Older Adults with HIV

To address our questions on social networks in this population, we used data from the study 'Research on Older Adults with HIV (ROAH)'. Details of participant recruitment, inclusion criteria, and procedures have been reported elsewhere [27]. The study protocol was approved by the Copernicus Group Institutional Review Board, and written informed consent was obtained from study participants. The sample consisted of 640 men, 264 women, and 10 transgender persons. The average age was 55.5 years (range 50–78 years). Half were non-Hispanic Black, a third Hispanic, and 14% non-Hispanic White. Two-thirds self-identified as heterosexual, 9% as bisexual, and 24% as homosexual. Seventy percent lived alone. The education level was similar to the general population of New York City; 30% had high school degrees, 27% had attended college, and 22% reported college degrees and/or post-graduate education [3]. Over three-quarters reported inadequate incomes, and 46% had a history of incarceration. They had been living with HIV for 12.6 years on average (range 3 months to 26 years), 51% had received an AIDS diagnosis and 13% reported CD4 counts below 200. Most experienced at least one (91.4%) comorbid illness, and the average number of comorbidities was 3.3 [6].

### *Measures and Data Analysis*

Standardized measures were employed in the ROAH study. Single items were used to assess participants' age, gender, sexual identity, race/ethnicity, education, employment status, income adequacy, living arrangement, and history of incarceration. Single items assessed time since HIV diagnosis, prior AIDS diagnosis, CD4 count, history and number of comorbid conditions obtained from a checklist of 23 physical and mental health problems experienced in the previous year.

Detailed information regarding the network size, composition, and frequency of contact was assessed with measures used in previous large-scale studies of social networks among older adults [9, 28]. The presence, number, and contact frequency with 5 network support elements (i.e., parents, children, siblings, other relatives, and friends) were included. The frequency of both in-person and telephone contact for each network element was measured using a 5-level, Likert-type scale (daily, weekly, monthly, several times a year, once a year or less). When assessing social networks, it is important to distinguish between the presence of individuals in the social network versus those who could be reasonably expected to provide assistance when needed, namely, functional supports. In 2 large-scale studies of older adults and other work on social networks of older adults with HIV [9, 23, 24, 28], a functional support element was defined as someone who was in contact with sufficient regularity that expectations of support were warranted (i.e., seen face-to-face at least monthly or talked to at least weekly by phone). This definition was employed in the current study.

Participants were asked to indicate the types of help they had received during the previous month from family and friends, respectively, using items from previous social network studies of older adults [9, 28]. Items included 5 types of instrumental help (i.e., shop/run errands, keep house/prepare meals, take or drive places, mail/correspondence, manage money/pay bills) and 3 types of emotional support (give advice on a big decision, talk when feeling down/low, talk about personal/family problem). Responses were on a 6-point scale (i.e., from every day to never), which were dichotomized for analysis (i.e., yes (at least monthly) or no). Two indices were created for the number of ways family or friends helped, respectively (range 0–8). Four items assessed the availability and adequacy of informal network support [9, 28]. Two identical items provided separate ratings of instrumental and emotional support availability, 'do you have someone you can count on to help you with (type of support)?' on a 4-point scale (i.e., not at all, only occasionally, some of the time, or most of the time). Adequacy of support assessed independent ratings for emotional and instrumental support needs; 'in the past year, how much more help or assistance with (type of support) did you need?' (i.e., needed a lot more, needed some more, or needed a little more help, or got all the help needed).

Loneliness was assessed with the UCLA Loneliness Scale version 3 [29], a 20-item measure with high internal consistency (coefficient $\alpha = 0.89–0.94$) and acceptable test–retest reliability after 1 year ($r = 0.73$). There are 11 negatively worded items and 9 positively worded items. Participants responded to items with a 4-level scale (never, rarely, sometimes, always). The 9 positively worded items are reverse coded, and scores from all 20 items are summed. Scores range from 20 to 80, and higher scores indicate greater degrees of loneliness. Cronbach's alpha for this measure in the ROAH sample was 0.90 indicating a high degree of internal consistency. Depressive symptomatology was measured by the Center for Epidemiologic Studies Depression Scale [30], a 20-item self-report scale. Responses are summed to obtain a total symptom score with a range of 0–60; higher scores indicate greater depressive symptomatology. In the ROAH sample, the Cronbach's alpha for the CES-D was 0.87. Ryff [31] theoretically-derived scales assessed psychological well-being. Each of the six 9-item scales (e.g., autonomy, environmental mastery, personal growth, positive relations with others, purpose in life, and self-acceptance) utilize a 6-point scale ranging from 'strongly agree' to 'strongly disagree' to assess well-being, with scores ranging from 9 to 54. Higher scores indicate greater well-being in each dimension. Only 2 scales were significantly related to the social network typology described below and were retained for analysis; personal growth ($\alpha = 0.70$) and autonomy ($\alpha = 0.65$).

The HIV Stigma Scale (Berger, Ferrans and Lashley, 2001), a 40-item instrument, was used to assess perceived stigma [32]. Analyses from previous studies of diverse samples of people living with HIV identified 4 factors in this measure (e.g., personalized stigma, disclosure concerns, negative self-image, and concern with public attitudes toward people with HIV). Personalized stigma relates to the personal consequences of others knowing that one has HIV, such as the loss of friends. Disclosure concerns relate to the control of information around one's HIV status, such as keeping one's serostatus a secret. Negative self-image is defined as negative self-perception due to one's HIV status, such as feeling 'dirty' or not as good as other people. Concern with public attitudes assesses the dimension of stigma regarding other people's attitudes towards someone with HIV, such as assuming flaws in the person's character. Higher scores indicate greater perceived stigma. Inter-item reliability of the subscales were high in the ROAH sample (i.e., personalized stigma $\alpha = 0.95$, disclosure concerns $\alpha = 0.83$, negative self-image $\alpha = 0.89$, concern with public attitudes $\alpha = 0.94$).

To develop a social network typology, we used 2-stage cluster analysis (SPSS version 16.0), using variables that conceptually affect social network composition and interaction. These included social network factors (i.e., living arrangements, degree of face-to-face and telephone contact with social network members, religious participation, whether religious participation was affected by HIV diagnosis), sociodemographic characteristics (e.g., employment, language, history of incarceration), and health-related factors (e.g., length of time since HIV diagnosis). Based on the initial clustering analysis, a number of covariates were dropped from the analysis (i.e., employment, language, history of incarceration, religious participation affected by HIV diagnosis, length of time since HIV diagnosis) because they did not significantly vary between individuals. The final cluster analysis identified 3 groups that were significantly different based on chi-square tests with a Bonferroni adjustment for multiple comparisons. To test if this typology would be related to the receipt of social support from family and friends, and perceptions of support availability and adequacy, we used chi-square tests for categorical variables and one-way analysis of variance (ANOVA) for continuous variables. Multivariate ANOVAs (MANOVAs) were used to test the 4 psychosocial variables (loneliness, depression, personal growth, and autonomy) and the 4 HIV stigma subscales for significant relationships to the social network typology. LSD post-hoc tests were used to examine pair-wise group differences in the ANOVAs and MANOVAs.

## The Typology of Social Networks of Older Adults with HIV

Table 1 presents social support and engagement variable differences between the 3 social network types. We present data on functional social network members as these variables indicate both the presence of the social network member as a frequent contact and being available to provide support. In the first group termed *'Isolated'* (31%), about one-third had at least one functional child, but had little contact with other family members, there was an absence of functional friends, and they reported low levels of participation in their religious congregations. The next group, *'Friend-centered'* (35%) was well-endowed with functional friends, but did not have functional children. The level of contact with other family members was low and similar to the *Isolated* group, as was the relatively low degree of religious participation (40% and 41%,

**Table 1.** Social support and engagement factors by social network type

| | Isolated, % | *Friend-centered*, % | Integrated, % |
|---|---|---|---|
| Functional parent*** | 22.1 | 23.0 | 36.6 |
| Functional child*** | 34.7 | 0.0 | 79.4 |
| Functional sibling*** | 36.8 | 33.9 | 60.8 |
| Functional other relative*** | 20.0 | 20.1 | 53.6 |
| Functional friend*** | 0.4 | 96.8 | 94.8 |
| Regularly attend religious services*** | 40.9 | 40.0 | 58.2 |
| Living arrangements*** | | | |
| Alone | 70.9 | 82.4 | 60.1 |
| Spouse/partner | 14.4 | 8.9 | 19.0 |
| Child | 3.5 | 0.0 | 7.2 |
| Other person | 11.2 | 8.6 | 13.7 |

Total (n = 914); Isolated (n = 285); *Friend-centered* (n = 313); Integrated (n = 306). Valid percentages.
* $p < 0.05$, ** $p < 0.01$, *** $p < 0.001$.

respectively). Group 3, labeled '*Integrated*' (34%), had the broadest spectrum of functional relationships, including children, family, friends, and the highest levels of religious participation. Demographic differences between groups were in line with the typologies identified. Two-thirds of the *Friend-Centered* group reported a gay or bisexual orientation, typically associated with friend-dominated social networks, as compared to 19% in the *Isolated* and 13% in the *Integrated* groups. The *Integrated* group reported the highest proportion of women (45%) who are most likely to have children, as compared with 26% of the *Isolated* and 15% of the *Friend-Centered* groups. These latter groups were also the most likely to report living alone (82% and 71%, respectively), as compared with 60% of those with *Integrated* networks. Those with *Integrated* networks were the most likely to live with a spouse/partner (19%) compared to their peers (14% of the *Isolated* and 9% of the *Friend-Centered* groups). Living with a child in the household was infrequent, even for those in the *Integrated* group (7%).

*Informal Assistance and Social Network Types*

The differences in social network composition between the 3 social network types were apparent in the examination of help received from these 2 sources of social support (table 2). Overall, those with *Friend-Centered* networks were the least likely to receive both instrumental and emotional support from family members, which can be attributed to the absence of functional children who tend to provide the greatest amount of familial support, and low proportions reporting functional siblings and other relatives. The *Isolated* group received lower levels of family assistance compared with the *Integrated* group, especially with regard to emotional support, which was similar to the *Friend-Centered* group. The *Integrated* group was the most likely to receive instrumental help from family members (e.g., 52% had help with shopping or running

**Table 2.** Receipt of assistance from family and friends by social network type

| | Isolated, % | *Friend-Centered*, % | Integrated, % |
|---|---|---|---|
| Help from family, % | | | |
| Shop or run errands*** | 31.9 | 20.8 | 51.6 |
| Keep house/prepare meals*** | 27.0 | 17.3 | 44.1 |
| Take or drive you places*** | 21.8 | 15.7 | 44.1 |
| Mail or correspondence*** | 24.2 | 16.6 | 32.0 |
| Manage money or pay bills*** | 22.8 | 13.7 | 28.8 |
| Give advice*** | 35.4 | 38.0 | 57.5 |
| Talk when feeling down/low*** | 48.4 | 51.1 | 71.9 |
| Talk about personal/family problem*** | 42.1 | 48.2 | 71.6 |
| Help from friends, % | | | |
| Shop or run errands*** | 17.9 | 30.4 | 48.7 |
| Keep house/prepare meals*** | 11.6 | 23.0 | 25.8 |
| Take or drive you places*** | 11.9 | 23.0 | 46.4 |
| Mail or correspondence** | 10.2 | 16.9 | 19.9 |
| Manage money or pay bills* | 10.2 | 15.3 | 17.0 |
| Give advice*** | 16.5 | 61.7 | 59.5 |
| Talk when feeling down/low*** | 26.3 | 73.8 | 75.8 |
| Talk about personal/family problem*** | 17.9 | 76.0 | 74.2 |
| Number of ways family helps**, mean ± SD | 2.5±2.7 | 2.2±2.4 | 4.0±2.6 |
| Number of ways friends help***, mean ± SD | 1.2±2.2 | 3.2±2.2 | 3.7±2.4 |

Total (n = 914); Isolated (n = 285); *Friend-Centered* (n = 313); Integrated (n = 306). MANOVA: $F(2, 1802) = 65.2$, $p < 0.001$. Post-hoc tests: help from family (Integrated significantly different from *Friend-Centered* and Isolated groups); help from friends (all 3 groups significantly different). * $p < 0.05$, ** $p < 0.01$, *** $p < 0.001$.

errands) and were also the most likely to receive family emotional support, particularly when feeling down or low, or needing to discuss a personal problem (72%), as compared to about one-half of those with *Isolated* or *Friend-Centered* networks.

With regard to friend assistance, the *Friend-Centered* group was more likely to report both instrumental help and emotional support from friends as opposed to family members (table 2). As might be expected, given the low prominence of friends in their networks, those with *Isolated* network types reported assistance from friends infrequently. Older adults with HIV having *Integrated* networks were the most likely to report instrumental help and emotional support from friends, and seemed to at an advantage compared to both *Isolated* and *Friend-Centered* network types. This was further illustrated in the indices of family and friend support. Those with *Integrated* networks reported significantly more types of assistance from family (M = 4.0), compared to either the *Isolated* or *Friend-Centered* groups (M = 2.5 and 2.2, respectively). With regard to help from friends, all 3 groups were significantly different, with the *Integrated* group reporting more types of assistance on average (3.7), followed by the *Friend-Centered* group (3.2) and the *Isolated* (1.2) group. Thus, although friends form

**Table 3.** Perceptions of social support sufficiency by social network type

| | Isolated, % | *Friend-Centered*, % | Integrated, % |
|---|---|---|---|
| Availability instrumental support*** | | | |
| Not at all | 32.5 | 20.8 | 19.1 |
| Only occasionally | 17.3 | 24.4 | 17.2 |
| Sometimes | 24.2 | 23.7 | 29.4 |
| Most/all the time | 26.0 | 31.2 | 34.3 |
| Adequacy instrumental support | | | |
| Need a lot more | 14.0 | 10.5 | 8.0 |
| Need some more | 16.6 | 17.7 | 19.7 |
| Need a little more | 28.8 | 29.2 | 30.4 |
| Got all help needed | 40.6 | 42.6 | 41.8 |
| Availability emotional support*** | | | |
| Not at all | 20.4 | 6.1 | 8.9 |
| Only occasionally | 17.6 | 13.8 | 13.2 |
| Sometimes | 29.0 | 28.9 | 23.4 |
| Most/all the time | 33.3 | 50.8 | 54.6 |
| Adequacy emotional support* | | | |
| Need a lot more | 22.5 | 19.0 | 18.5 |
| Need some more | 22.5 | 24.2 | 19.5 |
| Need a little more | 24.7 | 26.1 | 24.4 |
| Got all help needed | 30.2 | 30.6 | 37.6 |

Total (n = 914); Isolated (n = 285); *Friend-Centered* (n = 313); Integrated (n = 306). Valid percentages.
* $p < 0.05$, ** $p < 0.01$, *** $p < 0.001$, chi-square tests of association.

the backbone of social networks of the *Friend-Centered* group, the levels of assistance they provide do not compensate for the lack of support from family. Those in the *Integrated* group receive the highest levels of support from both family and friends.

*Social Network Type and Perceptions of Social Support Sufficiency*

Social network type was significantly related to the availability of instrumental support, and the availability and adequacy of emotional support. The *Isolated* network type was the most likely to report that instrumental support was unavailable (33%) as compared to 21% of the *Friend-Centered* group and 19% of the *Integrated* group (table 3). Furthermore, only 26% of the *Isolated* group said instrumental support was available all or most of the time, as compared with approximately one-third of the older adults with HIV in the other 2 groups. Social network type was not significantly related to instrumental support adequacy. With regard to emotional support, 20% of the *Isolated* group reported that such support was not available, more than twice the proportion found in the *Friend-Centered* or *Integrated* groups (6 and 9%, respectively). Over half of the *Integrated* (55%) and *Friend-Centered* groups (51%) indicated that emotional support was available all or most of the time in comparison to one-third of those in the *Isolated* Group. Those in the *Integrated* group were significantly

**Table 4.** MANOVAs on psychosocial well-being and HIV stigma by social network type

| | Isolated, mean ± SD | *Friend-Centered,* mean ± SD | Integrated, mean ± SD |
|---|---|---|---|
| Psychosocial measures | | | |
| UCLA loneliness*** | 47.6±10.13 | 43.18±10.79 | 41.08±9.93 |
| CES-D depression** | 21.72±10.21 | 18.79±10.77 | 19.13±10.65 |
| Personal growth*** | 38.41±8.07 | 42.12±7.63 | 41.71±7.95 |
| Self-acceptance*** | 36.63±7.93 | 38.10±9.11 | 39.84±8.14 |
| Berger stigma scale | | | |
| Disclosure** | 25.4±6.5 | 24.0±5.8 | 24.0±5.9 |
| Personal*** | 40.8±12.9 | 37.8±11.1 | 36.6±10.9 |
| Public*** | 47.8±13.4 | 44.6±11.4 | 43.6±11.2 |
| Self-image*** | 28.3±8.8 | 25.1±7.5 | 25.2±7.4 |

Well-being MANOVA: F(8, 1720) = 10.84, p < 0.001. Isolated (n = 271); *Family-Centered* (n = 301); Integrated (n = 293). Post-hoc tests (i.e., p < 0.05); UCLA loneliness, all groups different from each other; CES-D depressive symptoms, isolated different from Friend-Centered and Integrated: personal growth, isolated different from *Friend-Centered* and Integrated; self-acceptance, all groups different from each other. Berger stigma MANOVA: F(8, 1764) = 4.60, p < 0.001. Post-hoc tests: Isolated different than *Friend-Centered* and Integrated on all scales at $p < 0.02$ or greater. * $p < 0.05$, ** $p < 0.01$, *** $p < 0.001$.

more likely to report they had received adequate emotional support; 38% reported receiving all the emotional support needed in the past year as compared to 30% of the *Isolated* and 31% of the *Friend-Centered* groups.

*Social Network Types, Psychosocial Factors and Stigma*

As illustrated in table 4, social network type was significantly related to HIV stigma and psychosocial indicators. Older adults with HIV in the *Isolated* group reported the highest average loneliness scores (47.6) as compared to either the *Friend-Centered* or *Integrated* group (43.2 and 41.1, respectively). Post-hoc analysis revealed all 3 groups were significantly different from each other with regard to loneliness. The *Isolated* group also reported significantly greater depressive symptoms on average (21.7) compared to the *Friend-Centered* or *Integrated* groups (18.8 and 19.1, respectively), with post-hoc analysis finding no significant differences between the latter 2 groups. The reverse pattern was true with regard to psychological well-being measures of personal growth and self-acceptance in terms of average scores in the *Friend-Centered* (42.1 and 38.1, respectively) and *Integrated* groups (41.7 and 39.8, respectively) relative to the *Isolated* group (38.4 and 36.6, respectively). Post-hoc analyses found the *Isolated* group significantly different from both of the other groups in terms of personal growth, while all 3 groups were significantly different from each other on self-acceptance. With regard to HIV stigma, the *Isolated* group reported the highest average levels of stigma in all 4 domains of disclosure concerns, personal stigma, public

attitudes, and self-image compared to those with *Friend-Centered* or *Integrated* networks (table 4). Post-hoc analysis found significant differences between the *Isolated* group members and the other 2 groups, but no significant differences between the *Friend-Centered* and *Integrated* groups on the 4 dimensions of HIV stigma.

## Conclusions

Our empirical investigation has helped to clarify the nature of social network characteristics among older adults with HIV. Cluster analysis of social network characteristics identified 3 distinct social network types in this population. These data are in line with earlier research that described fragile and friend-dominated social networks of older adults with HIV, showing a greater reliance on friends rather than spouses/partners, children and other family members [23, 24, 33]. However, our typology suggests that a more nuanced description of these social networks is warranted, as for some (*Isolated* type) friends are nearly absent and provide little support, while for others (*Integrated* type) there are substantial levels of family involvement and receipt of familial assistance.

We found that social network types were significantly related to receiving assistance from family and friends, and perceptions of availability and adequacy of instrumental and emotional support. As might be expected, those with *Friend-Centered* network types received most of their assistance from friends, while the *Isolated* group with few friends received greater assistance on balance from family, but still less than the *Integrated* group who had reported a greater variety of functional family members. However, for those with *Friend-Centered* networks, the amount of assistance received from friends did not compensate for the lack of family support, and is congruent with past reports that indicate friends do not typically provide the same level of support as do family members, particularly with regard to instrumental assistance [9].

Older adults with HIV with *Isolated* network types were the most likely to report that both instrumental and emotional supports were not available, and the most likely to indicate that the emotional support they received in the previous year was inadequate. These findings support known network dynamics which show that social isolation among older adults with HIV will interfere with their ability to access informal caregiving and other forms of assistance as they age. As a consequence, these older adults report low levels of perceived adequacy and availability of instrumental and emotional supports, especially in comparison to other older adult populations [33]. Interestingly, social network characteristics (i.e., type) were not related to the perceived adequacy of instrumental help. This may reflect the relatively young age of this sample (i.e., 56 years on average), such that their needs for informal assistance at present may not be acute. However, it is likely that these older adults with HIV will need increased informal support and caregiving as they age.

Our hypothesis that social network types would relate to psychosocial measures and perceived HIV stigma was also supported, and is congruent with past research finding that those with higher perceptions of social support sufficiency, namely, the *Integrated* and *Friend-Centered* groups, report lower levels of psychological distress (i.e., loneliness, depression) and greater psychological well-being (i.e., personal growth and self-acceptance). We also observed that those with *Isolated* network types reported the highest levels of perceived HIV stigma. Given the cross-sectional nature of these data, it is not possible to determine if stigma was causal with regard to social isolation through rejection by other network members and/or self-protective withdrawal, or if social isolation exacerbated feelings of HIV stigma. These data suggest that *Friend-Centered* and *Integrated* network types offer similar advantages with regard to psychosocial functioning and act to buffer the effects of stigma.

*Strengths and Limitations*

As is typical of most studies on people living with HIV, our empirical investigation employed a convenience sample. However, the demographic profile of ROAH respondents parallels epidemiological data on older adults with HIV living in New York City at the time data were collected [3]. Also, because social network data were self-reported, the objective nature of the size and frequency of contact on which the social network typology was based cannot be validated. An additional limitation is the cross-sectional nature of these data, thereby limiting our ability to make causal inferences; hence, longitudinal studies are needed. These network typologies in this chapter may also not be generalizable to other populations with HIV given the diversity of social structures and cultures that affect social network dynamics from a global perspective. A major strength was the large sample size, the use of measures with established reliability and validity, and the use of multivariate statistical analyses.

*Implications for Practice*

To address the needs of older adults living with HIV, it is essential to understand the physical and disease-related factors. However, to achieve optimal health outcomes the psychosocial circumstances of these individuals must be identified and considered in developing plans for treatment and care. Rates of depression are higher in the HIV-positive older adults in this study compared to other groups of older adults [34], and are strongly related to HIV stigma [7]. Thus, each of these factors is a separate, albeit inter-related, phenomenon and may have different implications for policy, planning, and service provision.

Older adults with HIV lacking social support in resource-rich settings such as the US and Western Europe will likely have to turn to formal community-based support systems for care [23, 35]. Prior research finds that older adults with HIV (50 years of age or older) use more services than non-infected older adults 65 and older (3.6 vs. 1), and greater service needs are associated with accessing more community-based supports in the HIV-positive older adults [9, 35]. As the population with HIV ages, they will increasingly access community-based services, particularly if they are socially isolated. However, there are fewer options for government and community-based support in resource-poor setting such as most countries in sub-Saharan Africa; innovative policy and programs need to be developed to address this issue in these regions to ensure older adults with HIV in these areas receive sufficient support.

The present findings illustrate the pervasive impact of having an HIV diagnosis, and the implications of such a diagnosis on bio-psycho-social functioning. Many older adults with HIV present with numerous vulnerabilities, including multimorbidity, social isolation, low psychological well-being, greater depression and loneliness, and an intensified experience of HIV stigma. Stigma remains one of the most insidious aspects in the lives of this population, fueling both social isolation and having a profoundly negative impact on health and psychological functioning. As the population with HIV over 50 burgeons, there is a need to carefully consider how best to empower these older adults to achieve their maximum levels of psychosocial functioning in their communities, given available personal and social resources. HIV-positive older adults, with the help of modern medicine, can look forward to a longer life. But will this longer life be one of impenetrable isolation, or will it be as a functioning, integrated member of society?

## Acknowledgements

We thank R. Andrew Shippy and the late Marjorie H. Cantor for their contributions to early versions of this work. This research was entirely supported by the generous contributions of our supporters at ACRIA.

## References

1 Harrison KM, Song R, Zhang X: Life expectancy after HIV diagnosis based on national HIV surveillance data from 25 states, United States. J Acquir Immune Defic Syndr 2010;53:124–130.
2 Effros RB, Fletcher CV, Gebo K, Halter JB, Hazzard WR, Horne FM, Huebner RE, Janoff EN, Justice AC, Kuritzkes D, Nayfield SG, Plaeger SF, Schmader KE, Ashworth JR, Campanelli C, Clayton CP, Rada B, Woolard NF, High KP: Aging and infectious diseases: workshop on HIV infection and aging: what is known and future research directions. Clin Infect Dis 2008;47:542–553.
3 Karpiak SE, Brennan M: Aging with HIV: implications and future directions; in Brennan M, Karpiak SE, Shippy RA, Cantor MH (eds): Research on Older Adults with HIV: An In-Depth Examination of an Emerging Population. New York, Nova Science Publishers, 2009, pp 1–12.
4 Centers for Disease Control and Prevention: Diagnoses of HIV infection among adults aged 50 years and older in the United States and dependent areas, 2007–2010. HIV Surveillance Supplemental Report 2013; 18(No. 3). http://www.cdc.gov/hiv/pdf/statistics_2010_HIV_Surveillance_Report_vol_18_no_3.pdf (retrieved February 21, 2014).
5 Chesney MA, Chambers DB, Taylor JM, Johnson LM: Social support, distress, and well-being in older men living with HIV infection. J Acquir Immune Defic Syndr 2003;33(suppl 2):S185–S193.
6 Havlik RJ, Brennan M, Karpiak SE: Comorbidities and depression in older adults with HIV. Sex Health 2011;8:551–559.
7 Grov C, Golub SA, Parsons JT, Brennan M, Karpiak SE: Loneliness and HIV-related stigma explain depression among older HIV-positive adults. AIDS Care 2010;22:630–639.

8 Wallach I, Brotman S: Ageing with HIV/AIDS: a scoping study among people aged 50 and over living in Quebec. Ageing and Society 2013;33:1212–1242.
9 Cantor MH, Brennan M: Social Care of the Elderly: The Effects of Ethnicity, Class and Culture. New York, Springer, 2000.
10 Cantor MH, Mayer M: Factors in differential utilization of services by urban elderly. J Gerontol Soc Work 1978;1:47–61.
11 Kara M, Mirici A: Loneliness, depression, and social support of Turkish patients with chronic obstructive pulmonary disease and their spouses. J Nurs Scholarsh 2004;36:331–336.
12 Cornwell EY, Waite LJ: Social disconnectedness, perceived isolation, and health among older adults. J Health Soc Behav 2009;50:31–48.
13 Miller JF: Assessment of loneliness and spiritual well-being in chronically ill and healthy adults. J Prof Nurs 1985;1:79–85.
14 Emlet CA: 'You're awfully old to have this disease': experiences of stigma and ageism in adults 50 years and older living with HIV/AIDS. Gerontologist 2006;46:781–790.
15 Lichtenstein B, Laska MK, Clair JM: Chronic sorrow in the HIV-positive patient: issues of race, gender, and social support. AIDS Patient Care STDS 2002;16:27–38.
16 Chenard C: The impact of stigma on the self-care behaviors of HIV-positive gay men striving for normalcy. J Assoc Nurses AIDS Care 2007;18:23–32.
17 Reece M, Tanner AE, Karpiak SE, Coffey K: The impact of HIV-related stigma on HIV care and prevention providers. J HIV AIDS Soc Serv 2007;6:55–73.
18 Courtenay-Quirk C, Wolitski RJ, Parsons JT, Gómez CA: Is HIV/AIDS stigma dividing the gay community? Perceptions of HIV-positive men who have sex with men. AIDS Educ Prev 2006;18:56–67.
19 Poindexter CC, Shippy RA: HIV diagnosis disclosure: stigma management and stigma resistance. J Gerontol Soc Work 2010;53:366–381.
20 Brennan M: Spirituality and religiousness predict adaptation to vision loss among middle-age and older adults. Int J Psychol Relig 2004;14:193–214.
21 Emlet CA, Fredriksen-Goldsen KI, Kim HJ: Risk and protective factors associated with health-related quality of life among older gay and bisexual men living with HIV disease. Gerontologist 2013;53:963–972.
22 Nichols JE, Speer DC, Watson BJ, Watson M, Vergon TL, Vallee CM, Meah, JM: Aging with HIV: Psychological, Social, and Health Issues. San Diego, Calif., Academic Press, 2002.
23 Shippy RA, Karpiak SE: The aging HIV/AIDS population: fragile social networks. Aging Ment Health 2005;9:246–254.
24 Shippy R, Karpiak S: Perceptions of support among older adults with HIV. Res Aging 2005;27:290–306.
25 Emlet CA: An examination of the social networks and social isolation in older and younger adults living with HIV/AIDS. Health Soc Work 2006;31:299–308.
26 Brennan M, Applebaum A: Loneliness among older adults with HIV; in Brennan M, Karpiak SE, Shippy RA, Cantor MH (eds): Research on Older Adults with HIV: An In-Depth Examination of an Emerging Population. New York, Nova Science Publishers, 2009, pp 75–78.
27 Brennan M, Karpiak SE, Shippy RA, Cantor MH: Older Adults with HIV: An In-Depth Examination of an Emerging Population. New York, Nova Science Publishers, 2009.
28 Cantor MH: Neighbors and friends: an overlooked resource in the informal support system. Res Aging 1979;1:434–463.
29 Russell DW: UCLA loneliness scale (version 3): reliability, validity, and factor structure. J Pers Assess 1996;66:20–40.
30 Radloff LS: The CES-D scale: a self-report depression scale for research in the general population. Appl Psych Meas 1977;1:385–401.
31 Ryff CD: Happiness is everything, or is it? Explorations on the meaning of psychological well-being. J Pers Soc Psychol 1989;57:1069–1081.
32 Berger BE, Ferrans CE, Lashley FR: Measuring stigma in people with HIV: psychometric assessment of the HIV stigma scale. Res Nurs Health 2001;24:518–529.
33 Cantor MH, Brennan M, Karpiak SE: The social support networks of older people with HIV; in Brennan M, Karpiak SE, Shippy RA, Cantor MH (eds): Research on Older Adults with HIV: An In-Depth Examination of an Emerging Population. New York, Nova Science Publishers, 2009, pp 1–12.
34 Applebaum A, Brennan M: Mental health and depression; in Brennan M, Karpiak SE, Shippy RA, Cantor MH (eds): Research on Older Adults with HIV: An In-Depth Examination of an Emerging Population. New York, Nova Science Publishers, 2009, pp 1–12.
35 Brennan-Ing M, Seidel L, London AS, Cahill S, Karpiak SE: Service utilization among older adults with HIV: the joint association of sexual identity and gender. J Homosex 2014;61:166–196.

Mark Brennan-Ing, PhD
ACRIA, ACRIA Center on HIV and Aging
575 Eighth Avenue, Suite 502
New York, NY 10018 (USA)
E-Mail mbrennan@acria.org

Brennan-Ing M, DeMarco RF (eds): HIV and Aging. Interdiscipl Top Gerontol Geriatr.
Basel, Karger, 2017, vol 42, pp 173–186 (DOI: 10.1159/000448562)

# Remediating HIV-Associated Neurocognitive Disorders via Cognitive Training: A Perspective on Neurocognitive Aging

David E. Vance · Shameka L. Cody · Linda Moneyham

The University of Alabama School of Nursing, University of Alabama at Birmingham (UAB), Birmingham, Ala., USA

**Abstract**

Over 50% of adults with HIV exhibit some form of HIV-associated neurocognitive disorder, ranging from mild asymptomatic neurocognitive impairment to HIV-associated dementia. As adults age with HIV and become susceptible to cardiovascular and metabolic comorbidities, the prevalence and severity of such neurocognitive disorders are likely to increase. With compromised renal and hepatic functioning often accompanying HIV, pharmaceutical interventions to address such neurocognitive disorders may not be the best strategy and are not without risks. Fortunately, as noted in the geriatric literature, cognitive training strategies have been shown to improve targeted neurocognitive domains and everyday functioning. A review of some of these cognitive training strategies, especially as they relate to aging with HIV, are highlighted and explained in the context of neuroAIDS, aging, and neurocognitive reserve. Implications for practice and research are provided.



By 2017, 70% of adults with HIV will be aged 50 and older [1]. The pharmaceutical advancements that can keep the HIV virus from replicating have by and large contributed to aging of the population with HIV, such that normal lifespans are now projected for those with HIV who have access to such HIV medications [2]. Using data from the national Dutch ATHENA cohort of +10,000 HIV patients, Smit et al. [3] project that by 2030, 73% of those with HIV will be 50 and older. However, they also project that 84% of this population will develop at least one additional comorbidity, and 28% will develop at least 3; this is in contrast to only 19% of their HIV-negative counterparts who will also develop at least 3 comorbidities. Driving such comorbidities will be cardiovascular disease (78%), diabetes (17%), and malignancies (17%)

which reflect current studies, suggesting greater prevalence of such conditions in those with HIV [4]. Concomitant treatments of comorbidities along with HIV medications will undoubtedly increase concerns over polypharmacy; in fact, Smit et al. [3] also project 53% will experience adverse drug interactions. In an aging population such as this which also has higher rates of renal and hepatic dysfunction, such comorbidities will produce additional burden not only on the body, but also on brain health and neurocognitive functioning [5].

The purpose of this article is to highlight how cognitive training exercises may be used to improve or remediate neurocognitive functioning in adults with HIV, particularly, when they age. To accomplish this, HIV-associated neurocognitive disorders (HANDs) and their causes are summarized in the context of neurocognitive reserve. A brief review of selective cognitive training exercises is provided, followed by implications for practice and research.

## Neurocognitive Reserve

Brain reserve, often called neurocognitive reserve, refers to the concept that the stronger, more sophisticated, and healthier the connections between neurons and various brain regions, the better one can weather neurological damage (e.g., head trauma, HIV, etc.) by rewiring to remaining functional neurological circuits and still maintain optimal neurocognitive functioning [6]. The degree of neurocognitive reserve depends on 2 processes: positive neuroplasticity and negative neuroplasticity. Positive neuroplasticity encapsulates those factors (i.e., engagement in neurocognitively stimulating activities) that promote such strong connections through continued use and learning; negative neuroplasticity includes those factors (i.e., lack of neurocognitive engagement) that atrophies and weakens such connections through disuse. Neurobiologically, such engagement with learning and neurocognitively stimulating activities is known to produce changes in brain-derived neurotrophic and other growth factors that increase neuronal connectivity and produce morphological changes in cortical and subcortical structures [6]. Such changes can result in improved neurocognitive reserve and neurocognitive functioning.

Exemplifying this process, in a sample of 181 community-dwelling older adults, Stine-Morrow et al. [7] conducted a randomized control trial using experimental and control conditions. Those in the experimental condition engaged with others in their group to solve problems as a team in weekly meetings; meanwhile, the control condition received no such neurocognitive engagement. After 20 weekly sessions, the researchers observed that older adults in the actively engaged, experimental group experienced improved neurocognitive functioning compared to controls. The study supports the efficacy of positive neuroplasticity in increasing or maintaining neurocognitive reserve. The findings of other studies likewise show that older adults who engage in more education, learn how to play a musical instrument, or other such behaviors that encourage positive neuroplasticity likewise increase neurocognitive functioning and delay or mitigate age-related neurocognitive impairments and dementia [6, 8, 9].

## HIV-Associated Neurocognitive Disorder

Unfortunately, a diagnosis of HIV can directly and indirectly weaken neurocognitive reserve, resulting in poorer neurocognitive functioning. While the HIV virus does not directly infect neurons, the virus infects macrophages which can cross the blood–brain barrier. Once in the brain, the HIV virus infects microglial cells. Microglial cells normally support neuronal functioning, but once infected with HIV, the virus replicates within these cells which secrete several neurotoxic substances (e.g., TAT, IL-6, TNF-α) as they eventually die (i.e., apoptosis). This process creates a neurotoxic environment, which either kills neurons or impairs their function; this is reflected in MRIs in which adults with HIV display more atrophy in cortical and subcortical gray matter areas and reduced integrity of white matter tracts connecting such gray matter areas [10].

Indirectly, a number of factors (e.g., substance abuse, hepatitis C, heart disease) associated with HIV may also contribute to reduced neurocognitive reserve and increased neurocognitive impairment. Two such factors are mood disturbances and lack of neurocognitive engagement. Mood disturbances are quite common for those with HIV; in one sample of ~1,500 adults with HIV, approximately 40 and 20% had depression or anxiety, respectively [4]. Given the high degree of stress, stigma, and corresponding mood disorders associated with HIV, such distress can stimulate the hypothalamus-pituitary-adrenal axis that can increase cortisol levels that over the long-term, can cause neuroinflammation, compromising neurocognitive reserve [11].

Lack of neurocognitive engagement, such as those observed with social withdrawal or lack of employment, represents negative neuroplasticity and may contribute to poorer neurocognitive reserve. In fact, in one study of those with HIV, 40% were continuously unemployed over a 30-month period while only 20% engaged continuously in employment during the same time [12]. The high rate of unemployment is unfortunate because there are numerous documented neurocognitive benefits of being employed, including having a steady routine that regulates health behaviors (e.g., sleep schedule), having purposeful and productive activity, being socially engaged and working as a team, and continuously learning new skills and competencies [13]. Emphasizing this point, Fazeli et al. [14] examined whether engagement in certain lifestyle factors predicted HAND in 139 adults with HIV ($M_{age}$ = 48.7 years). The lifestyle factors included engagement in full-time or part-time employment (yes/no), and whether they were socially active (yes/no) and physically active (yes/no). The researchers observed that as these participants engaged in more of the lifestyle factors,

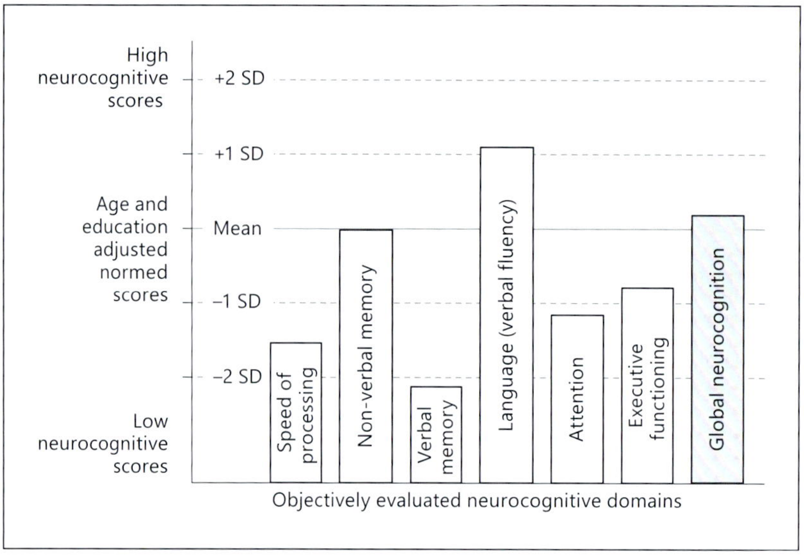


**Fig. 1.** This is an example of a case classification of HAND. In this example, the patient is performing less than one SD on a normed measure of speed of processing and attention, and more than 2 SD on a normed measure of verbal memory. Using the Frascati criteria, this patient would be diagnosed as possibly having either asymptomatic neurocognitive impairment or mild neurocognitive impairment, depending on the degree to which such impairment interferes with everyday functioning and quality of life. Note that language is 1 SD above the normed mean and global neurocognition functioning is also at the mean/average level; this suggests that certain neurocognitive domains may be more resistant to some neurocognitive decline than others, and yet, some patients may actually appear to be cognitively intact as exhibited by the overall good global functioning but in fact experience neurocognitive impairments in one or more cognitive domains.

the prevalence of HAND significantly decreased, reflecting better neurocognitive reserve.

Unfortunately, once neurocognitive reserve declines and the brain is unable to compensate, neurocognitive impairments emerge. In adults with HIV, neurocognitive impairments can be observed in a number of neurocognitive domains. In fact, HAND is diagnosed and classified using what is referred to as the Frascati criteria [15], where a series of standardized neurocognitive tests are administered to a patient with HIV. These tests measure at least 5 different neurocognitive domains (e.g., verbal fluency, verbal memory) and are normed by age and education (fig. 1). Norming is essential because age and education are known to influence performance on these neurocognitive tests (likely due to neuroplasticity and biological reasons, but this is a discussion beyond the scope of this review). For example, a 30-year-old patient with a PhD probably has better memory and speed of processing abilities than an 80-year-old patient with a 5th grade education. These normed neurocognitive tests have been validated across larger populations to determine how people of different ages and education levels perform on these tests. Within each group, say adults 50–55 years with a master's degree, the mean and SD are determined for the group so that clinicians can evaluate how a particular patient is performing within his/her reference group along the normal distribution – whether he/she is performing at the mean, higher, or lower compared to his/her reference group (fig. 1).

Based on the battery of normed neurocognitive tests administered to the patient, the level of HAND is determined. The 3 levels of HAND range from least severe to most severe, and include: asymptomatic neurocognitive disorder, mild neurocognitive disorder, and HIV-associated dementia. Asymptomatic neurocognitive disorder is diagnosed when patients score less than 1 SD below their adjusted norm within 2 neurocognitive domains; in figure 1, this is observed for speed of processing and psychomotor ability. With this diagnosis, the patient may be unaware that he/she is experiencing such neurocognitive impairments, and it may not interfere with his/her everyday functioning. For a diagnosis of mild neurocognitive disorder, the same neurocognitive criteria are used; however, such neurocognitive impairments interfere mildly to moderately with everyday functioning (e.g., driving, medication adherence) and may be noticeable and troubling to the patient. Finally, HIV-associated dementia is diagnosed when the patient performs 2 or more SD below his/her adjusted norm within at least 2 neurocognitive domains, and such neurocognitive impairments severely interfere with everyday functioning and are troubling to the patient and the caregivers. In figure 1, this patient performed less than 2 SD on verbal memory but does not qualify for HIV-associated dementia; however, if she would have performed a little worse on speed of processing such that her score was under 2 SD, then a diagnosis of HIV-associated dementia would be considered.

Although there are a number of nuances in making such neurocognitive diagnoses (not discussed here), based on these criteria, the prevalence of HAND ranges from 52 to 59% of the adult HIV population [16, 17]. Within this broad classification, approximately 33% have asymptomatic neurocognitive impairment, 12% have mild neurocognitive impairment, 5% have a confounded neurocognitive disorder, and 2% have HIV-associated dementia.

However, as the HIV-infected population continues to age, it is possible that the prevalence of HAND in this population will be ever greater. In a study of 182 adults with HIV, Valcour et al. [18] observed that HIV-associated dementia occurred 3 times more often in older participants. Likewise, in comparing performance on several neurocognitive tests in 162 older (50+) and younger (18–49) adults with and without HIV, Vance et al. [19] observed that in general, older adults with HIV performed the worst, while younger adults without HIV performed the best. These and other studies suggest that there may be either accentuation or acceleration of the neurocognitive aging process for many adults with HIV [20]. Given these concerns, rehabilitating, stabilizing, or compensating for these neurocognitive impairments are important to improve and protect the quality of life and everyday functioning for patients and caregivers.

## Cognitive Training Strategies

Cognitive training strategies often focus on delivering exercises and activities designed to improve either a specific neurocognitive domain (i.e., executive functioning) or a combination of neurocognitive domains (i.e., executive functioning and speed of processing) that may improve the overall global neurocognitive functioning. There are numerous cognitive training strategies described in the literature, but for the sake of brevity, this section provides a few specific examples of cognitive training strategies that either focus on improving a specific neurocognitive domain or global cognition. Surprisingly, only a few studies have investigated cognitive training strategies in those with HIV. Yet, it is reasonable to assume that if such cognitive training protocols can improve cognition in older adults without HIV, such protocols could possibly benefit older adults with HIV. Fortunately, many such cognitive training protocols are conveniently computerized, which allows them to be delivered in a variety of venues and allows for standardization of protocols [21].

Lampit et al. [22] provided an excellent summary and meta-analysis of the published research using computerized cognitive training interventions with older adults. They evaluated 52 cognitive training interventions for their efficacy in improving the targeted neurocognitive ability. Pooling the effect sizes across studies with a control group, they found significant small to moderate training gains (i.e., effect sizes) in cognitive training interventions designed to improve speed of processing ($g = 0.31$), visuospatial skills ($g = 0.30$), nonverbal memory ($g = 0.24$), working memory ($g = 0.22$), and verbal memory ($g = 0.08$). Interestingly, they did not observe significant improvements in effect sizes for cognitive training interventions designed to improve attention and executive functioning. Although beyond the scope of the current literature review, Lampit et al. [22] also examined the influence of modifiers of training such as dose (less than 20 vs. 20+ h), training session length, and frequency of training (once/week vs. >3 sessions/week) on the effect size for each type of training protocol. Some of these modifiers are important considerations and are interjected as examples of the cognition training interventions mentioned in the next section.

### *Speed of Processing Training*

Speed of processing training has been employed extensively in the geriatric population to improve the neurocognitive ability. In the Advanced Cognitive Training for Independent and Vital Elderly (ACTIVE) Study, 2,802 community-dwelling older adults were randomized to one of the training conditions: (1) speed of processing; (2) reasoning; (3) memory; and (4) no-contact control [23]. With as little as 10-hours of cognitive training, robust gains were observed in the speed of processing and reasoning training groups, with results lasting over several years. Furthermore, over time those in the speed of processing training group had fewer at-fault crashes, less depressive symptomatology, and better self-rated health, health-related quality of life, and locus of control than those in the control group [24]. These additional benefits are particularly appealing for older adults with HIV in who depression, health-related quality of life, and locus of control are of concern due to the physical and social-emotional characteristics of this disease.

Building on the ACTIVE Study, Vance et al. [25] randomized 46 middle-aged and older adults (40 and older) to either a speed of processing or a no-contact control group. Those in the speed of processing group engaged in up to 10 h of computerized exercises designed to increase the speed at which complex stimuli were detected within one's visual field on a screen. Stimuli were presented and remained on the computer screen for varying numbers of milliseconds; after each presentation, participants responded indicating what stimuli they just observed by touching choices on the screen. If they responded correctly, the next presentation speed was faster; if they responded incorrectly, the next presentation speed was slower. Using this basic algorithm, the speed of the participants' perceptual threshold was always at their maximum level, thus forcing them through neuroplastic changes to gradually increase the speed at which they processed information. Compared to the no-contact control group at 5–6 weeks post-test, those in the speed of processing group experienced significant gains on the Useful Field of View test, a measure of visual speed of processing. In fact, those who improved on the Useful Field of View measure were statistically more likely to rate that engaging in the speed of processing training improved their mental abilities [26]. Furthermore, this training also translated to significant improvement on the Instrumental Activities of Daily Living (IADL) test, which is a timed measure in which participants perform everyday activities such as counting out change, looking up a phone number, and reading medication labels.

In a follow-up study, Cody et al. [27] used a within-group design to examine the response of 20 middle-aged and older adults (40+ years; $M_{age}$ = 50.22 years) with HIV to the speed of processing training installed on their home computers. Without weekly prompts by investigators, participants engaged in the home-based training 8.20 h (SD 3.43; range 0–11) on average. Compared to baseline performance, significant post-test improvements were observed on the Useful Field of View test and the Timed IADL test. Likewise, on a scale from 1 (not at all) to 5 (extremely), on average participants indicated that they felt this training moderately improved their overall mental abilities, memory, speed of processing, and attention. The findings support the idea that cognitive training can successfully be conducted in the privacy of one's home, which may be particularly relevant for those older adults with HIV who may be less likely to venture out to a clinic due to perceived stigma [28].

Such cognitive training has been shown to improve the visual speed of processing, which is an important neurocognitive ability needed for driving. In a related study, Vance et al. [29] examined the relationship between driving simulator performance and neurocognitive functioning in 26 middle-aged and older adults (40+) with HIV. They found that poorer visual speed of processing, as measured by the Useful Field of View test, was related to slower reaction time in a driving simulator. This finding was particularly relevant given that slower reaction time was significantly related to the number of actual self-reported accidents within the past 2 years. With both the aging of the HIV population and the propensity for neurocognitive disorders, it is likely that many older adults with HIV may also experience problems with driving. Fortunately, the speed of processing training shows promise for improving the neurocognitive abilities needed for safe driving.

*Reasoning/Executive Training*

A type of executive training, referred to as reasoning training, has been used in the ACTIVE Study cited above, and shown to improve this neurocognitive ability even 10 years after initial training [30]. Such training consists of providing group exercises whereby participants practice strategies to recognize patterns in groups of numbers, words, letters, and everyday life (e.g., bus schedules, medication regimens). Although in their meta-analysis of cognitive training interventions, Lampit et al. [22] concluded that the effects of such training are not significant; the ACTIVE Study by Rebok et al. [30] was not included in this meta-analysis. Although this cognitive training intervention has not been tested in adults with HIV, this approach may be of value.

*Memory Training*

People tend to notice impairments in memory first, even though other neurocognitive abilities such as reasoning or speed of processing may also have declined. Complaints about memory impairment are common with age and can be most distressing because of obvious conscious reliance on memory in everyday life (e.g., Where did I put my keys?), which are often focused on verbal memory (What is his name? What was the name of that movie?). Such memory complaints can interfere with everyday functioning and negatively impact quality of life. As noted previously, Lampit et al. [22] found that the effect size for nonverbal memory training interventions (g = 0.24) and working memory training interventions (g = 0.22) were higher than for verbal memory training interventions (g = 0.08). Despite documented memory impairments in many older adults with HIV [19], to date few neurocognitive interventions to improve memory have been conducted in this population; fortunately, there are several in the gerontological literature. For example, Cohen-Mansfield et al. [31] randomized 44 older adults with memory complaints into either a health promotion, a patient-centered, or a cognitive (memory) training condition. Using intervention strategies derived from the ACTIVE Study to improve verbal episodic memory, over a 10-week period participants were taught practical strategies for recalling short text and remembering lists of words such as using method of loci or using visual images and mental associations to recall and remember such verbal information. Compared to other conditions, those in the memory training condition reported fewer memory complaints.

In a related study of 10 older adults with HIV experiencing neurocognitive impairment, Neundorfer et al. [32] used a combination of mnemonic (i.e., posted reminders, lists, calendars) and the spaced-retrieval method. The spaced-retrieval method is a well-established strategy for recalling a discrete unit of information (e.g., a phone number, a medication schedule) over increasingly longer periods of time, ideally ~16 min, until that information is consolidated into one's long-term memory. The researchers observed that a combination of these cognitive training and compensatory strategies were effective in improving activities such as remembering clinic visits or taking medication as prescribed.

*Global Cognitive Training*

Global neurocognitive function is considered an overall combination of one's neurocognitive abilities including attention, memory, speed of processing, and others [33]; in fact, such global neurocognitive assessments such as the Mini-Mental Status Exam or the Montreal Cognitive Assessment have individual test items that assess functioning in such individual domains. Many adults with HIV often report declines in their overall neurocognitive functioning, likely due to deficits in a number of other neurocognitive domains or the inability to discern what particular neurocognitive domain(s) is impaired due to metacognitive deficits (i.e., thinking about thinking, anosognosia) [34]. Thus, cognitive training interventions that focus on improving multiple neurocognitive domains simultaneously may be efficacious in improving global neurocognitive function.

Although not tested with older adults with HIV, Boivin et al. [35] administered a computerized global cognitive training protocol to Ugandan children with HIV. Sixty children were randomized to either the experimental condition where they received 10 sessions of training exercises called Captain's Log, which focused on building attention and memory skills, or to the control, no intervention condition. Children in the experimental condition displayed better performance on measures of simple attention and speed in a learning task, reflective of global neurocognitive functioning. This study showed excellent adherence (95%) to the protocol.

Likewise, in a mixed sample of 60 adults with and without HIV, Becker et al. [36] assigned these participants to either receive a cognitive training intervention called SmartBrain or not. Those randomized to SmartBrain were instructed to engage in 14 exercise modules targeting attention, memory, executive functioning, and knowledge over a 24-week period. Neurocognitive improvements were not observed; however, adherence was poor as only 54% of those assigned to the intervention used the program more than once, which may account for the lack of neurocognitive improvement.

Fortunately, the gerontological literature is replete with a variety of cognitive training interventions that have been shown to improve global neurocognitive functioning across multiple neurocognitive domains. For example, in a pre-post experimental design, Stine-Morrow et al. [7] assigned 181 community-dwelling older adults to either a no-contact control group or an experimental group. In the experimental group, called the Odyssey program, participants were grouped in teams of 5–7 members whereby they met for 20 weekly meetings to interact and solve convergent and divergent puzzles and tasks as a group, often playing off each other's ideas, working quickly, and taking risks. Relative to controls, the researchers observed that those in the Odyssey program experienced improvements in speed of processing, inductive reasoning, and divergent thinking. Other studies with older adults demonstrate improved overall global neurocognitive functioning as exhibited by improvement in several neurocognitive domains, using strategies such as non-action video games [37] and theatre training protocols [38], to name a few.

## Implications for Practice and Research

Given the efficacy of many cognitive training strategies with demonstrated improvements in neurocognitive and everyday functioning, the cognitive training approaches offer opportunities for practice and/or research. First, cognitive training may be used to improve specific neurocognitive deficits in adults with HIV; in fact, it may alter the diagnosis of HAND by improving such cognitive functioning. Second, cognitive training may improve everyday functioning such as driving and engagement/re-engagement in employment, and extend independent living for older adults with HIV. Finally, cognitive training strategies may have maximum outcomes when combined with other multi-modal approaches that may make the brain more receptive to and increase the benefits of such cognitive training.

*Altering the Diagnosis of HAND*

As noted, a HAND diagnosis is determined by performance deficits in 2 or more neurocognitive domains. Yet, it may be possible to change the diagnosis by applying targeted cognitive training to areas in which particular deficits lend themselves to the diagnostic criteria. As exemplified by the patient in figure 1, deficits below 1 SD are observed for the speed of processing and executive functioning. If a domain-specific cognitive training regimen such as speed of processing can improve the neurocognitive functioning for this patient so that he/she is no longer functioning below 1 SD for his/her age and education level, such a diagnosis may no longer be applicable when reassessed with a battery of neurocognitive tests. Although yet to be studied extensively, cognitive training provides a potentially useful approach for reducing the incidence and prevalence of HAND. Likewise, those with a diagnosis of HIV-associated dementia or mild neurocognitive disorder may be particularly motivated to engage in cognitive training because they do not want to be labeled as having such a diagnosis or to avoid common cognitive declines.

*Improved Everyday Functioning*

Independent of improving neurocognitive functioning, an essential implicit goal of cognitive training is to improve everyday functioning and quality of life, and reduce caregiver burden. As observed in the ACTIVE Study, the reasoning and speed of processing training reduced self-reported difficulty with IADLs at 10 years post-training [30]. As already mentioned, speed of processing training in particular has been shown to improve the speed and accuracy at which adults with HIV perform IADLs [25]. Likewise, other studies in non-HIV older samples have shown that the speed of processing training can improve driving safety by decreasing at-fault crashes, and it has been shown to protect older adults from depressive symptomatology and support better self-rated health, health-related quality of life, and locus of control [24].

Another area in which such cognitive training may be relevant is employment. By some estimates, many (~40%) adults with HIV are continuously unemployed over a 30-month period [12]. Many individuals may not benefit from the neurocognitive stimulation provided by employment and be at-risk for neurocognitive impairment; conversely, some individuals may stop working due to poorer health and neurocognitive impairment [13]. Albeit, for those with some neurocognitive impairments which may interfere with their ability to find or engage in an employment setting, targeting specific neurocognitive abilities needed for certain employment tasks may be helpful. This approach is particularly relevant for many older adults with HIV who may lack a satisfactory retirement income and may need to augment their income with part-time work.

Unfortunately, in some circumstances the brain may not be neuroplastic enough to reap the benefits of cognitive training. Fortunately, there are several mnemonic and compensation strategies that can be used when neurocognitive functioning cannot be improved or rehabilitated. Vance et al. [39] categorized such compensation strategies for adults with HIV into low-tech and high-tech mnemonics. Low-tech mnemonics include such strategies as: (1) using a weekly pill box to help with medication adherence; (2) journaling to keep track of events; and (3) deploying redundant systems such as multiple sets of keys in case one misplaces a set. High-tech mnemonics include strategies such as: (1) use of a 30/30 app (similar to an egg timer) to allocate enough time to devote to tasks since a sense of timing is distorted for some; (2) use of the Mint app to help organize and keep track of finances; and (3) use of alarms on cell phones to provide medication reminders. Such compensation strategies are supported by the findings of a recent study of 42 younger and 46 older adults with HIV, which showed that working memory impairments in older adults were mitigated by employing higher-level mnemonics [40].

*Combination Approaches*

The efficacy of cognitive training techniques may be augmented further by combination, multimodal approaches. One example of a combination/multimodal approach is by blending cognitive training with transcranial direct current stimulation (tDCS). tDCS delivers an electrical current to the scalp that alters (excites or inhibits) the action potential of neurons below the surface that may facilitate certain changes in mood, behavior, or cognition [41]. Combining tDCS with cognitive training has been shown to accentuate the therapeutic effects of such training. In a sample of 96 adults, Clark et al. [42] placed a positive (anodal) electrode on the scalp over the right inferior frontal cortex and a negative (cathodal) electrode on the upper left shoulder; placing electrodes over this area is thought to excite neurons responsible for executive functioning, attention, and allocating neurocognitive resources. These researchers examined whether 30 min of various current intensities, while playing a virtual reality environment training program called 'DARWARS Ambush!', would improve the performance to detect bombs. Participants exposed to 2 milliamps displayed significantly better learning, as exhibited by detecting more bombs compared to those who received only 0.1 milliamps. In fact, those assigned to receive only 0.1 milliamps reported feeling a tingling sensation which they attributed to being electrically stimulated; however, no therapeutic benefit was observed, which makes this dosage an idea sham/control condition.

Currently, sponsored by a grant from the National Institute of Aging (NIH/NIA PI: Fazeli – K99AG048762) titled 'A Novel Neurorehabilitation Approach for Cognitive Aging with HIV', Fazeli et al. [14] are combining speed of processing training with tDCS in older adults with HIV aged 50 and older. Participants are randomized into one of 2 groups: (1) speed of processing training + tDCS (experimental group), or (2) speed of processing training + sham tDCS (standard group), which are administered in a laboratory setting. All participants receive 10 one-hour training sessions using a computerized game already shown to improve speed of processing [25]. Those in the standard condition also received 20 min of tDCS at 0.1 milliamps delivered over the right orbitofrontal cortex; as previously, this amount of electricity is not considered to be of any therapeutic value. Those in the experimental condition are administered the same protocol but with tDCS at 2.0 milliamps which, based on previous studies, has been shown to have therapeutic value. Thus, it is hypothesized that based on the placement of electrodes and the dosage of electricity applied (i.e., amount of milliamps and time it is applied), those in the experimental group will exhibit larger training gains from this multimodal intervention, including improved everyday functioning as measured by driving simulator performance.

Other multimodal approaches may consist of pairing cognitive training protocols with lifestyle activities that support the overall health and brain functioning, thus making the brain more receptive for learning. For example, research findings suggest that older adults prescribed a Mediterranean diet rich in either olive oil or nuts experienced better neurocognitive functioning over time compared to a control group [43]. Similarly, engagement in physical activity may also improve the neurocognitive and functional status in older adults [14]. As these strategies support overall brain health, combining cognitive training with such strategies may boost neurocognitive gains.

## Conclusion

Not all older adults with HIV will develop neurocognitive impairments; in fact, many will successfully age, even neurocognitively. Yet for those who need help with neurocognitive functioning, psychopharmacological approaches with lithium, modafinil, and methylphenidate have been shown to be somewhat effective in improving neurocognitive functioning in adults with HIV [44]. Unfortunately, such approaches may not be appropriate in an already heavily medicated population prone to hepatic and renal dysfunction [4]. Non-psychopharmacological approaches, such as cognitive training, will be needed to bolster neurocognitive reserve and remediate in lieu of functional loss in particular neurocognitive domains.

## Acknowledgment

This article was supported by a NIH/NIMH R01-award (R01MH106366-01A1) titled 'An RCT of Speed of Processing Training in Middle-aged and Older Adults with HIV'.

## References

1 United States Senate Special Committee on Aging: Hearing: Older Americans: The Changing Face of HIV/AIDS in America. Washington, One Hundred Thirteenth Congress, First Session, 2013.

2 Rodger AJ, Lodwick R, Schechter M, Deeks S, Amin J, Gilson R, Paredes R, Bakowska E, Engsig FN, Phillips A; INSIGHT SMART, ESPRIT Study Groups: Mortality in well controlled HIV in the continuous antiretroviral therapy arms of the SMART and ESPRIT trials compared with the general population. AIDS 2013;27:973–979.

3 Smit M, Brinkman K, Geerlings S, Smit C, Thyagarajan K, Sighem Av, de Wolf F, Hallett TB; ATHENA Observational Cohort: Future challenges for clinical care of an ageing population infected with HIV: a modelling study. Lancet Infect Dis 2015;15:810–818.

4 Vance DE, Mugavero M, Willig J, Raper JL, Saag MS: Aging with HIV: a cross-sectional study of comorbidity prevalence and clinical characteristics across decades of life. J Assoc Nurses AIDS Care 2011;22: 17–25.

5 Vance DE, Cody SL: Predictions of geriatric HIV in 2030. Lancet Infect Dis 2015;15:753–754.

6 Vance DE, Roberson AJ, McGuiness T, Fazeli PL: Protecting cognitive functioning across the lifespan: a multifactorial perspective on neuroplasticity and cognitive reserve. J Psychosoc Nurs Ment Health Serv 2010;48:23–30.

7 Stine-Morrow EA, Parisi JM, Morrow DG, Park DC: The effects of an engaged lifestyle on cognitive vitality: a field experiment. Psychol Aging 2008;23:778–786.

8 Seinfeld S, Figueroa H, Ortiz-Gil J, Sanchez-Vives MV: Effects of music learning and piano practice on cognitive function, mood and quality of life in older adults. Front Psychol 2013;4:810.

9 Wilson RS, Boyle PA, Yu L, Barnes LL, Schneider JA, Bennett DA: Life-span cognitive activity, neuropathologic burden, and cognitive aging. Neurology 2013;81:314–321.

10 Vance DE, Cody SL, Batey DS: HIV-related cognitive dysfunction: implications for aging and social work. Social Work Mental Health 2015;13:553–570.

11 Sartori AC, Vance DE, Slater LZ, Crowe M: The impact of inflammation on cognitive function in older adults: implications for healthcare practice and research. J Neurosci Nurs 2012;44:206–217.

12 Rabkin JG, McElhiney M, Ferrando SJ, van Gorp W, Lin SH: Predictors of employment of men with HIV/AIDS: a longitudinal study. Psychosom Med 2004; 66:72–78.

13 Vance DE, Cody SL, Yoo-Jeong M, Jones GL, Nicholson WC: The role of employment on neurocognitive reserve in adults with HIV: a review of the literature. J Assoc Nurses AIDS Care 2015;26:316–329.

14 Fazeli PL, Woods SP, Heaton RK, Umlauf A, Gouaux B, Rosario D, Moore RC, Grant I, Moore DJ; HNRP Group.: An active lifestyle is associated with better neurocognitive functioning in adults living with HIV infection. J Neurovirol 2014;20:233–242.

15 Woods SP, Moore DJ, Weber E, Grant I: Cognitive neuropsychology of HIV-associated neurocognitive disorders. Neuropsychol Rev 2009;19:152–168.

16 Bonnet F, Amieva H, Marquant F, Bernard C, Bruyand M, Dauchy FA, et al; S CO3 Aquitaine Cohort: Cognitive disorders in HIV-infected patients: are they HIV-related? AIDS 2013;27:391–400.

17 Heaton RK, Clifford DB, Franklin DR Jr, Woods SP, Ake C, Vaida F, et al; CHARTER Group: HIV-associated neurocognitive disorders persist in the era of potent antiretroviral therapy: CHARTER Study. Neurology 2010;75:2087–2096.

18 Valcour V, Shikuma C, Shiramizu B, Watters M, Poff P, Selnes OA, Grove J, Liu Y, Abdul-Majid KB, Gartner S, Sacktor N: Age, apolipoprotein E4, and the risk of HIV dementia: the Hawaii aging with HIV cohort. J Neuroimmunol 2004;157:197–202.

19 Vance DE, Fazeli PL, Gakumo CA: The impact of neuropsychological performance on everyday functioning between older and younger adults with and without HIV. J Assoc Nurses AIDS Care 2013;24: 112–125.

20 Pathai S, Bajillan H, Landay AL, High KP: Is HIV a model of accelerated or accentuated aging? J Gerontol A Biol Sci Med Sci 2014;69:833–842.

21 Vance DE, McNees P, Meneses K: Technology, cognitive remediation, and nursing: directions for successful cognitive aging. J Gerontol Nurs 2009;35:50–56.

22 Lampit A, Hallock H, Valenzuela M: Computerized cognitive training in cognitively healthy older adults: a systematic review and meta-analysis of effect modifiers. PLoS Med 2014;11:e1001756.

23 Ball KK, Ross LA, Roth DL, Edwards JD: Speed of processing training in the ACTIVE study: how much is needed and who benefits? J Aging Health 2013; 25(8 suppl):65S–84S.
24 Vance DE, Humphrey SC, Nicholson WC, Jablonski-Jaudon R: Can speed of processing training ameliorate depressive symptomatology in adults with HIV? Ann Depress Anxiety 2014;1:pii:1013.
25 Vance DE, Fazeli PL, Ross LA, Wadley VG, Ball KK: Speed of processing training with middle-age and older adults with HIV: a pilot study. J Assoc Nurses AIDS Care 2012;23:500–510.
26 Kaur J, Dodson JE, Steadman L, Vance DE: Predictors of improvement following speed of processing training in middle-aged and older adults with HIV: a pilot study. J Neurosci Nurs 2014;46:23–33.
27 Cody SL, Fazeli PL, Vance DE: Feasibility of a home-based speed of processing training program in middle-aged and older adults with HIV. J Neurosci Nurs 2015;47:247–254.
28 Slater LZ, Moneyham L, Vance DE, Raper JL, Mugavero MJ, Childs G: The multiple stigma experience and quality of life in older gay men with HIV. J Assoc Nurses AIDS Care 2015;26:24–35.
29 Vance DE, Fazeli PL, Ball DA, Slater LZ, Ross LA: Cognitive functioning and driving simulator performance in middle-aged and older adults with HIV. J Assoc Nurses AIDS Care 2014;25:e11–e26.
30 Rebok GW, Ball K, Guey LT, Jones RN, Kim HY, King JW, Marsiske M, Morris JN, Tennstedt SL, Unverzagt FW, Willis SL; ACTIVE Study Group: Ten-year effects of the advanced cognitive training for independent and vital elderly cognitive training trial on cognition and everyday functioning in older adults. J Am Geriatr Soc 2014;62:16–24.
31 Cohen-Mansfield J, Cohen R, Buettner L, Eyal N, Jakobovits H, Rebok G, Rotenberg-Shpigelman S, Sternberg S: Interventions for older persons reporting memory difficulties: a randomized controlled pilot study. Int J Geriatr Psychiatry 2015;30:478–486.
32 Neundorfer MM, Camp CJ, Lee MM, Skrajner MJ, Malone ML, Carr JR: Compensating for cognitive deficits in persons aged 50 and over with HIV/AIDS. J HIV AIDS Soc Serv 2004;3:79–97.
33 Vance DE, Graham MA, Fazeli PL, Heaton K, Moneyham L: An overview of nonpathological geroneuropsychology: implications for nursing practice and research. J Neurosci Nurs 2012;44:43–53.
34 Vance DE, Farr KF, Struzick T: Assessing the clinical value of cognitive appraisal in adults aging with HIV. J Gerontol Nurs 2008;34:36–41.
35 Boivin MJ, Busman RA, Parikh SM, Bangirana P, Page CF, Opoka RO, Giordani B: A pilot study of the neuropsychological benefits of computerized cognitive rehabilitation in Ugandan children with HIV. Neuropsychology 2010;24:667–673.
36 Becker JT, Dew MA, Aizenstein HJ, Lopez OL, Morrow L, Saxton J, Tárraga L: A pilot study of the effects of internet-based cognitive stimulation on neuropsychological function in HIV disease. Disabil Rehabil 2012;34:1848–1852.
37 Ballesteros S, Prieto A, Mayas J, Toril P, Pita C, Ponce de León L, Reales JM, Waterworth J: Brain training with non-action video games enhances aspects of cognition in older adults: a randomized controlled trial. Front Aging Neurosci 2014;6:277.
38 Noice H, Noice T, Staines G: A short-term intervention to enhance cognitive and affective functioning in older adults. J Aging Health 2004;16:562–585.
39 Vance DE, Nicholas N, Cody SL: HIV neurocognitive impairment and aging: perspectives on neurocognitive reserve and behavioral remediation/compensation strategies. Austin J Neuropsychiatry Clin Neurosci 2015;1:1002.
40 Woods SP, Weber E, Cameron MV, Dawson MS, Delano-Wood L, Bondi MW, Grant I; HIV Neurobehavioral Research Center (HNRC) Group: Spontaneous strategy use protects against visual working memory deficits in older adults infected with HIV. Arch Clin Neuropsychol 2010;25:724–733.
41 Vance DE, Fazeli PL, Cody SL, Bell TR, Pope CN: A description and critical analysis of the therapeutic uses of transcranial direct current stimulation: Implications for clinical practice and research. Nurs Res Rev, in press.
42 Clark VP, Coffman BA, Mayer AR, Weisend MP, Lane TD, Calhoun VD, Raybourn EM, Garcia CM, Wassermann EM: TDCS guided using fMRI significantly accelerates learning to identify concealed objects. Neuroimage 2012;59:117–128.
43 Valls-Pedret C, Sala-Vila A, Serra-Mir M, Corella D, de la Torre R, Martínez-González MÁ, Martínez-Lapiscina EH, Fitó M, Pérez-Heras A, Salas-Salvadó J, Estruch R, Ros E: Mediterranean diet and age-related cognitive decline: a randomized clinical trial. JAMA Intern Med 2015;175:1094–1103.
44 Vance DE: Prevention, rehabilitation, and mitigation strategies of cognitive deficits in aging with HIV: implications for practice and research. ISRN Nurs 2013;2013:297173.

David E. Vance, PhD, MGS
The University of Alabama School of Nursing, Room 2M024
1701 University Boulevard, University of Alabama at Birmingham (UAB)
Birmingham, AL 35294-1210 (USA)
E-Mail devance@uab.edu

Brennan-Ing M, DeMarco RF (eds): HIV and Aging. Interdiscipl Top Gerontol Geriatr.
Basel, Karger, 2017, vol 42, pp 187–203 (DOI: 10.1159/000448564)

# Mental Health, Psychosocial Challenges and Resilience in Older Adults Living with HIV

Perry N. Halkitis[a–d] • Kristen D. Krause[a, b] • Dorice L. Vieira[b, e]

[a]Center for Health, Identity, Behavior and Prevention Studies, [b]College of Global Public Health, [c]Department of Population Health, Langone Medical Center, [d]Department of Applied Psychology, Steinhardt School, [e]NYU Health Sciences Library, Langone Medical Center, New York University, New York, N.Y., USA

## Abstract

In addition to physical health challenges, older people living with HIV/AIDS (PLWHA) experience mental health burdens and challenges to their social well-being that diminish their overall health. These health states are synergistic and are driven by HIV and HIV treatments, the aging process itself, and psychosocial and structural conditions of their lives. However, resilience, which we understand as both a trait and a process, may serve to buffer the effects that HIV/HIV treatments, aging, and social/structural conditions may have on the overall well-being of the individual. In this chapter, we examine the extant literate on the mental health and psychosocial challenges experienced by older PLWHA as elements of the total health of the individual. We also provide a contextualization and conceptualization for understanding the significant role that resilience may play in empowering individuals to enact processes which buffer health from the stressors. In this perspective, the health of older PLWHA must be viewed through a lens of power and strength rather than one of deficit. We conclude by outlining a theoretical paradigm for the role of resilience in the health of older HIV-positive adults, which may serve as a guide to clinicians, public health practitioners, and researchers working with this population. 

## Introduction

As the population of adults living with HIV/AIDS (PLWHA) in the United States and globally continues to age, entering middle age and beyond, individuals within the population confront a growing number of health issues. Health challenges naturally emerge for individuals as they enter the later stages of their lives; but for older adults living with HIV, the process of aging may be fraught with health complications that are wide and varied due to the aging process itself, due to HIV/AIDS and HIV treatments, and due to the interaction of aging with HIV/AIDS [1–3]. Psychosocial and structural drivers may exacerbate these conditions and also further diminish health [4, 5].

For many older PLWHA, the inability to decipher the source of their ailments (i.e., whether it is due to aging, HIV, or an interaction of both) may increase anxiety and potentially compromise their overall well-being. This idea is presented in *The AIDS Generation: Stories of Survival and Resilience* [6], where the life experiences of 15 older HIV-positive gay men, are examined. One of these men summarizes the emotional state related to the ailments experienced in older age as follows: 'all I know is that it takes a lot longer to heal. Like my back. When I used to pull it, it'd be fine in a day. Now it's five days – and cuts and colds. That's the problem of getting older. Or maybe it's because I'm poz. I dunno' [6].

Regardless of the roots of these health burdens, the fact remains that older PLWHA face myriad health complications. The most common of these health challenges include depression, coronary artery disease, hypertension, erectile dysfunction, diabetes, peripheral neuropathy, hepatitis C, and renal disease [7]. Indeed as has often been stated, HIV-positive individuals are living longer and fuller lives since the implementation of effective antiretroviral treatment (ART) in or about 1995/1996. However, aging with HIV is associated with numerous additional challenges including but not limited to age-related comorbidities, ongoing HIV trauma, potentially fragile social networks, multiple experiences of stigma, uncertainty, and confusion, all of which results in a 'novel chronic disease that will span several decades' [2]. The trauma emanates from a lifetime of living with HIV, especially in the early days of the epidemic when there was little hope for survival (i.e., prior to 1995/1996), which led to seemingly endless loss of those in one's social circle [6]. To this point, the health challenges faced by members of this population extend beyond the physical domain and encompass the emotional and social domains.

Unfortunately, the health and well-being of PLWHA, including older adults, is often predicated on physical health, specifically HIV-related health, and the ability of ART to maintain viral suppression [8]. This approach to care is directed by the fact that a viremia results in a decreased likelihood of developing opportunistic infections [9] and transmitting the virus. Treating PLWHA with the goal of reducing HIV viral load in the population is one element in a constellation of biomedical approaches to prevention, known as 'Treatment as Prevention' [10]. While the effective uptake and adherence to ART are critically important, care for older adults living with HIV cannot be defined solely by the containment of the virus and HIV-related health. Care for this population must attend equally to emotional and social health in addition to physical health, encompassing a holistic approach to care [11], namely a biopsychosocial perspective. 'HIV is more than an infection with a pathogen' [6]. In this perspective, successful aging with HIV consists of multiple components including length of life, biological health, mental health, cognitive efficiency, social competence, productivity, personal control, and life satisfaction [12].

In addition to embracing such a holistic approach to understanding the well-being of older PLWHA, it is critical we recognize that many of these individuals have survived and thrived despite the most dire circumstances. This situation is particularly true for those infected and diagnosed prior to the implementation of ART. However, within the population of older PLWHA, which is overrepresented by individuals who are racial, ethnic, and sexual minorities, it is also likely that many of these individuals have navigated the realities of homophobia, sexism, racial/ethnic discrimination, and economic discrimination. Despite these conditions, many have demonstrated fortitude, grit, and determination that have empowered them to enact adaptive processes to confront these social conditions, and which likely equips them to effectively address the realities associated in aging with HIV. This quality and its associated processes have come to be understood as resilience. Deciphering resilience may also provide us with a lens upon which healthcare providers may build their delivery of care.

It is with these conceptions of a biopsychosocial perspective and resilience that we approach the ideas presented in this chapter. Throughout the last decade, there has been a vast literature examining the physical complications of aging with HIV [13]. In this chapter, we seek to look beyond the physical aspects of health and attend to the psychological and emotional realities of older adults living with HIV. First, we examine the literature to date regarding the mental health and psychosocial challenges of these adults. Thereafter, we consider the relationships and synergistic effects of mental health with physical and social health. We conclude our work by considering resilience among older PLWHA and by examining the buffering effects of this characteristic on the psychological, physical, and social health of older adults living with HIV; we present an overall paradigm for understanding the total health of the population. With no cure for HIV/AIDS and ongoing incidence of this disease in new generations, what we understand and know about the psychological and overall health, and the resilience embodied by members of this first generation of adults aging with HIV will have long lasting implications as HIV-positive individuals in the United States and around the world continue to age with HIV for the foreseeable future.

## Mental Health and Psychosocial Challenges in Older Adults Living with HIV

Older PLWHA confront myriad mental health burdens and psychosocial challenges. For example, Warren-Jeanpiere et al. [14] reported that among 23 women participating in the Washington DC Women's Interagency HIV Study, 22 had at least one comorbid disease, more than half noted three or more conditions, and depression was noted in approximately one-quarter of the women. Similarly, Chambers et al. [15] found that depression is a key health challenge for older PLWHA.

Depression, stigma, ageism, and diminished social capital are among the most common mental health issues and/or psychosocial challenge factors affecting populations aging with HIV. The mental health of PLWHA is also shaped by experiences of anger, anxiety, frustration, fear, and loss of hope as members of the population enter older adulthood [6]. Moreover, the medical comorbidities that accompany aging with HIV create clusters of symptoms that include synergies between anxiety, disruptions in interpersonal relationships, stigma, overt discrimination, and/or violence [16].

Vance et al. [12] identified the level of depression as a key factor explaining the cognitive efficiency, mental health, and productivity of older PLWHA, with heightened depression being associated with less successful aging. In particular, depression, in combination with stress, anxiety, and constant thinking about HIV, also referred to as rumination, were shown to have a negative impact on aging successfully. As part of the Veterans Aging Cohort 5-Site Study, Justice et al. [17] found a higher prevalence of depressive symptomatology among older PLWHA veterans as compared to age-matched HIV-negative veterans. Data from the Research on Older Adults with HIV Study indicate that approximately 40% of 914 New York City-based older female and male PLWHA meet the criteria for severe depressive symptomatology [5], while another study of 83 older PLWHA reported 25% of the sample of 83 with severe or moderate levels of depression [18]. Corroborating these findings, Halkitis et al. [19] identified depressive symptoms in 20% of a sample of HIV-positive MSM aged 50 and over, a high level of association between depressive symptoms and post traumatic stress disorder (PTSD), and depression as one part of a constellation of interlocking health problems faced by older PLWHA. Depression, as part of a syndemic [19], is supported by the work of Illangasekare et al. [20] which found that intimate partner violence and substance use was associated with depression in HIV-positive African-American women. Such heightened levels of depression in older PLWHA indicate the need for psychological support, coupled with information about the management of HIV and aging [21].

The mental health of older PLWHA is highly linked to psychosocial challenges associated with HIV and aging, ageism and other forms of stigma and diminished social capital, including higher levels of loneliness [5, 15]. It has been noted that older PLWHA who endorse more psychological symptoms also report more HIV-related life-stressor burden and less support from friends [18]. In this regard, loneliness and social isolation are often amplified due to the added burden of HIV/AIDS resulting in the fear of disclosure of serostatus [22], which may undermine access to care and compromise the overall well-being. Such conditions may be exacerbated further by experiences of ageism [23]. Besides ageism, the psychological health of older PLWHA is negatively impacted by experiences of stigma related to sexual orientation (homonegativity) as a result of a heterosexist and antigay society, which are further heightened among racial and ethnic minorities [24].

Lack of social support, experiences of stigma, and loneliness are associated with negative consequences [22, 23, 25–28]. Such life circumstances may function to exacerbate mental health burdens in older PLWHA and undermine the overall well-being of these individuals.

### Mental Health and Associated Comorbidities in Older Adults Living with HIV

The World Health Organization conceptualizes health as 'a state of complete physical, mental and social well-being and not just the absence of disease or infirmity' [29]. Both mental health and psychological well-being are critical to ensure that a strong overall physical health status is met and maintained. The National Institute of Mental Health reports that 15.3% of adults aged 50 and over are living with a mental illness in the United States [30], and prevalence is even higher in older PLWHA [31, 32]. In fact, older PLWHA demonstrate higher levels of affective distress than both older and younger HIV-negative counterparts (although equivalent rates to younger PLWHA) [3]. Among 144 PLWHA screened at an outpatient clinic in Brazil, over one-quarter met the criteria for depression [33]. Differences in mental health states such as depression may be higher among female PLWHA than male PLWHA [34] and are indicative of the unique challenges that may be faced by seropositive women [35].

Higher prevalence rates of mental disorders such as depression are also noted among individuals living with other long-term conditions including cardiovascular disease [36], chronic obstructive pulmonary disease [37], and diabetes [38]. The interactive effects between physical health conditions and mental health have been observed in the literature. For example, Herbst et al. [36] demonstrate the association between depression/dysthymia and coronary heart disease.

Diminished psychological health may function to compromise the overall health of PLWHA by interfering with consistent access to care. In a study of 503 HIV-infected gay/bisexual men, 47% screened positive for anxiety disorder, 22% screened positive for depressive mood disorder, and 19% had elevated substance use [39]. Importantly, only 33% of those with anxiety disorder, 50% of those with depressive mood disorder, and a mere 9% of those with substance abuse symptoms, were identified as utilizing primary care, potentially compromising their overall health and well-being. Similarly, Israelski et al. [39] found that of 210 HIV-positive participants, 56% met symptom criteria for at least one mental health disorder, and 35% reported use of psychotropic medications. Among those who met the screening criteria for depression, acute stress disorder, and/or PTSD, 43% had not received any mental healthcare treatment. Given the elevated rates of mental health problems in PLWHA, it is critical for healthcare providers to ensure that they are properly screening patients for psychological disorders and the social circumstances that may diminish both mental and physical health [35]. In effect, optimal care for older PLWHA cannot be viewed as a single disease issue but must address the mental health and other comorbidities associated with HIV [14].

The mental health of PLWHA is highly associated with HIV disease indicators. Specifically, depression, trauma, and chronic stress have been implicated in HIV disease progression. A review of the extant literature [40] has shown that depression, ongoing trauma, and chronic stress are associated with decreases in CD4 counts, increases in HIV viral load, and a greater risk for clinical decline and mortality. In a cross-sectional study conducted at the Washington University HIV outpatient clinic, Taniguchi et al. [41] also found that as symptoms of depression increased, there was a linear decline in CD4 counts. This association may have been confounded by the fact that adherence to ART was suboptimal in those who had severe depressive symptoms. Similarly, in a sample of PLWHA in West Africa, those who met criteria for depression demonstrated a 2.3 greater odds of having CD counts <50 cells/μl [41]. Working with a sample of HIV-positive women, Evans et al. [34] suggested a mechanism by which depression affects HIV-related health, such that depression is proposed to decrease natural killer cell activity and lead to an increase in activated CD8 T lymphocytes and viral load. The association between depression and HIV-related health may explain mortality rates detected by Ickovics et al. [42]. Over a seven-year period, HIV-positive women with depressive symptoms were two times more likely to die than those with limited or no depressive symptoms.

It is likely that the effects of mental health burdens on HIV-related health, in part, are mediated by adherence to ART. In our own study of HIV-positive MSM aged 50 and over, adherence, failing to take HIV medications based on schedule and following medication instructions, were both associated with higher levels of depression [43]. Interestingly, Ghidei et al. [44] found that adherence to ART was stronger among older PLWHA compared to their younger counterparts. Such a finding points to the fact that despite the myriad physical, mental health, and psychosocial challenges faced by older PLWHA, the population of aging PLWHA is also resilient in their own right.

## Resilience in Older Adults Living with HIV

As has been demonstrated in the previous sections of this chapter, older PLWHA face a variety of complex psychological and psychosocial burdens that may compromise their mental health and potentially impact their overall health. Not attending to these mental health issues may seriously compromise the overall well-being of older PLWHA [45]. These conditions support a biopsychosocial model of healthcare for older PLWHA, which attends to all aspects of health and is not confined solely to the common denominators of suppressed viral load and elevated CD4 counts. While these are clinically significant markers regarding the course of viral infection, such biomarkers are insufficient to assure overall health integrity of individuals. Robert Espinoza summarizes this ides as follows:

> Yet aging with HIV can be especially difficult. Older adults with HIV report high levels of isolation, yet few community spaces embrace their full identities as older people, people with HIV and, in most cases, given the epidemic's prevalence, LGBT and people of color. Additionally, medical research has found multiple health concerns related to aging with HIV – and the psychological dimensions of living with HIV, or a new diagnosis, can spur its own storms. Without a large-scale,

dedicated response, the 'younger' end of this older adult spectrum, including Don [the author's friend], will join their older peers over the next decade in entering an aging system unprepared to meet their unique needs, despite their overwhelming numbers [46].

The circumstances described in Espinoza's editorial are indicative of the current state of care for many older adults living with HIV. In addition to the physical and psychological aspects that characterize the lives of PLWHA, psychosocial challenges, including isolation and financial hardships, add stress to the already overburdened lives [47]. Thus, it would appear, based on one perspective in the existing literature to date [5, 18, 48], that the outlook for older PLWHA is bleak, despite the benefits bestowed by ART which transforms the disease to one that is chronic, with which one can have a near-normal life expectancy. However, there is another approach to understand the life experiences of older PLWHA – an approach that focuses on strength and not on deficit, namely resilience [6]. This perspective aligns with the trends in psychology over the last several decades that have shifted focus from deficit-based models to strength-based models [49].

## Contextualizing Resilience in Older Adults Living with HIV/AIDS

The AIDS Generation is defined as those who came of age during the bleakest period of the epidemic, prior to the implementation of ART in the mid- to late-1990s [6]. This concept is rooted in the work of Strauss and Howe, and describes a generation as encountering key historical events and social trends while occupying the same phase of life [50]. These historians purport that members of a generation are shaped in lasting ways by the eras they encounter as children and young adults. All individuals who came of age in this period, including those who are currently older PLWHA, are members of the AIDS Generation. This notion of a generational effect is supported further by epidemiological findings which indicate the highest prevalence of HIV in gay men born between 1960 and 1964 [51].

This digression into the conception of the AIDS Generation is critical to our understanding of the role that resilience may play in the lives of the current cohort of older adults living with HIV. More than any other generation that has followed HIV-positive individuals of the AIDS Generation are those who confronted a disease that was, at the time of their diagnosis, associated with mortality within a short period of time. Halkitis [6] delineates the workings of resilience in HIV-positive gay men who were members of the AIDS Generation and suggests that proactivity and attendance to the physical, psychological, and social aspects of one's health was indicative of the determination and grit, the resilience that may have been key to the survival of these men. Resilience may have not been sufficient in preventing mortality, but it is a characteristic that many who have survived over the course of the last few decades while living with HIV appear to embody.

Before further delving into the concept of resilience and the role that it may play in buffering complex and interconnected health issues, it is also critical to nest the life experiences of the current generation of older adults living with HIV within a socio-political context. The epidemiological landscape of the aging HIV-positive population in the United States suggests that sexual and racial/ethnic minorities are overrepresented, both in terms of prevalence and incidence of HIV infection [52]. For almost all of these individuals, the fight for civil liberties and rights defined the periods of childhood and adolescence. In fact, the 1960s and 1970s was the time when gay men, African Americans, and women were fighting for their place within American society. For many of the current cohort of older adults living with HIV, the disease was simply another in a long series of battles that defined their lives – perhaps a critical component in understating the development of the quality of resilience in this population. Thus, resilience may be a trait that evolves and manifests over time [53]. While it is beyond the scope of this chapter to examine the development and origins of resilience, these aforementioned ideas are presented to consider the role that life circumstances and environmental influence, including tools bestowed by parents, caregivers, and communities, in addition to developmental and biogenetic factors, may play in understanding the resilient nature of some individuals [6, 53–55].

### Conceptualizing Resilience in Older Adults Living with HIV/AIDS

There is no one consistent definition for resilience in the extant literature [56, 57]. Generally, resilience is understood both as a trait and as a dynamic adaptive process [58]. As a trait, it refers to hardiness, grit, resourcefulness, strength of character, and determination – an innate ability or temperament that allows one to meet the challenges of life. As an adaptive process, resilience refers to a dynamic feedback loop of actions and coping mechanisms, whereby individuals are empowered to manage adversities and traumas in life. Through actions and cognitive strategies that promote psychological health, resilience equips individuals to adapt to stressful life events and maintain a sense of normality in terms of overall functioning and well-being [59, 60]. Healthier outcomes are the result of the adaptation and management of life circumstances afforded by resilience and resilient processes. Regardless of how resilience is conceptualized, there is a general consensus that resilience involves positive adaptation in light of adverse circumstances [56]. Hence, living, surviving, and thriving with HIV and the trauma of the AIDS crisis is evocative of resilience [61].

In our conceptualization of the construct in older adults living with HIV, resilience is viewed in 2 ways. First, we view resilience as a trait or temperament; secondly we understand the adaptive actions or approaches undertaken by individuals to cope and manage adversity as resilient processes. It has been suggested that for long-term survivors of HIV, engaging coping strategies that attend to their physical and socio-emotional health, even in the absence any effective therapies, were demonstrative of resilience [6]. To this point, resilient individuals are capable of enacting strategies that are protective against challenging life circumstances, and these strategies emanate from an innate trait. The behaviors and cognitive strategies used to adapt to adversity are manifestations of the person's resilient nature. One of the men portrayed in Halkitis' book defined resilience as follows:

> Resilience means making the choice, after months and months of vomiting, diarrhea, and being in pain and finally crawling back out of the hole, only to find yourself once again attacked and struck down even further, to take the step-by-step push to get back on top, even though you know that, physically, the top of the mountain is not possible. But you strive on [6].

This perspective exemplifies the notion that a resilient person enacts processes that are demonstrative of his/her resilient nature. The processes and actions are the manifest elements of resilience that are born from the latent trait. In short, we know a person to be resilient by the actions and cognitive strategies the individual enacts to manage the negative effects of adversity in his/her life.

Our conceptualization of resilience aligns with most of the current views that consider both the trait and process characterization of the construct. Taken together, resilience is both a constellation of characteristics [62] and a dynamic process of adaptability [60]. In the model proposed, we do not view these conceptions of resilience as conflicting but rather complementary. In short, we believe that resilience is a trait possessed by some older PLWHA that empower these individuals to undertake adaptive processes in response to life stressors; and when successfully used, serve to reinforce the resilient nature of these individuals.

For older PLWHA, resilience helps to counter the many life challenges these individuals face including but not limited to the realities of aging with disease, HIV-related stigma [63], ageism [4], and for many, sexual stigma and homophobia [64], racism [65], and/or discrimination due to socioeconomic status, position, and social class [66]. The adversities faced by many HIV-positive older adults, over and above HIV itself, necessitate actions that buffer against these adverse conditions, namely resilient processes. Managing HIV and coping with aging, coupled with psychosocial and structural burdens, create challenges in the lives of older PLWHA. Those who possess resilience react to the challenges brought on by these conditions by invoking processes which mitigate the impact of these adverse life circumstances on their health.

To date, literature addressing resilience in older PLWHA incorporates both the trait and process-oriented characterizations of the construct. While there is a lack of consistency in terminology used, all point to similar understandings in the population of older PLWHA, namely that many older adults living with HIV possess resilient natures which enable them to enact resilient processes in the light of adversities such as those noted above. Emlet et al. [67] delineate seven qualities that are indicative of resilience that include both trait and process conceptions: self-acceptance, optimism, will to live, generativity, self-management, relational living, and independence. These ideas complement those of Barroso, in which resilience is understood more in relation to processes than as a trait, and which include normalizing, focusing on living, taking care of one's self, being in relation with others, and triumphing as the foundations for surviving AIDS [68, 69]. Halkitis' understanding of resilience in this population also centers on processes – the will to live, the efforts undertaken to live, and the adoption of strategies to empower one's physical, emotional, and social well-being, even in the light of the most dire conditions [6]. Regardless of how it is defined in the population of older PLWHA, resilience is highly related to positive emotionality [70]; and, thus, the trait of resilience is likely to empower the individual to enact processes or actions which bestow beneficial effects on emotional, physical, and social health.

As has been described earlier, the aging process itself, HIV, HIV treatments, and the complex interaction of the aforementioned, are critical drivers of the health of older adults living with HIV. It is posited that these psychosocial and structural burdens impact all aspects of well-being. In this light, resilience can be understood as a quality that empowers individuals to enact processes which provide buffering effects against these sets of interlocking adverse conditions, in effect ameliorating the negative sequelae of these drivers. As such, resilience has been demonstrated across socioeconomic strata [71]. It has been noted in gay older men who have lived through the early days of the AIDS crisis [72] and in those who actually do age and grow older living with HIV [28]. Moreover, this view of resilience aligns with the meta-model of stress, emotions, and performance [73] in which it is proposed that the personal characteristics of some individuals enable them to enact processes that mitigate the impacts of stress.

The mediating (i.e., buffering) effects afforded by the processes enacted by resilient older PLWHA have been documented in the literature. Based on cross-sectional data drawn from a sample of 299 older PLWHA, researchers demonstrated that resilient processes in the form of coping self-efficacy, active coping, social support, and a resilient trait in the form of hope/optimism, reduced the negative impact of life stressors on the physical, emotional, and functional well-being [74–76]. Such beneficial effects were also demonstrated in a comparison of HIV positive and HIV-negative adults in San Diego [27]. While HIV-positive individuals reported poorer successful aging, psychosocial stress, physical, and mental health than their seronegative counterparts, the groups did not differ with regard to the traits of resilience and optimism, and the process of personal mastery, all of which were found to be related to self-reported successful aging regardless of serostatus. With this in mind, Vance et al. [61] suggest that hardiness (i.e., resilience viewed as trait) functions to mitigate the effects of HIV. Specifically, it is proposed that health outcomes and resilient processes, namely cognitive efficiency, social competency, productivity, personal control, and life satisfaction would be compromised in the absence of hardiness among older adults living with HIV. This perspective suggests our own understanding of the resilient trait, which gives rise to resilient processes in the presence of adversity, which in turn are protective of health in older adults living with HIV.

## Modeling the Role of Resilience on the Health of Older Adults Living with HIV/AIDS

Despite the diversity terminology used to describe and define resilience, the terms point to one overriding concept of resilience, namely a characteristic that enables the individual to enact effective actions that mediate and buffer against challenging life conditions. For older PLWHA, these challenges include living with and managing HIV, aging, and the psychosocial stressors many of these individuals face. Because of the health benefits, which may be afforded by resilience, the Office on AIDS Working Group on HIV and aging has identified understanding resilience in some individuals and methods by which resilience may be developed in others as a priority area of research [77].

To understand the buffering effects of resilience on the well-being of older PLWHA, we must accept the proposition that the health needs of older PLWHA are multidimensional and require that we attend to mental health and social health in addition to the physical and HIV-related health of the population, in effect adapting a biopsychosocial and holistic perspective [19]. Successful aging does incorporate all of these domains and necessitates active engagement with life, maximization of high cognitive and physical functioning, prevention of disease and disability, and spirituality in the context of developmental processes [78]. In recent years, numerous models have been proposed that encompass this biopsychosocial concept of well-being and multiple health challenges faced by older adults living with HIV. Havlik et al. [11] consider the interconnectedness of 4 dimensions of aging within this population, namely depression, HIV and other health risks, multiple morbidity and adherence to HIV and other treatments, while Vance et al. [61] illustrate the impact that hardiness may have on successful aging with HIV. Justice [8], while primarily focused on physical health, suggests a paradigm by which HIV, viral hepatitis and substance use, in combination with aging are conceptualized to drive immune deterioration. Halkitis et al. [19] propose a multilevel model of aging in gay men, regardless of serostatus, in which physical, mental, social and sexual health, and heath care utilization, are proposed to be directed by micro-, meso- and macro-level factors. Finally, O'Brien et al. [79] conceptualize the experiences of episodic disability that may be experienced by individuals living with HIV.

It is with this conception of health we put forth a theoretical model which delineates the role of resilience in relation to the overall health of older adults living with HIV (fig. 1). In this view, the health of older PLWHA is operationalized as physical and socio-emotional health; and these health states are mutually reinforcing and synergistic, creating a concept of total health. Health of older PLWHA is, in turn, directed by three sets of stressors: (1) HIV and HIV treatments, (2) aging and aging processes, and (3) psychosocial and structural burdens. These three sets of factors individually and interactively direct and may compromise the health of older adults living with HIV. In the model, resilience is viewed as an innate, latent trait of older adults living with HIV that endows them to enact effective strategies to buffer against the

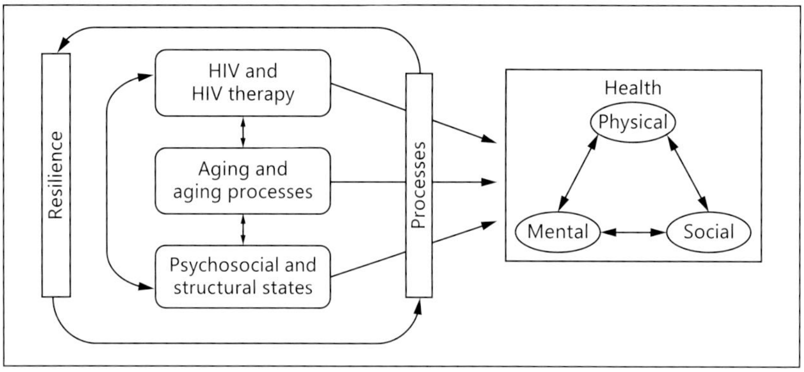


**Fig. 1.** Resilience and health paradigm for older PLWHA.

effects of stressors on the overall health. These resilient processes are envisioned as buffers dampening the impact of the life stressors on health by empowering the individuals to enact actions to manage these life stressors, rather than shields which provide complete protection from the impacts of these stressors on health [80].

In this paradigm, resilience is manifested in the actions and processes undertaken by an individual to create the buffering effects. If an older PLWHA is one who possesses this trait, the individual is more empowered to take control of these life circumstances, face adversities 'head on', and enact approaches, which may mitigate the negative effects that these life circumstances may have on one's health. The processes are understood as active and proactive steps one takes to confront these challenges. In this proposed model, resilience is understood in this manner, namely the actions invoked by older PLWHA to enhance their health by managing aging, HIV, and psychosocial stressors in their lives. Because this conception of resilience is rooted in tangible actions and processes, it empowers us to document these resilient processes, and enables us to develop them in others who do not possess this innate ability of resilience.

A critical component of the model indicates a feedback loop between the trait of resilience and resilient processes. It is posited that individuals who enact successful processes in response to challenging circumstances further bolster confidence in their own resilient natures. It has been proposed that such positive experiences may be critical in the development of resilience [80]. This understanding further supports the notion that resilience may be developed over time as the individual effectively, and over numerous interactions with the environment, enacts adaptive strategies to control life struggles [81]. In fact, it has been proposed that adversity in childhood and protective mechanisms enacted by children in response to these conditions may promote resilience in adulthood [82]. In this regard, many older PLWHA, most of whom are members of marginalized populations (i.e., racial and ethnic minorities, sexual minorities, and women), likely experience numerous psychosocial stressors during their lifetimes which necessitated the enactment of resilient processes, even at very young ages – conditions which may have helped to further reinforce the resilient nature of these individuals over the course of their lives. For many older HIV-positive gay men, HIV was another in a long list of struggles that they combatted in their lifetimes [6]. Like a muscle that strengthens and tones with optimal and effective use, resilience may also be enhanced when the processes that emanate from this trait lead to successful outcomes. This idea aligns with the crisis competence model first articulated by Kimmel [83]. As is shown in figure 1, we propose that the trait of resilience of the older adult living with HIV/AIDS enables an individual to enact resilient processes to ameliorate the impact of life stressors on the overall health; implied in this loop is that as these processes bestow beneficial effects on health, the resilient nature of the individual is further bolstered.

## Conclusions

The resilience model that we propose has implications for both individuals and populations. In effect, the basic tenets of the model effect may be used to inform how healthcare providers work with their patients and how public health practitioners and policy makers address the needs of an ever-growing population of older adults living with HIV in the United States and globally. In addition, the model provides a testable tool for researchers.

For clinicians working with older PLWHA, two important elements of our model inform working with patients. First, there needs to be recognition that the health of patients must be understood as more than the management of physical well being, and that approaches to care should address both physical and socio-emotional conditions. Second, by understanding the successful processes enacted by patients with higher levels of resilience, practitioners may utilize their patient's own adaptive strategies in formulating effective programs of care that build on patient strength. Finally, through this understanding, practitioners can document adaptive strategies to help provide tools for those patients with less resilient natures. By delineating and documenting concrete and tangible strategies used by those with more resilience, clinicians may be able to provide behavioral and cognitive strategies for managing the adversities of aging with HIV for others who are less resilient. Consecutively, the successful enactment of these processes (i.e., yielding optimal results) may also serve to further build the individual's innate resilience. Such an approach to treatment helps redirect care from being focused on deficit to being focused on strength.

With regard to public health, a resilience-based model, as the one we propose, may help to frame messaging and programming that focuses on what is working well, rather than dwelling on what is failing. This approach may inspire and support the many who are aging with HIV, who experience isolation and may help to further the development of 'community' within this population. Such a system of social support in which the more able function to support and elevate the less able, which leads to the development of a community that cares for its own, was the underlying premise of The Buddy Program developed by Gay Men's Health Crisis at the onset of the epidemic – a program that recently has been re-envisioned as one for supporting aging HIV-positive individuals.

Finally, the model of resilience that we have put forth is highly testable, and thus provides researchers with a paradigm for examining the proposed constructs that constitute the model and the protection bestowed by a resilient nature and resilient processes on the health of older HIV-positive adults. Specifically, by operationalizing resilience in relation to processes, researchers may be able to effectively operationalize and measure the workings of this latent state and determine the extent to which the processes actually function to mediate the relationship between life adversities and health or PLWHA; and, moreover, determine which strategies serve to bestow the greatest protection, with an eye that different processes may emerge as beneficial across the diverse sub-populations of older adults living with HIV.

In the end, the proposed resilience paradigm is a starting point in our attempt to further understand the role that resilience plays in the health of aging PLWHA specifically, and more broadly for all individuals living with challenging health conditions. It is also our expectation that the proposed model provides another element in the conversation regarding the care of older adults with HIV – a discussion that will be ongoing for the foreseeable future as new generations emerge into older adulthood living with HIV.

## Acknowledgements

The authors wish to acknowledge Dr. Farzana Kapadia and Christopher Stults for their support and insights.

## References

1 Bhatia R, Ryscavage P, Taiwo B: Accelerated aging and human immunodeficiency virus infection: emerging challenges of growing older in the era of successful antiretroviral therapy. J Neurovirol 2012; 18:247–255.

2 Deeks SG, Lewin SR, Havlir DV: The end of AIDS: HIV infection as a chronic disease. Lancet 2013;382: 1525–1533.

3 Rodriguez-Penney AT, Iudicello JE, Riggs PK, Doyle K, Ellis RJ, Letendre SL, Grant I, Woods SP; The HIV Neurobehavioral Research Program HNRP Group: Co-morbidities in persons infected with HIV: increased burden with older age and negative effects on health-related quality of life. AIDS Patient Care STDS 2013;27:5–16.

4 Emlet CA: 'You're awfully old to have this disease': experiences of stigma and ageism in adults 50 years and older living with HIV/AIDS. Gerontologist 2006;46:781–790.

5 Grov C, Golub SA, Parsons JT, Brennan M, Karpiak SE: Loneliness and HIV-related stigma explain depression among older HIV-positive adults. AIDS Care 2010;22:630–639.

6 Halkitis PN: The AIDS Generation: Stories of Survival and Resilience. Oxford University Press, 2013.

7 Heckman TG, Halkitis PN: Biopsychosocial aspects of HIV and aging. Behav Med 2014;40:81–84.

8 Justice AC: HIV and aging: time for a new paradigm. Curr HIV/AIDS Rep 2010;7:69–76.

9 Kaplan JE, Benson C, Holmes KK, Brooks JT, Pau A, Masur H; Centers for Disease Control and Prevention (CDC); National Institutes of Health; HIV Medicine Association of the Infectious Diseases Society of America: Guidelines for prevention and treatment of opportunistic infections in HIV-infected adults and adolescents. MMWR Recomm Rep 2009;58:1–207.
10 Montaner JS, Lima VD, Barrios R, Yip B, Wood E, Kerr T, Shannon K, Harrigan PR, Hogg RS, Daly P, Kendall P: Association of highly active antiretroviral therapy coverage, population viral load, and yearly new HIV diagnoses in British Columbia, Canada: a population-based study. Lancet 2010;376:532–539.
11 Havlik RJ, Brennan M, Karpiak SE: Comorbidities and depression in older adults with HIV. Sex Health 2011;8:551–559.
12 Vance DE, McGuinness T, Musgrove K, Orel NA, Fazeli PL: Successful aging and the epidemiology of HIV. Clin Interv Aging 2011;6:181–192.
13 Deeks SG: HIV infection, inflammation, immunosenescence, and aging. Annu Rev Med 2011;62:141–155.
14 Warren-Jeanpiere L, Dillaway H, Hamilton P, Young M, Goparaju L: Taking it one day at a time: African American women aging with HIV and comorbidities. AIDS Patient Care STDS 2014;28:372–380.
15 Chambers LA, Rueda S, Baker DN, Wilson MG, Deutsch R, Raeifar E, Rourke SB; Stigma Review Team: Stigma, HIV and health: a qualitative synthesis. BMC Public Health 2015;15:848.
16 Cook PF, Sousa KH, Matthews EE, Meek PM, Kwong J: Patterns of change in symptom clusters with HIV disease progression. J Pain Symptom Manage 2011; 42:12–23.
17 Justice AC, McGinnis KA, Atkinson JH, Heaton RK, Young C, Sadek J, Madenwald T, Becker JT, Conigliaro J, Brown ST, Rimland D, Crystal S, Simberkoff M: Psychiatric and neurocognitive disorders among HIV-positive and negative veterans in care: veterans aging cohort five-site study. AIDS 2004;18(suppl 1):S49–S59.
18 Heckman TG, Heckman BD, Kochman A, Sikkema KJ, Suhr J, Goodkin K: Psychological symptoms among persons 50 years of age and older living with HIV disease. Aging Ment Health 2002;6:121–128.
19 Halkitis PN, Kupprat SA, Hampton MB, Perez-Figueroa R, Kingdon M, Eddy JA, Ompad DC: Evidence for a syndemic in aging HIV-positive gay, bisexual, and other MSM: implications for a holistic approach to prevention and health care. Ann Anthropol Pract 2012;36:365–386.
20 Illangasekare SL, Burke JG, McDonnell KA, Gielen AC: The impact of intimate partner violence, substance use, and HIV on depressive symptoms among abused low-income urban women. J Interpers Violence 2013;28:2831–2848.
21 Nokes KM, Chew L, Altman C: Using a telephone support group for HIV-positive persons aged 50+ to increase social support and health-related knowledge. AIDS Patient Care STDS 2003;17:345–351.
22 Chambers LA, Wilson MG, Rueda S, Gogolishvili D, Shi MQ, Rourke SB: Evidence informing the intersection of HIV, aging and health: a scoping review. AIDS Behav 2014;18:661–675.
23 Grodensky CA, Golin CE, Jones C, Mamo M, Dennis AC, Abernethy MG, Patterson KB: 'I should know better': the roles of relationships, spirituality, disclosure, stigma, and shame for older women living with HIV seeking support in the South. J Assoc Nurses AIDS Care 2015;26:12–23.
24 Slater LZ, Moneyham L, Vance DE, Raper JL, Mugavero MJ, Childs G: The multiple stigma experience and quality of life in older gay men with HIV. J Assoc Nurses AIDS Care 2015;26:24–35.
25 Bland SE, Mimiaga MJ, Reisner SL, White JM, Driscoll MA, Isenberg D, Cranston K, Mayer KH: Sentencing risk: history of incarceration and HIV/STD transmission risk behaviours among black men who have sex with men in Massachusetts. Cult Health Sex 2012;14:329–345.
26 Webel AR, Higgins PA: The relationship between social roles and self-management behavior in women living with HIV/AIDS. Womens Health Issues 2012; 22:e27–e33.
27 Moore RC, Moore DJ, Thompson WK, Vahia IV, Grant I, Jeste DV: A case-controlled study of successful aging in older HIV-infected adults. J Clin Psychiatry 2013;74:e417–e423.
28 Roger KS, Mignone J, Kirkland S: Social aspects of HIV/AIDS and aging: a thematic review. Can J Aging 2013;32:298–306.
29 Constitution of the World Health Organization: Am J Public Health Nations Health 1946;36:1315–1323.
30 Any Mental Illness (AMI) Among Adults. Bethesda, National Institute of Mental Health, 2014. https://www.nimh.nih.gov/health/statistics/prevalence/any-mental-illness-ami-among-adults.shtml.
31 Bing EG, Burnam MA, Longshore D, Fleishman JA, Sherbourne CD, London AS, Turner BJ, Eggan F, Beckman R, Vitiello B, Morton SC, Orlando M, Bozzette SA, Ortiz-Barron L, Shapiro M: Psychiatric disorders and drug use among human immunodeficiency virus-infected adults in the United States. Arch Gen Psychiatry 2001;58:721–728.
32 Schumacher JE, McCullumsmith C, Mugavero MJ, Ingle-Pang PE, Raper JL, Willig JH, You Z, Batey DS, Crane H, Lawrence ST, Wright C, Treisman G, Saag MS: Routine depression screening in an HIV clinic cohort identifies patients with complex psychiatric co-morbidities who show significant response to treatment. AIDS Behav 2013;17:2781–2791.

33 Troncoso FT, Conterno Lde O: Prevalence of neurocognitive disorders and depression in a Brazilian HIV population. Rev Soc Bras Med Trop 2015;48: 390–398.
34 Evans DL, Ten Have TR, Douglas SD, Gettes DR, Morrison M, Chiappini MS, Brinker-Spence P, Job C, Mercer DE, Wang YL, Cruess D, Dube B, Dalen EA, Brown T, Bauer R, Petitto JM: Association of depression with viral load, CD8 T lymphocytes, and natural killer cells in women with HIV infection. Am J Psychiatry 2002;159:1752–1759.
35 Durvasula R: HIV/AIDS in older women: unique challenges, unmet needs. Behav Med 2014;40:85–98.
36 Herbst S, Pietrzak RH, Wagner J, White WB, Petry NM: Lifetime major depression is associated with coronary heart disease in older adults: results from the national epidemiologic survey on alcohol and related conditions. Psychosom Med 2007;69:729–734.
37 Wagena EJ, Arrindell WA, Wouters EF, van Schayck CP: Are patients with COPD psychologically distressed? Eur Respir J 2005;26:242–248.
38 Doherty AM, Gaughran F: The interface of physical and mental health. Soc Psychiatry Psychiatr Epidemiol 2014;49:673–682.
39 O'Cleirigh C, Magidson JF, Skeer MR, Mayer KH, Safren SA: Prevalence of psychiatric and substance abuse symptomatology among HIV-infected gay and bisexual men in HIV primary care. Psychosomatics 2015;56:470–478.
40 Leserman J: Role of depression, stress, and trauma in HIV disease progression. Psychosom Med 2008;70: 539–545.
41 Kaharuza FM, Bunnell R, Moss S, Purcell DW, Bikaako-Kajura W, Wamai N, Downing R, Solberg P, Coutinho A, Mermin J: Depression and CD4 cell count among persons with HIV infection in Uganda. AIDS Behav 2006;10(4 suppl):S105–S111.
42 Ickovics JR, Hamburger ME, Vlahov D, Schoenbaum EE, Schuman P, Boland RJ, Moore J: Mortality, CD4 cell count decline, and depressive symptoms among HIV-seropositive women: longitudinal analysis from the HIV epidemiology research study. JAMA 2001;285:1466–1474.
43 Halkitis PN, Perez-Figueroa RE, Carreiro T, Kingdon MJ, Kupprat SA, Eddy J: Psychosocial burdens negatively impact HIV antiretroviral adherence in gay, bisexual, and other men who have sex with men aged 50 and older. AIDS Care 2014;26:1426–1434.
44 Ghidei L, Simone MJ, Salow MJ, Zimmerman KM, Paquin AM, Skarf LM, Kostas TR, Rudolph JL: Aging, antiretrovirals, and adherence: a meta analysis of adherence among older HIV-infected individuals. Drugs Aging 2013;30:809–819.
45 Emlet CA: Current knowledge and future directions on aging and HIV research. Behav Med 2014;40: 143–148.
46 Espinoza R: HIV, Aging, and LGBT People: A Metamorphosis. The Huffington Post, 2014.
47 Rueda S, Law S, Rourke SB: Psychosocial, mental health, and behavioral issues of aging with HIV. Curr Opin HIV AIDS 2014;9:325–331.
48 Sankar A, Nevedal A, Neufeld S, Berry R, Luborsky M: What do we know about older adults and HIV? A review of social and behavioral literature. AIDS Care 2011;23:1187–1207.
49 Richardson GE: The metatheory of resilience and resiliency. J Clin Psychol 2002;58:307–321.
50 Howe N, Strauss W: Generations: The History of America's Future, 1584 to 2069. Harper Collins, 1992.
51 Chan G, Bennett A, Buslin S, Dombrowski G, Golden M: Dramatic declines in lifetime HIV risk and persistence of racial disparities among men who have sex with men (MSM) in King County, Washington, USA. IAS; Vancouver, BC, Canada 2015, July 21.
52 Centers for Disease Control; National Center forHealth and PreventionL Viral Hepatitis, STD, and TB Prevention: HIV among People Aged 50 and Older 2015. http://www.cdc.gov/hiv/pdf/group/age/olderamericans/hiv-older-americans-fact-sheet-508.pdf.
53 Rutter M: Resilience: some conceptual considerations. J Adolesc Health 1993;14:626–631.
54 Simeon D, Yehuda R, Cunill R, Knutelska M, Putnam FW, Smith LM: Factors associated with resilience in healthy adults. Psychoneuroendocrinology 2007;32:1149–1152.
55 Ungar M: The importance of parents and other caregivers to the resilience of high-risk adolescents. Fam Process 2004;43:23–41.
56 Fletcher D, Sarkar M: Psychological Resilience: A Review and Critique of Definitions, Concepts, and Theory, 2014.
57 Davydov DM, Stewart R, Ritchie K, Chaudieu I: Resilience and mental health. Clin Psychol Rev 2010;30: 479–495.
58 Zautra AJ, Hall JS, Murray KE: Resilience: a new definition of health for people and communities; in Reich JW, Zautra, AJ, Hall JS (eds): Handbook of Adult Resilience. New York, The Guilford Press, 2010, pp 3–34.
59 Bonanno GA: Loss, trauma, and human resilience: have we underestimated the human capacity to thrive after extremely aversive events? Psychol Trauma 2008;S:101–113.
60 Luthar SS, Cicchetti D, Becker B: The construct of resilience: a critical evaluation and guidelines for future work. Child Dev 2000;71:543–562.
61 Vance DE, Struzick TC, Masten J: Hardiness, successful aging, and HIV: implications for social work. J Gerontol Soc Work 2008;51:260–283.

62 Connor KM, Davidson JR: Development of a new resilience scale: the Connor-Davidson Resilience Scale (CD-RISC). Depress Anxiety 2003;18:76–82.
63 Sayles JN, Ryan GW, Silver JS, Sarkisian CA, Cunningham WE: Experiences of social stigma and implications for healthcare among a diverse population of HIV positive adults. J Urban Health 2007;84:814–828.
64 Herek GM, Gillis JR, Cogan JC: Internalized stigma among sexual minority adults: insights from a social psychological perspective. J Couns Psychol 2009;56:32–43.
65 Ford CL, Daniel M, Earp JA, Kaufman JS, Golin CE, Miller WC: Perceived everyday racism, residential segregation, and HIV testing among patients at a sexually transmitted disease clinic. Am J Public Health 2009;99(suppl 1):S137–S143.
66 Bird ST, Bogart LM, Delahanty DL: Health-related correlates of perceived discrimination in HIV care. AIDS Patient Care STDS 2004;18:19–26.
67 Emlet CA, Tozay S, Raveis VH: 'I'm not going to die from the AIDS': resilience in aging with HIV disease. Gerontologist 2011;51:101–111.
68 Barroso J: Social support and long-term survivors of AIDS. West J Nurs Res 1997;19:554–573; discussion 573–582.
69 Barroso J: Focusing on living: attitudinal approaches of long-term survivors of AIDS. Issues Ment Health Nurs 1996;17:395–407.
70 Tugade MM, Fredrickson BL: Resilient individuals use positive emotions to bounce back from negative emotional experiences. J Pers Soc Psychol 2004;86:320–333.
71 Wagnild G: Resilience and successful aging. Comparison among low and high income older adults. J Gerontol Nurs 2003;29:42–49.
72 Genke J: Resistance and resilience: the untold story of gay men aging with chronic illnesses. J Gay Lesbian Soc Serv 2004;17:81–95.
73 Fletcher D, Fletcher J: A meta-model of stress, emotions and performance: conceptual foundations, theoretical framework, and research directions. J Sports Sci 2005;23:157–158.
74 Fang X, Vincent W, Calabrese SK, Heckman TG, Sikkema KJ, Humphries DL, Hansen NB: Resilience, stress, and life quality in older adults living with HIV/AIDS. Aging Ment Health 2015;19:1015–1021.
75 Beasley M, Thompson T, Davidson J: Resilience in response to life stress: the effects of coping style and cognitive hardiness. Pers Indiv Differ 2003;34:77–95.
76 Friborg O, Hjemdal O, Rosenvinge JH, Martinussen M, Aslaksen PM, Flaten MA: Resilience as a moderator of pain and stress. J Psychosom Res 2006;61:213–219.
77 High KP, Brennan-Ing M, Clifford DB, Cohen MH, Currier J, Deeks SG, Deren S, Effros RB, Gebo K, Goronzy JJ, et al: HIV and aging: state of knowledge and areas of critical need for research. A report to the NIH Office of AIDS Research by the HIV and Aging Working Group. J Acquir Immune Defic Syndr 2012;60(suppl 1):S1–S18.
78 Parker MW, Bellis JM, Bishop P, Harper M, Allman RM, Moore C, Thompson P: A multidisciplinary model of health promotion incorporating spirituality into a successful aging intervention with African American and white elderly groups. Gerontologist 2002;42:406–415.
79 O'Brien KK, Ibáñez-Carrasco F, Solomon P, Harding R, Cattaneo J, Chegwidden W, Gahagan J, Baxter L, Worthington C, Gayle P, Merritt B, Baltzer-Turje R, Iku N, Zack E: Advancing research and practice in HIV and rehabilitation: a framework of research priorities in HIV, disability and rehabilitation. BMC Infect Dis 2014;14:724.
80 Rutter M: Resilience concepts and findings: implications for family therapy. J Fam Ther 1999;21:119–144.
81 Galli N, Vealey RS: 'Bouncing Back' from adversity: athletes' experiences of resilience. Sport Psychol 2008;22:316–335.
82 Luecken LJ, Gress, JL: Early adversity and resilience in emerging adulthood; in Reich JW, Zautra, AJ, Hall, JS (eds): Handbook of Adult Resilience. New York, The Guilford Press, 2010, pp 238–257.
83 Kimmel DC: Adult development and aging: a gay perspective. J Soc Issues 1978;34:113–130.

Prof. Perry N. Halkitis
Center for Health, Identity, Behavior and Prevention Studies
College of Global Public Health and Langone School of Medicine, New York University
41 East 11th Street, Seventh Floor, New York, NY 10003 (USA)
E-Mail perry.halkitis@nyu.edu

Brennan-Ing M, DeMarco RF (eds): HIV and Aging. Interdiscipl Top Gerontol Geriatr.
Basel, Karger, 2017, vol 42, pp 204–221 (DOI: 10.1159/000448563)

# Medical, Social and Supportive Services for Older Adults with HIV

Lisa E. Cox[a] • Mark Brennan-Ing[b]

[a] School of Social and Behavioral Sciences, Stockton University, Social Work Program, Galloway, N.J., and
[b] ACRIA, Center on HIV and Aging, New York University College of Nursing, New York, N.Y., USA

**Abstract**

Older people living with HIV are increasingly requiring formal supportive community-based services. Supportive services are essential to medical care and treatment for older people living with HIV/AIDS. This chapter considers Andersen's behavioral model of health services, and explores the predisposing, enabling, and need factors that affect service utilization among the older HIV population. The Andersen model provides a lens to understand the need for supportive services to go beyond primary medical care. Examples of such services and referrals typically include medical and non-medical case management, clinical provider referrals, mental health and substance use treatment, housing assistance, legal services, nutrition, transportation, home care, emergency assistance, patient education support groups, and other programs such as the AIDS Drug Assistance Program and secondary prevention services. Barriers to assistance and support, and consequences and resources for caregivers are addressed. Aspects surrounding structural inequities, multiple-minority status, and HIV stigma are examined with the goal of offering insight and advocacy ideas for community-based providers and policy makers. In future, the healthcare and supportive services infrastructure must be better equipped to manage the distinctive treatment and care needs of HIV-positive older adults.



Worldwide trends suggest a 'graying' of the HIV epidemic with an increasing proportion of people with HIV aged 50 years or older. This demographic shift is not limited to resource-rich settings: one 2014 study in sub-Saharan Africa reported the greatest number of people with HIV 50 years of age or older being enrolled in HIV programs to-date [1]. By 2020, more than 70% of Americans with HIV are expected to be age 50 and older [2]. Currently, life-saving treatment in the form of highly active antiretroviral therapy (HAART) has transformed HIV from a terminal illness it was decades ago into a chronic, albeit serious, condition, and dramatically increased life expectancy of older people with HIV (OPWH).

However, new challenges have accompanied this success. While we witness a burgeoning number of OPWH, this population also faces high levels of comorbidities portending greater caregiving needs as they grow older. But many OPWH lack sufficient informal social support resources, and it is not clear how existing informal and formal support mechanisms will be able to address the complex needs of this growing population in the future [3, 4]. To complicate further, older people living with HIV must also cope with normative age-related changes in physical functioning that are unrelated to HIV, and often diminished vitality, poor financial situations, and social role loss. These individuals also cope with ostracism, fear, and stigma that still accompany HIV [5], and the taboos around sexuality and older adults that still pervade society [6, 7].

This chapter examines formal, community-based services and their role in supporting aging individuals with HIV. Formal services are distinguished from informal social supports, in that the latter is typically obtained from the social network of family, friends, and neighbors, is voluntary, and for the most part, unpaid [8]. Informal caregivers perform tasks to help OPWH remain healthy and active in their communities through assisting with instrumental and personal activities of daily living, including help with medication, housekeeping (cooking, cleaning), providing rides or escorts to medical appointments, financial management, advice, and vital emotional support [9].

In contrast, formal supports include services provided by professionally trained paid employees, such as the personal care assistant who may help with bathing, or providers such as case managers. Formal caregivers include health professionals, behavioral health specialists, and social workers who are trained and compensated for their work. The trained volunteers associated with AIDS service organizations (ASOs), AIDS care teams, and hospice programs also fall into this category. In many cases, formal support is accessed when the needs of the older individual outstrip the ability of informal caregivers with regard to time, resources, or skills (e.g., nursing care) [8].

Both formal and informal supports play a role in the lives of OPWH, and both types matter. Formal and informal support networks often work in tandem, and both are needed to help an older person thrive and maintain their independence in the community [8]. Therefore, optimal supports for older adults occur when these 2 systems work together. For example, without a personal care assistant (formal support), an older client's informal caregiver (a partner or child) who has a job, may need to miss work or find a creative way to assist the OPWH in his/her care.

#### Using the Andersen Model to Understand Service Use among Older Adults with HIV

Andersen proposed a conceptual model to explain utilization of health services, which has been generalized to examine formal service use in a variety of domains [10, 11]. The Andersen model contains 3 sets of predictive factors: predisposing, enabling, and

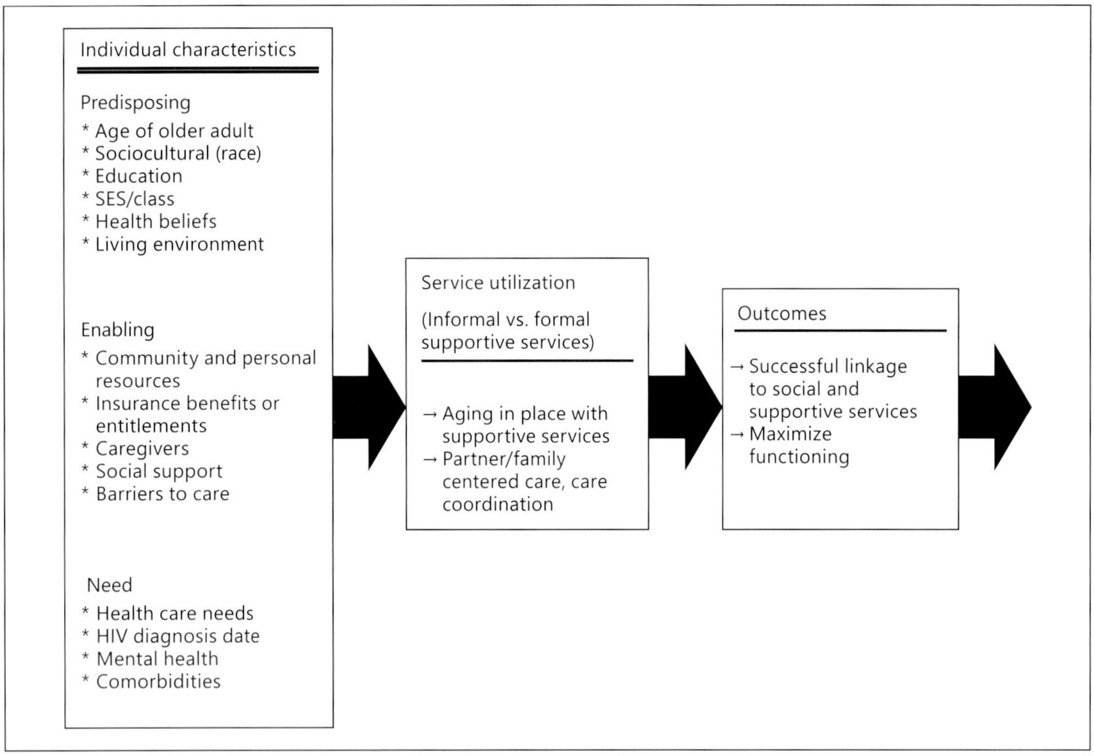


**Fig. 1.** Access to and use of supportive services among older adults living with HIV/AIDS (Andersen [10]).

need. Figure 1 portrays components of the Andersen model and envisions what formal service providers must consider to best help older people living with HIV/AIDS [3, 10]. When assessing and helping older people living with HIV/AIDS, these multiple individual characteristics require consideration.

Predisposing factors comprise demographic, social, and cultural characteristics, such as age, race/ethnicity, education level, class/socioeconomic status, health beliefs, and living environs (e.g., at home, in a long-term care or correctional setting, etc.). Such factors influence individuals to seek (or not seek) formal services to help them address their needs. Enabling factors are described by Andersen as one's community and personal resources (e.g., are they eligible for entitlements? who is the caregiver? how viable is their informal social network?), and barriers to care (e.g., lack of transportation) which can inhibit or promote service use. Need factors typically drive service utilization, such as health status (e.g., length of HIV and/or AIDS diagnosis, extent and severity of comorbidities), behavioral health needs (e.g., to what extent do co-occurring disorders exist, such as problem substance use, mental illness, etc.), and non-medical service needs (e.g., socialization, recreation, entitlement help). Applying the Andersen model to understand service utilization among OPWH, we will examine the predisposing, enabling, and need factors that characterize this population.

*Predisposing Factors*

Despite increasing rates of HIV among older people, this group continues to be unseen and marginalized in data collection, instruments, education and prevention programs, and treatment studies, to name a few. OPWH have been referred to as the 'overlooked epidemic', 'hidden population', and 'invisible epidemic' [12, 13]. Typically, older adult in the context of HIV infection is defined differently from the designation of old age in the general population. The Centers for Disease Control and Prevention (CDC) [14] categorizes older adults with HIV as being aged 50 or older. A person's life stage is always a consideration when providing supportive services due to changes in physiology, life circumstances, and emotional needs across the life span. Although the aging process for people with HIV is inadequately researched, OPWH on HAART can currently expect near-normal life expectancies [15]. However, their life stage may not always reflect their chronological age. OPWH may self-identify as older because they feel marginalized in society by age, as the US is extremely youth-oriented [16].

Many OPWH are members of historically disadvantaged groups, including gay/bisexual men and transgender women (GBT). Among those over 50 who are living with HIV, approximately 60% are GBT [14], sometimes referred to as men who have sex with men (MSM). As a group, lesbians have not manifested the same disproportionate rates of HIV infection as compared to other sexual and gender minorities, though it is important to note the historic role they have played in the epidemic with regard to advocacy and addressing the caregiving needs of those who are HIV positive. A subset of MSM does not embrace a gay or bisexual identity. Due to societal changes in attitudes and acceptance of homosexuality, it may be more common for older MSM to be married to or have been married to a woman than it is for younger MSM. Some MSM may seek sex in casual relationships or have dual lives, one as a married man and the other as a gay man [17].

Sexual and gender minorities tend to suffer from health disparities that result in higher levels of illness, disability, and premature death than observed in the general population [18]. In a large national US study of older lesbian, gay, bisexual and transgender (LGBT) adults, 50% had disability, 33% reported depression, and about 33% did not have a will or durable healthcare power of attorney [19]. Most research about the older gay and bisexual population has been conducted with Caucasians, thereby leaving critical gaps in provider's understanding, 'including potential models from communities in which the older LGBT population is well integrated' [20]. Thus, the literature on older gay/bisexual men along with transgender women remains underdeveloped, particularly for bisexual and transgender groups. Within this literature, diversity with regard to race/ethnicity, income and education is extremely under-researched, and the intersection of multiple disadvantaged and stigmatized identities among older LGBT individuals is not well understood. However, one study on service utilization among older HIV-infected adults found that sexual identity and gender were not strongly related to service utilization [3].

Little empirical research focuses on the service needs of older adults who are LGBT. These populations must often be creative in accessing supportive services and rely on chosen family (i.e., non-kin) rather than risk the possibility of being discriminated against by homophobic and transphobic service providers [3, 20–23]. Knochel et al. [20] found the lesbian and gay population to be incredibly invisible in both the gerontology literature and in the planning and provision of senior services. Mental health and substance use treatment utilization is low in this population [23].

Often providers fail to recognize and treat the person when they disclose their sexual orientation. Consequently, medical and social service providers may not fully understand the lifelong experiences of discrimination of these clients who came of age in an era of homophobia prior to the 1969 Stonewall Rebellion and the advent of the HIV/AIDS epidemic in the 1980s [20]. This lack of cultural competence on the part of service providers and clients' fear of discrimination often keeps individual caregivers, be it LGBT themselves or caring for LGBT people, from accessing services [22]. As a result, caregivers of older LGBTs may shoulder a greater amount of responsibility for a longer time than other caregivers [24].

Unfortunately, these negative life experiences of abuse and stigma have conditioned many OPWH who require supportive services to be mistrustful of mainstream institutions, including medical and social service providers. For example, treatment in long-term care and home health care settings is a major concern for older LGBT people due to unintended or unwanted disclosure of sexual orientation and/or gender identity to home health care workers, with concomitant fear of discrimination or retaliation [25]. Discrimination against LGBT older adults is well-documented; 13% of older LGBT adults had been denied healthcare or received inferior care and over 20% did not disclose their sexual or gender identities to their physician in one study [19].

According to the CDC, 40% of OPWH in the US are heterosexual cisgender men and women [14]. An egregious myth is to consider HIV to be a 'gay' disease that does not affect heterosexuals. However, heterosexual intercourse is now responsible for numerous transmissions worldwide. In particular, older Black men represent 68% of all heterosexually acquired HIV cases among US men in 2011 [14], and heterosexual transmission has become increasingly frequent since the start of the epidemic [26]. Financial challenges affect people aging with HIV, especially African Americans [27]. Many older adults may experience economic disparity; however, minorities, especially African American women, have disproportionately been affected by poverty and HIV [14, 28, 29].

*Enabling Factors*

According to Andersen [10, 11], enabling factors are those that can either facilitate or serve as barriers to service utilization. Many barriers to service utilization for OPWH are structural and arise from the composition and dynamics of the formal service sector. Barriers to assistance and supportive services in the US include inadequate funding and human resources, inappropriate policies, inadequate and unresponsive services, poor service coordination, and negative attitudes, abuse, and stigma. People who require supportive services are usually more vulnerable than those who do not. OPWH have needs for which assistance and supportive services are not neatly packaged into what a single provider can offer.

Furthermore, many OPWH lack informal social support resources, which may facilitate greater reliance on formal, community-based services. Many OPWH, including heterosexuals, often rely on chosen families of lovers, friends, and acquaintances rather than their families of origin (i.e., blood relatives) similar to the social network dynamics observed in LGBT communities [30]. Reliance on chosen families has the potential to stir up challenging issues regarding legal recognition of decision-making by non-kin caregivers, such as power of attorney or healthcare proxies [31]. Research has characterized how the social networks of OPWH may be characterized as fragile, given the lack of family involvement, poor perceived availability and adequacy of social support, and high degrees of social isolation [32]. This network fragility can drive formal service use as described by Cantor's Hierarchical Compensatory Theory of Social Support. According to this theory, when older people need assistance they prefer kin, first turning to close family such as spouses and children [8, 33]. When close family are not available, more distant relatives, friends, and neighbors are engaged. When these latter supports are not available, formal services are accessed. Formal services may also be utilized when the capacity of informal caregivers exceeds the needs of the older adult, for example, when advanced medical care in the home is required [8].

HIV stigma can inhibit the use of formal services. Cahill and Valadez [34] have aptly noted how HIV-positive people aged 50 years or older are typically more socially isolated than their younger counterparts. This isolation typically occurs because they may still be trying to conceal their HIV status, or they have sustained relentless social stigma associated with AIDS. HIV stigma, which refers to discrediting and discrimination directed towards people thought to have HIV, is a complicated process. Emlet's 2006 qualitative study used 25 in-depth interviews, to examine whether OPWH experienced both ageism and HIV stigma [35]. He discovered that 68% of respondents did experience both; however, the experiences were often distinct. Nine themes emerged from Emlet's study; interviewees reported experiencing rejection, stereotyping, fear of contagion, violations of confidentiality, and internalized ageism.

Whether an older adult has contracted HIV from sexual activity or injection drug use [36, 37], both modes of transmission are laced with stigma and may alter one's access to supportive services. Unfortunately, because of the ongoing misperception that HIV is a gay disease, people who are homophobic perpetuate stigma and discriminate against people. OPWH are affected differentially by stigma, depending on their sexual orientation, gender, and social networks. In reality, older adults who live with HIV may experience multiple stigmatizing attributes [34]. Newly diagnosed/infected people, even older people, are more likely to report feelings of stigma and 'blame' for their disease, and need help to adjust their medication regimen.

Because medical, social, and supportive service providers have not received adequate training, they may continue to be ageist and stigmatize the LGBT community [38], which presents barriers to OPWH who are sexual minorities. Fredriksen-Goldsen and Muraco [18] studied aging in non-heterosexual populations and found that predictors of poor mental health included experiences of discrimination by healthcare providers, loneliness, living alone, low self-esteem, internalized homophobia, and being victimized because of either their sexual orientation or gender identity/expression. Jessup and Dibble emphasize how the intersection of ageism and heterosexism is causing sexual minority elders to have 'fewer resources in the community and within healthcare systems for prevention, earlier diagnosis and assessment and treatment, thereby keeping them from accessing or seeking help' [23].

The problem of HIV stigma goes beyond those identified as gay or bisexual; all OPWH may face stigma-related lack of access to testing, treatment, and care. Due to HIV stigma, heterosexuals may be challenged to access supportive services simply because an HIV diagnosis can associate them with homosexual and/or drug use behaviors. As a result, medical, social, and supportive care services go unaddressed. Examples of 'unattended to needs' include mental health services for depression, anxiety or substance use, unstable housing, food insecurity, lack of economic and employment opportunities, assistive living, home healthcare, and so on [39–43]. Older heterosexuals, including those who are injection drug users, experience a high degree of HIV stigma and ageism. Consequently, this group may perceive less social support, and feel less in control of their life circumstances.

*Need Factors*

OPWH present with myriad needs, and seek community-based services to meet those needs [3]. The older adult population with HIV has a median age of 58 years, a chronological age that does not reflect the functional age of this population. Older adults with HIV are developing clinical symptoms of multimorbidity, namely multiple comorbid conditions, occurring 15–20 years earlier than expected [44–54]. A 2015 study of older adults with HIV details a spectrum of geriatric syndromes found in a sample whose average age was 57 [55]. In fact, the number of reports finding the typically geriatric-associated syndrome of frailty in HIV patients in their 5th and 6th decades of life is increasing [56–64]. Thus, the functional age of this older adult population is at least 20–25 years greater than their chronological age.

The mental and physical health of older adults with multiple minority status are affected by psychiatric symptoms and structural inequities in systems that find it continually easy to stigmatize and scapegoat those with HIV [60]. Thus, it is not surprising that OPWH are not typical of the aging population without HIV. Rates of depression are up to 5 times higher in OPWH compared to the general population [65], and OPWH evidence higher rates of suicidal ideation that contribute to reduced health outcomes. Rates of substance use are also increasing in the over 50 population, thereby highlighting the need for provider's attention to mental and physical health outcomes that require supportive services [23]. As they age, many OPWH use alcohol, tobacco, and other substances often as a self-medication strategy, further compromising their health [32]. They report difficulties with tasks of daily living, including housekeeping, transportation, meal preparation, employment, finances, and accessing entitlements [3]. Given their lack of informal social resources and social isolation, it is not surprising that the greatest reported services need among OPWH is opportunities for socialization [3]. Consequently, the provision of medical, social, and supportive services is essential for ensuring a decent quality of life for OPWH. If individual characteristics and service utilization aspects are understood, then the expected outcome for the older person living with HIV/AIDS would be that they would be successfully linked to medical and social/supportive services, and have the resources to maximize their physical and emotional functioning.

### Medical and Social Supportive Services for OPWH

The preceding review of the predisposing, enabling, and need factors that characterize the burgeoning population of OPWH underscores the importance of providing needed supportive services that span the bio-psycho-social spectrum of care. One can roughly divide service providers into those addressing medical and healthcare needs and those characterized as social services. However, in reality, these services exist on a continuum and may address multifaceted and overlapping needs. For example, in some instances ASOs may provide clinical medical services and social services at the same site. As another example, HIV case management programs may provide referrals for housing or employment opportunities to address social needs, but these may be in service of addressing medical needs such as strengthening care engagement and adherence to HAART [66]. Geriatric and gerontological care models and principles provide a valuable perspective on the service delivery system for OPWH as they emphasize considering the client in their environment with the goal of maximizing function through leveraging available personal and social resources [67]. Innovation is required on the part of providers, and segregated service settings may not be conducive to optimal client outcomes. Person-centered services, as prescribed by geriatric care models, can be very beneficial by allowing OPWH to be involved in decision-making and choose among supportive services they receive.

Medical assistance and social supportive services are complex because they are provided by diverse sources, funded in different ways, and delivered in many different locations. The cost of formal care and supportive services may be met with increased state and national government funding, insurance, charitable or voluntary sector, or through out-of-pocket payment from clients. Most likely, a combination of funding methods will be required to meet a growing demand for services in light of flat or reduced government support.

**Table 1.** Examples of formal supportive services for older people living with HIV/AIDS

| |
|---|
| *Support services for old (50–64), old-old (65–84) and oldest-old (≥85) HIV-infected people are varied:* |
| Home care |
| Aging in place with caregivers (family, friends, neighbors; informal support) |
| Aging in place with formal home healthcare |
| Teletherapies (supportive-expressive or coping group) |
| Medical/long-term care |
| Continuing care communities and assisted living |
| Intermediate care facilities (ICF level of care or assisted living) |
| Skilled nursing facilities (SNF level of care – long-term care) |
| Examples of community-based care |
| Adult day healthcare (ADHC) |
| Family-based services (FBS) |
| Job training program (JTP) |
| Legal advocacy services |
| Outreach to homeless |
| Prevention program for sex workers (e.g., project voice: housingworks.org HEAL) |
| Health library |
| Needle exchange and overdose prevention program |
| Mental health and substance abuse counseling (e.g., MALE center, Boston MA – for gay/bisexual men – aac.org) |
| Peer support – delivered by PLWH, provides individual and group support programs to reduce isolation and improve client's ability to manage their health. |
| Rental and utility assistance – deliver short-term emergency assistance to PLWH who face eviction, unaffordable housing, and high utility bills. |
| HOPWA |
| Volunteer-based support services: grocery shopping and small errands assistance; respite care Computer assistance; friendly visits; reassurance phone calls; minor home repairs; meals on wheels; discounted/access to medical alert devices; education, training and support groups; transportation. |
| Dental care assistance |
| Insurance continuation assistance program |
| HRSA part B support services – Ryan White Care Act |
| Faith-based organizations or pastoral care services |

Types of medical care and social/supportive services are depicted in table 1 with examples of existing formal supportive services available to OPWH. If OPWH have medical and/or social service needs, an array of programs may be accessed whether the older person resides in their own home, in a continuing care or assisted living community, or in a residential long-term care setting.

*Medical and Healthcare-Related Supportive Services*

Medical supportive services in this chapter refer to formal services that come from paid healthcare providers and social service providers (e.g., medical case management) that are embedded in medical care organizations.

The changing demographics of the HIV epidemic, along with the growing complexity of medical care, have created major challenges for healthcare professionals who provide curative and palliative care. For people receiving medical care services, decisions must still be made about when to start HAART, which drug combinations to use, and how to manage viral resistance and drug-specific toxicities. Therapeutic regimens often must be modified for people who are homeless and those with comorbidities, such as mental illness and chemical dependence [39, 40]. Early intervention services are available in many regions. The goal of such programs is to keep HIV-positive men and women healthier for longer periods. Physicians, knowledgeable in the latest HIV treatment guidelines, provide specialty appointments in infectious disease clinics.

Government-sponsored service delivery has traditionally focused on institutional care, such as hospitals or skilled nursing facilities (nursing homes) that are reimbursed through Medicaid and/or Medicare. Governments have also provided community-based services such as home healthcare or adult day care. As HIV-infected people age, the need for personal assistance services appears to be increasing. Paid personal care, for example, has traditionally and predominantly been provided by women, and often older women of low social status [68]. Little research has explored to what extent OPWH, many of whom cope with inadequate incomes, are receptive to caregivers who are themselves financially disadvantaged. When remaining at home is no longer an option due to complex health needs such as frailty, institutional-based care may be accessed, including palliative and/or hospice care.

In addition to physical healthcare needs, behavioral healthcare to address mental health issues are also provided by this sector. To manage physical limitations, grief from loss, and legal or financial difficulties, counseling and psychotherapeutic services may be helpful to OPWH. Some HIV-infected people may frequently experience depression or problematic substance use, but may be unable to access supportive services to manage these challenges [69]. Given the high rates of mental distress reported by OPWH [65], this is one arena where provider innovation is essential. Some innovations developed to-date involve the mechanism for delivering services. Research has been conducted on the utility of telephone-administered supportive-expressive group therapy or coping effectiveness training to reduce depressive symptoms in HIV-infected older adults [70]. Heckman et al. [70] noted how HIV-infected older adults have complex medical and mental health needs, tend to be diagnosed later in the course of their HIV disease, experience greater cognitive dysfunction, have lower CD4 cell counts and higher viral loads, and survive for shorter periods of time after progressing to AIDS. Because the same OPWH have comorbid health conditions and significant concerns about confidentiality or are geographically isolated from traditional mental health resources, teletherapy, especially supportive, expressive group therapy, may be much more practical than face-to-face interventions and may help to lessen depression, psychiatric symptoms (e.g., anxiety, hostility, somatization), and to decrease unprotected intercourse and increase immune function [70].

OPWH and their families often require care services that can be coordinated by medical case management, community-based medical care management, and nursing care management services [3]. Medical social workers assist people with HIV by addressing their most immediate needs and connecting them with ongoing case management services. Public health nurses and medical social workers team up to provide care management services to people with severely disabling HIV or AIDS, and their goal is to help clients remain independent and at home as long as safely possible. Basically, the healthcare team coordinates services including medical care, treatment adherence, attendant care, nutritional care, nutritional counseling, mental health, substance use treatment and home delivered meals. Clinic-based services may also include counseling, education and prevention services, and assistance with partner counseling, medication adherence counseling, and AIDS Drug Assistance Program (ADAP) certification.

Medical case managers provide support to people with HIV whose health status does not require the services of a nurse case manager. Also, medical case managers frequently collaborate with physicians and other providers to encourage adherence to the medical treatment plan. Services in the medical sector often target keeping the OPWH connected to the healthcare system. Medical social workers, outreach workers, nurses and healthcare navigators work as a team to support HIV patients in making and keeping appointments, understanding their medications and accessing necessary clinical and support services [32, 71]. Insofar as outreach and linkage to care, outreach and support services are available in some communities to support clients who are out-of-care. Outreach referrals are made for people who have broken medical appointments, are missing labs, or who need medication adherence support. Outreach is also provided to HIV-positive people who have never been connected to care. Outreach activities include home visits, phone calls, collateral contacts, case conferencing, and so on to locate clients.

These types of supportive services are absolutely essential to assure that healthcare works for people living with HIV/AIDS. The National HIV/AIDS Strategy for the United States (NHAS) released in July 2010, established 3 goals, thereby recognizing the healthcare needs of HIV-infected people. The goals are to: (1) reduce the number of people who become infected with HIV; (2) increase access to care and optimize health outcomes for people living with HIV; and (3) reduce HIV-related health disparities. Supportive services are instrumental in achieving these goals [72].

OPWH with limited financial resources may need to access entitlement programs to meet their medical care needs, such as ADAP. ADAP pays for the often costly medications needed to treat HIV. To be eligible for ADAP, a person must be HIV positive, a resident of a particular state, and be over 18, have limited or no prescription drug benefits, and meet financial eligibility requirements. ADAP is a carve-out of the Ryan White CARE Act that provides millions of dollars for HIV medications for people who are uninsured. More than '…70% of Ryan White HIV/AIDS program clients are people of color and in 2010, 39% of Ryan White HIV/AIDS Programs clients were MSM' [2].

Because each state government administers its own ADAP program, there are many variations [73]: (1) eligibility criteria for program participation varies from 125 to 500% of the federal poverty level; (2) the types of drugs covered varies, with some states having formularies that cover HAART medications only, while others have an open formulary covering any medication required by someone who is eligible for ADAP (e.g., cholesterol medications, mental health drugs, hepatitis treatments, etc.); (3) states vary in their requirement of co-pays for prescriptions; and (4) states differ in administration and distribution models, based on geography and demand for services. Historically, up to 9,000 people have been on ADAP waiting lists for life sustaining medications, and the ADAP Advocacy Association and other groups have pressured the US Congress to address this issue [74].

Some states offer health insurance premium payment programs that pay the monthly health insurance premiums for eligible residents with an HIV/AIDS diagnosis. These programs may be available to people with health insurance who are at risk of losing it, and to people currently without health insurance who would like to buy it. In these instances, medical social workers and other helping professionals can help clients with the application process and submit the completed application to the proper place. People who do not have private insurance can oftentimes call healthcare provider lines for free health advice or go to urgent care providers. However, those in rural areas may still have difficulties locating needed services. The Affordable Care Act (ACA) has expanded health coverage for millions of people nationwide, including OPWH, by eliminating insurance exclusions for pre-existing conditions such as HIV and expanding Medicaid eligibility for those with low incomes. The ACA offers protections such as not having being charged higher premiums because of an HIV diagnosis. People with HIV rely heavily on Medicaid – much more than the general population, 'due to high disability rates, multiple chronic conditions, and the low-income realities that qualify many people with HIV for Medicaid' [2]. Unfortunately, not all 50 states have expanded Medicaid under ACA.

*Social Supportive Services*

Social supportive services in this chapter will refer to assistance coming from non-medical providers that are frequently provided through governmental agencies or community-based organizations. Social and supportive services are numerous and address the needs of OPWH. Such services include transportation, support groups, nutritional support (prepared meals, food vouchers, and food pantries), recreational activities, socialization, personal hygiene assistance, harm reduction, mental health and substance use treatment, educational workshops, emergency cash assistance, financial and entitlement assistance, alternative therapies, housing services, budget management, legal services, HIV prevention and education, and so on. Therefore, when it comes to assessing the needs of HIV-infected older adults, helping professionals require knowledge of a person's bio-psycho-social well-being and supportive and social services that exist in a given community.

These services often supplement or supplant assistance from informal caregivers who provide emotional and practical support to friends and relatives living with HIV in line with Cantor's Hierarchical Compensatory Model [33]. For many OPWH, this type of non-medical assistance and supportive services are essential for maintaining social participation and remaining independent in the community. The lack of necessary support services can place extraordinary demands on primary informal caregivers (spouse/partners or family members) and can prevent both the OPWH and their informal helpers from becoming economically productive and socially involved. Globally, OPWH have significant unmet needs for supportive services, yet multiple policy and service gaps exist in low resource settings. Realistically, no one model of supportive services will work in all instances and meet everyone's needs and such assistance needs to be tailored to the specific context of OPWH.

Brennan-Ing et al. [3] examined service utilization among OPWH in New York City, a high resource setting that offers a wide variety of social services. This study classified supportive services into 4 main groups: (1) government agencies and programs; (2) HIV/AIDS programs; (3) health and long-term care services; and (4) senior services. Government agencies included offices for federal entitlement programs (e.g., Social Security, Medicaid) and city government agencies (New York City Housing Authority, Police Department). HIV/AIDS services comprised of entities such as ASOs, HIV Day Programs, the New York City Department of HIV/AIDS services, and non-medical case management. The last group of senior services included senior centers, nutritional support, and legal advice. Given the high level of need factors affecting OPWH, it is not surprising that they use a high volume of services. Brennan-Ing et al. [3] found that OPWH used 3 times as many non-HIV services on average as compared to community-dwelling older adults aged 65 and older.

The health and long-term care services domain has considerable overlap with the medical supportive services previously discussed. However, some services in this domain are provided by non-medical providers, for example, social work counseling. There can also be considerable overlap in the types of services provided in this sector. For example, mental health services such as counseling may be provided by general social service agencies, ASOs, or even faith-based settings. While multiple service venues are not necessarily undesirable, as they allow for multiple points of entry into the social service system, they do point to a need for service coordination and referral, as articulated in care coordination models.

One point of coordination and referral in the existing system are non-medical case management services provided through programs such as the Ryan White CARE Act. Case management has been called a metaservice that increases access to all manner of community-based service providers [75], and has been identified as a critical positive enabling factor with regard to service utilization among OPWH [3, 66]. Case management for those with HIV is largely focused on promoting medical care engagement and HAART adherence, by helping clients to navigate social services and facilitating resources, such as housing or mental healthcare, that support engagement and adherence goals [66]. Case management requires nonjudgmental assessments, thoughtful care plans and effective advocacy and monitoring on the part of case managers. When fragile social networks are evident, referrals to social services may be required. Referrals may also include clinical provider referrals, mental health and substance use treatment, housing assistance, legal services, food, transportation, home care, emergency assistance, patient education support groups, and other programs such as ADAP and prevention services. One study found that clients who received comprehensive case management evidenced significantly greater care engagement, and achieved parity in average CD4 T-cell counts with a non-case management comparator group [66].

One area where care coordination is problematic is between HIV/AIDS and senior service sectors who have not historically shared clients and are just beginning to develop collaborative relationships [76]. There are cultural barriers between these 2 service sectors. HIV services developed in a culture of activism and militant politics that was evidenced by groups such as Act Up [77], a results-oriented worldview that was fostered in the early days of the AIDS crisis. In contrast, the culture of senior service providers reflects many of the values of social work, with an emphasis on process, human dignity, and social justice [78]. Thus, the first step in coordinating services for OPWH is to have both HIV and senior service providers being able to communicate and work together effectively. A second barrier is the age of the 'older' person with HIV. At present, the vast majority of this population (75%) is 59 years or younger [14]. However, to be eligible for senior services funded through the Older Americans Act (e.g., senior center meals), clients must be aged 60 or older [79]. Thus, a large sector of senior services is presently unavailable to most OPWH due to this age restriction, although they present with many of the same service needs as those in older cohort of 60 years and above. While tying senior program eligibility requirements to chronological age seems objectively fair and simplifies intake, it fails to recognize that age in and of itself is not the best determinant of service needs and artificially proscribes valuable services from a population who would benefit by being able to access a variety of senior services.

## Conclusions and Future Directions

Growth in the population of OPWH, and their rates of disability influence supply and demand for medical and supportive services from the formal sector. Such supply and demand is also influenced by informal network composition, such as changes in family structure and friend-centered networks, and how such changes impact the ability of informal network members to be available, willing, and competent to provide the level of caregiving and assistance needed. The aging of OPWH, and their friends and family members, point to a greatly increased demand for supportive services provided through government or community sources. As the number of OPWH continues to increase in the US and worldwide, it is uncertain if existing supportive resources will be able to cope with this demographic shift in the HIV epidemic. However, given the prevalence of multimorbidity and numerous service needs, supportive services of all types will be needed, and the capacity of the system to provide such services must increase. While the current focus on preventing and curing HIV is essential to ending this epidemic, advocacy, policy and program planners must better address the needs for care in an aging HIV population, in a variety of high- and low-resource settings.

To best help OPWH gain access to these services, formal and informal caregivers must be skilled in negotiating and navigating formal supportive services and systems, modeling a person-centered perspective, and maintaining effective communication. Care managers and providers can best help OPWH when they exhibit the qualities of an affirming attitude, authenticity, integrity and honesty, a nonjudgmental attitude, and patience. Providers should also work to educate, inform, and empower the OPWH to become an active advocate and agent for their own service needs, for without the voice of the client in care decisions and planning, we are unlikely to provide the support necessary to promote healthy aging in this population.

## Acknowledgements

We would like to thank Liz Seidel, MSW for her assistance in the preparation of this manuscript.

## References

1 Eduardo E, Lamb MR, Kandula S, Howard A, Mugisha V, Kimanga D, Kilama B, El-Sadr W, Elul B: Characteristics and outcomes among older HIV-positive adults enrolled in HIV programs in four sub-Saharan African countries. PLoS One 2014; 9:e103864.
2 Diverse Elder Coalition: Eight policy recommendations for improving the health and wellness of older adults with HIV. 2014. http://www.diverseelders.org/resource/eight-policy-recommendations-for-improving-the-health-wellness-of-older-adults-with-hiv/ (retrieved May 5, 2016).
3 Brennan-Ing M, Seidel L, London AS, Cahill S, Karpiak SE: Service utilization among older adults with HIV: the joint association of sexual identity and gender. J Homosex 2014;61:166–196.
4 Furlotte C, Schwartz K, Koornstra JJ, Naster R: 'Got a room for me?' housing experiences of older adults living with HIV/AIDS in Ottawa. Can J Aging 2012; 31:37–48.
5 Carwein VL, Sabo CE, Berry DE: HIV infection in traditional rural communities. Nurs Clin North Am 1993;28:231–239.
6 Echenique M, Illa L, Saint-Jean G, Avellaneda VB, Sanchez-Martinez M, Eisdorfer C: Impact of a secondary prevention intervention among HIV-positive older women. AIDS Care 2013;25:443–446.
7 Linsk NL: Experience of older gay and bisexual men living with HIV/AIDS. J Gay Lesbian Bisexual Identity 1997;2:285–308.
8 Cantor MH, Brennan M: Social care of the elderly: the effects of ethnicity, class, and culture. New York, Springer, 2000.
9 Cantor MH, Brennan M, Karpiak SE: The social support networks of older people with HIV; in Brennan M, Karpiak SE, Shippy RA, Cantor MH (eds): Research on Older Adults with HIV: An In-Depth Examination of an Emerging Population, 2009, pp 61–74.
10 Andersen RM: Revisiting the behavioral model and access to medical care: does it matter? J Health Soc Behav 1995;36:1–10.
11 Andersen R, Newman JF: Societal and individual determinants of medical care utilization in the United States. Milbank Q 2005;83:1–28.
12 Whipple B, Scura KW: The overlooked epidemic: HIV in older adults. Am J Nurs 1996;96:23–28.
13 Emlet CA: HIV/AIDS in the elderly: a hidden population. Home Care Provid 1997;2:69–75.
14 Centers for Disease Control and Prevention (CDC): Diagnoses of HIV infection among adults aged 50 years and older in the United States and dependent areas, 2007–2010. HIV Surveillance Supplemental Report 2013:18(No. 3). http://www.cdc.gov/hiv/topics/surveillance/resources/reports/#supplemental.

15 Nakagawa F, May M, Phillips A: Life expectancy living with HIV: recent estimates and future implications. Curr Opin Infect Dis 2013;26:17–25.
16 Linsk NL: HIV among older adults: age-specific issues in prevention and treatment. AIDS Read 2000; 10:430–440.
17 Grettenberger S, Boudreau M: Over fifty and living with HIV; in Rowan D (ed): Social Work with HIV and AIDS: A Case-Based Guide, 2013, pp 214–234.
18 Fredriksen-Goldsen K, Muraco A: Aging and sexual orientation: a 25-year review of the literature. Res Aging 2010;32:372–413.
19 Fredriksen-Goldsen KI, Kim HJ, Emlet CA, Muraco A, Erosheva EA, Hoy-Ellis CP, Goldsen J, Petry H: The Aging and Health Report: Disparities and Resilience among Lesbian, Gay, Bisexual, and Transgender Older Adults. Seattle, Institute for Multigenerational Health, 2011.
20 Knochel KA, Quam JK, Croghan CF: Are old lesbian and gay people well served? Understanding the perceptions, preparation, and experiences of aging services providers. J Appl Gerontol 2011;30:370–389.
21 Knochel KA, Croghan CF, Moone RP, Quam JK: Training, geography, and provision of aging services to lesbian, gay, bisexual, and transgender older adults. J Gerontol Soc Work 2012;55:426–443.
22 Hughes AK, Harold RD, Boyer JM: Awareness of LGBT aging issues among aging services network providers. J Gerontol Soc Work 2011;54:659–677.
23 Jessup MA, Dibble SL: Unmet mental health and substance abuse treatment needs of sexual minority elders. J Homosex 2012;59:656–674.
24 Brotman S, Ryan B, Collins S, Chamberland L, Cormier R, Julien D, Meyer E, Peterkin A, Richard B: Coming out to care: caregivers of gay and lesbian seniors in Canada. Gerontologist 2007;47:490–503.
25 Jackson NC, Johnson MJ, Roberts R: The potential impact of discrimination fears of older gays, lesbians, bisexuals and transgender individuals living in small- to moderate-sized cities on long-term health care. J Homosex 2008;54:325–339.
26 Havlik RJ: Health status, comorbidities, and health-related quality of life; in Brennan M, Karpiak SE, Shippy RA, Cantor MH (eds): Research on Older Adults with HIV: An In-Depth Examination of an Emerging Population. New York, Nova Science, 2009, pp 13–25.
27 Longmire-Avital B, Golub SA, Parsons JT, Brennan-Ing M, Karpiak SE: Financial hardship and life satisfaction among aging African Americans with HIV. J HIV/AIDS Soc Serv 2012;11:363–374.
28 Linsk N: HIV and the elderly. Fam Soc 1994;756: 362–372.
29 Stafford F, Krell G: Gerontology for Health Professionals: A Practice Guide, ed 2. Washington, NASW Press, 1997.
30 Irving G, Bor R, Catalan J: Psychological distress among gay men supporting a lover or partner with AIDS: a pilot study. AIDS Care 1995;7:605–617.
31 Fredriksen-Goldsen KI, Ellis C: Caregiving with pride: an introduction. J Gay Lesbian Soc Serv 2007;18:1–13.
32 Shippy RA, Karpiak SE: The aging HIV/AIDS population: fragile social networks. Aging Ment Health 2005;9:246–254.
33 Cantor MH, Mayer M: Factors in differential utilization of services by urban elderly. J Gerontol Soc Work 1978;1:47–61.
34 Cahill S, Valadez R: Growing older with HIV/AIDS: new public health challenges. Am J Public Health 2013;103:7–15.
35 Emlet CA: 'You're awfully old to have this disease': experiences of stigma and ageism in adults 50 years and older living with HIV/AIDS. Gerontologist 2006;46:781–790.
36 Williams E, Donnelly J: Older Americans and AIDS: some guidelines for prevention. Soc Work 2002;47: 105–111.
37 Levy JA: AIDS and injecting drug use in later life. Res Aging 1998;20:776–797.
38 Emlet CA: Experiences of stigma in older adults living with HIV/AIDS: a mixed-methods analysis. AIDS Patient Care STDS 2007;21:740–752.
39 Zanjani F, Saboe K, Oslin D: Age difference in rates of mental health/substance abuse and behavioral care in HIV-positive adults. AIDS Patient Care STDS 2007;21:347–355.
40 Whitehead NE, Hearn LE, Burrell L: The association between depressive symptoms, anger, and perceived support resources among underserved older HIV positive Black/African American adults. AIDS Patient Care STDS 2014;28:507–512.
41 Sutton MY, Parks CP: HIV/AIDS prevention, faith, and spirituality among Black/African American and Latino communities in the United States: strengthening scientific faith-based efforts to shift the course of the epidemic and reduce HIV-related health disparities. J Relig Health 2011;52:514–530.
42 Vance DE, Brennan M, Enah C, Smith GL, Kaur J: Religion, spirituality, and older adults with HIV: critical personal and social resources for an aging epidemic. Clin Interv Aging 2011;6:101–109.
43 Wood AW, Conley AH: Loss of religious or spiritual identities among the LGBT population. Counse Value 2014;59:95–111.
44 Karpiak S: More Years with HIV/AIDS Can Mean Multimorbidity and Complex Care. Aging Today, 2013.
45 Kim DJ, Westfall AO, Chamot E, Willig AL, Mugavero MJ, Ritchie C, Burkholder GA, Crane HM, Raper JL, Saag MS, Willig JH: Multimorbidity patterns in HIV-infected patients: the role of obesity in chronic disease clustering. J Acquir Immune Defic Syndr 2012;61:600–605.

46 Smit M, Brinkman K, Geerlings S, Smit C, Thyagarajan K, Sighem Av, de Wolf F, Hallett TB; ATHENA Observational Cohort: Future challenges for clinical care of an ageing population infected with HIV: a modelling study. Lancet Infect Dis 2015;15:810–818.
47 Raffetti E, Albini L, Gotti D, Segala D, Maggiolo F, di Filippo E, Saracino A, Ladisa N, Lapadula G, Fornabaio C, Castelnuovo F, et al; MASTER Cohort: Cancer incidence and mortality for all causes in HIV-infected patients over a quarter century: a multicentre cohort study. BMC Public Health 2015;15:235.
48 Althoff KN, McGinnis KA, Wyatt CM, Freiberg MS, Gilbert C, Oursler KK, Rimland D, Rodriguez-Barradas MC, Dubrow R, Park LS, Skanderson M, et al; Veterans Aging Cohort Study (VACS): Comparison of risk and age at diagnosis of myocardial infarction, end-stage renal disease, and non-AIDS-defining cancer in HIV-infected versus uninfected adults. Clin Infect Dis 2015;60:627–638.
49 Palacios R, Pascual J, Cabrera E, Lebrón JM, Guerrero-León MA, del Arco A, Colmenero JD, Santos J: Lung cancer in HIV-infected patients. Int J STD AIDS 2014;25:239–243.
50 Hirschhorn LR, Kaaya SF, Garrity PS, Chopyak E, Fawzi MC: Cancer and the 'other' noncommunicable chronic diseases in older people living with HIV/AIDS in resource-limited settings: a challenge to success. AIDS 2012;26(suppl 1):S65–S75.
51 So-Armah K, Freiberg MS: Cardiovascular disease risk in an aging HIV population: not just a question of biology. Curr Opin HIV AIDS 2014;9:346–354.
52 Petoumenos K, Reiss P, Ryom L, Rickenbach M, Sabin CA, El-Sadr W, d'Arminio Monforte A, Phillips AN, De Wit S, Kirk O, Dabis F, et la; D:A:D Study Group: Increased risk of cardiovascular disease (CVD) with age in HIV-positive men: a comparison of the D:A:D CVD risk equation and general population CVD risk equations. HIV Med 2014;15:595–603.
53 Esser S, Eisele L, Schwarz B, Schulze C, Holzendorf V, Brockmeyer NH, Hower M, Kwirant F, Rudolph R, Neumann T, Reinsch N: Rates of cardiovascular events and deaths are associated with advanced stages of HIV-infection: results of the HIV HEART study 7, 5 year follow-up. J Int AIDS Soc 2014;17(4 suppl 3):19542.
54 Kebodeaux CD, Wilson AG, Smith DL, Vouri SM: A review of cardiovascular and renal function monitoring: a consideration of older adults with HIV. HIV AIDS (Auckl) 2013;5:263–274.
55 Greene M, Covinsky KE, Valcour V, Miao Y, Madamba J, Lampiris H, Cenzer IS, Martin J, Deeks SG: Geriatric syndromes in older HIV-infected adults. J Acquir Immune Defic Syndr 2015;69:161–167.
56 Onen NF, Overton ET: A review of premature frailty in HIV-infected persons; another manifestation of HIV-related accelerated aging. Curr Aging Sci 2011;4:33–41.
57 Piggott DA, Muzaale AD, Mehta SH, Brown TT, Patel KV, Leng SX, Kirk GD: Frailty, HIV infection, and mortality in an aging cohort of injection drug users. PLoS One 2013;8:e54910.
58 Pathai S, Gilbert C, Weiss HA, Cook C, Wood R, Bekker LG, Lawn SD: Frailty in HIV-infected adults in South Africa. J Acquir Immune Defic Syndr 2013;62:43–51.
59 Onen NF, Agbebi A, Shacham E, Stamm KE, Onen AR, Overton ET: Frailty among HIV-infected persons in an urban outpatient care setting. J Infect 2009;59:346–352.
60 Brothers TD, Rockwood K: Biologic aging, frailty, and age-related disease in chronic HIV infection. Curr Opin HIV AIDS 2014;9:412–418.
61 Brothers TD, Kirkland S, Guaraldi G, Falutz J, Theou O, Johnston BL, Rockwood K: Frailty in people aging with human immunodeficiency virus (HIV) infection. J Infect Dis 2014;210:1170–1179.
62 Erlandson KM, Schrack JA, Jankowski CM, Brown TT, Campbell TB: Functional impairment, disability, and frailty in adults aging with HIV-infection. Curr HIV/AIDS Rep 2014;11:279–290.
63 Desquilbet L, Jacobson LP, Fried LP, Phair JP, Jamieson BD, Holloway M, Margolick JB: A frailty-related phenotype before HAART initiation as an independent risk factor for AIDS or death after HAART among HIV-infected men. J Gerontol A Biol Sci Med Sci 2011;66:1030–1038.
64 Leng SX, Margolick JB: Understanding frailty, aging, and inflammation in HIV infection. Curr HIV/AIDS Rep 2015;12:25–32.
65 Havlik RJ, Brennan M, Karpiak SE: Comorbidities and depression in older adults with HIV. Sex Health 2011;8:551–559.
66 Brennan-Ing M, Seidel L, Rodgers L, Ernst J, Wirth D, Tietz D, Morretti A, Karpiak SE: The impact of comprehensive case management on HIV client outcomes. PLoS One 2016;11:e0148865.
67 Counsell SR, Callahan CM, Clark DO, Tu W, Buttar AB, Stump TE, Ricketts GD: Geriatric care management for low-income seniors: a randomized controlled trial. JAMA 2007;298:2623–2633.
68 Butler SS, Wardamasky S, Brennan-Ing M: Older women caring for older women: the rewards and challenges of the home care aide job. J Women Aging 2012;24:194–215.
69 Wohl AR, Carlos JA, Tejero J, Dierst-Davies R, Daar ES, Khanlou H, Cadden J, Towner W, Frye D: Barriers and unmet need for supportive services for HIV patients in care in Los Angeles County, California. AIDS Patient Care STDS 2011;25:525–532.

70 Heckman TG, Heckman BD, Anderson T, Lovejoy TI, Mohr D, Sutton M, Bianco JA, Gau JT: Supportive-expressive and coping group teletherapies for HIV-infected older adults: a randomized clinical trial. AIDS Behav 2013;17:3034–3044.
71 Bradford JB, Coleman S, Cunningham W: HIV system navigation: an emerging model to improve HIV care access. AIDS Patient Care STDSs 2007;21(suppl 4):S49–S58.
72 National HIV/AIDS Strategy: Overview: United States Department of Health and Human Services. https://www.aids.gov/federal-resources/national-hiv-aids-strategy/overview/ (retrieved May 5, 2016).
73 Kaiser Family Foundation: AIDS Drug Assistance Programs (ADAP) formularies, number of medications by drug class, as of December 31, 2009. http://www.statehealthfacts.org/comparetable.jsp?ind=551&cat=11 (retrieved May 10, 2016).
74 Russell RH, Rowan D: US AIDS policy: the shifting landscapea; in Rowan D (ed): Social Work with HIV and AIDS: A Case-Based Guide, 2013, pp 474–515.
75 London AS, LeBlanc AJ, Aneshensel CS: The integration of informal care, case management and community-based services for persons with HIV/AIDS. AIDS Care 1998;10:481–503.
76 Seidel L, Karpiak SE, Brennan-Ing M: Training senior service providers about HIV and aging: evaluation of a multi-year, multi-city initiative. Gerontol Geriatrics Educ 2015, Epub ahead of print.
77 Gould D: Life during Wartime: Emotions and the Development of Act Up. Mobilization: An International Quarterly, 2002, vol 7, pp 177–200.
78 Nigel P: Some thoughts on the relationship between theory and practice in and for social work. Brit J Soc Work 2000;304:449–463.
79 Fox-Grage W, Ujvari K: The Older Americans Act. Washington, AARP Public Policy Institute, 2014.

Lisa E. Cox, PhD, LCSW
Research Chair, Stockton Center on Successful Aging
Stockton University, 101 Vera King Farris Drive
Galloway, NJ 08205 (USA)
E-Mail lisa.cox@stockton.edu

Brennan-Ing M, DeMarco RF (eds): HIV and Aging. Interdiscipl Top Gerontol Geriatr.
Basel, Karger, 2017, vol 42, pp 222–233 (DOI: 10.1159/000448566)

# The Relevance of Palliative Care in HIV and Aging

Jacqueline Shorthill[a] · Rosanna F. DeMarco[b]

[a]Tigard, Oreg., and [b]Department of Nursing, College of Nursing and Health Sciences, University Massachusetts Boston, Boston, Mass., USA

**Abstract**

The connection between palliative care and HIV infection has deep and wide roots in the United States that go back to the time when many gay men in the early 1980s were dying from a disease we knew little about, and there was no way to help but to alleviate symptoms in hospice and end of life centers across the United States. More individuals (adults and children), families, and communities attribute the success of antiretroviral therapies and other therapeutic approaches to advancing quality of life and life itself today. The identity of HIV, like many 'life-threatening illness with no cure' has evolved as a 'chronic' condition with a longer time period to address physical, social, and emotional experiences that may concern those living with HIV infection. Chronic conditions create an opportunity for healthcare providers from all types of disciplines to rethink and retool their knowledge and skills, to have conversations with those affected by HIV infection as to what they would ideally want in addressing their care needs; care needs that are now complicated by comorbid conditions of aging and healthcare reimbursement that uniquely intersect with HIV infection. This chapter addresses the current relevance of palliative care in HIV history, both nationally and internationally, and offers ideas for health professionals to use a multidisciplinary integration of knowledge to not just cure but align 'cure and care' toward healing action while being present to others from their perspective and values.



## Defining Palliative Care in the Context of HIV Infection

According to the World Health Organization (WHO), palliative care is an approach that improves the quality of life of adults and children, and their families facing challenges associated with life-threatening illness [1]. This approach is taken by way of prevention and relief of suffering by means of early identification and assessment and treatment of pain and other problems, physical, psychosocial, and spiritual [1]. Palliative care includes, in particular: (1) relief from pain and other distressing symptoms; (2) affirmation of life and considering dying as a normal process; (3) integration of psychological and spiritual aspects of patient care; (4) offering a support system to help patients and families live actively until death; (5) use of a team approach; and (6) enhancing the quality of life [1]. Suggestive criteria for identifying candidates that may gain from palliation would include: the presence of a serious, chronic illness, multiple hospitalizations, declining ability to perform activities of daily living, difficulty controlling physical or emotional symptoms related to illness, patient/caregiver/MD uncertainty regarding prognosis, uncertainty regarding goals of care, advanced directive or DNR order conflicts, and/or psychological/spiritual distress which can be caused by all of the above. What is important to note, is the difference between palliative care and end of life care where palliation often begins during the early course of illness, in conjunction with other therapies. The trend of starting palliation earlier in chronic care conditions is encouraged, and is currently the norm to advance the benefits of the care to individuals, families, and communities earlier than later.

Palliative care is recognized by the WHO as an essential element of HIV care, from diagnosis to the end of life [2]. There is a long history of both the presence and active use of palliation and end of life care in the 1980s that was central to the standard of HIV care at the beginning of the epidemic, whereas just the opposite was the case for cancer patients [3]. Palliative care is part of the continuum of care. Following the initial diagnosis of the disease, the majority of patients seek out disease-modifying treatment to ward off symptoms and illness, which can include one or several surgeries, radiation, chemotherapy, medications, and adjuvant therapies, possibly successfully warding off disease for years. However, as the disease itself progresses, the modifying treatments can become less effective or more harmful as the number of treatment options diminishes. Goals of care can and do shift toward palliation, with goals of care involving symptom management and maximizing the quality of life [4, 5]. This 'change in focus' also applies to the treatment provided by healthcare providers, where it is recognized by both the patient and the provider that a return to 'normal' function may no longer be an option, and goals need to be changed to allow symptom relief and maximize independence – an important goal of patients with any advanced disease and represented in public health as secondary or tertiary prevention [6].

Palliative care is now better recognized and available in all arenas of healthcare, from outpatient clinics to in-hospital care to skilled nursing facilities to home health. The concept can be introduced to the patient at any point in the trajectory of any disease. Until recently, palliative care has mainly concentrated on those individuals with 'terminal diseases' such as cancer; however; palliative care can be used in any chronic illness at any stage, and needs to be further integrated into health and social services by improving knowledge, skills, and practice behavior to recognize when it is appropriate [7, 8].

Because HIV is no longer perceived as a terminal illness based on the success of antiretroviral therapies (ART) in many resource poor areas such as Africa and other developing areas of the world, HIV palliative care services are integrated in HIV specialty care services because of the common and chronic need to address the high burden of pain and physical, psychological, and social difficulties and many of the comorbidities that interface with living with HIV and aging. These symptom experiences and effects of not only HIV infection but also the cumulative layering of social determinants of health such as sexual orientation and race discrimination and ageism combined with poverty, can be managed effectively with the integration of palliative care throughout the trajectory of wellness and illness during a disease experience [9].

## HIV, Palliative Care, and Health Disparities

The challenge continues–most individuals, families, and communities that have the experience of living with HIV infections do not have access to the integration of palliation in the context of medical care for their disease. This is the case even though we know there is documented capacity for palliative care services to positively augment patients', families', and communities' health outcomes and boost adherence to antiretroviral treatments and life expectancy, in particular, at the individual patient level [3].

A growing body of research highlights that disparities exist around access to adequate healthcare in general, and palliative care in particular, especially in the context of medically underserved populations [10]. While 'medically underserved' may have many definitions, the term typically encompasses populations with inadequate access to healthcare and often includes elderly, poor, urban/rural-dwelling minorities or any group affected by discrimination and isolation [5], that is, groups disproportionately affected by HIV infection. While there is strong evidence that health disparities exist among racial and ethnic minorities living with chronic illnesses such as cancer, diabetes, heart disease that are associated with the aging process, living with HIV infection, and associated stigma and discrimination raises the double challenge of offering a trajectory of preventative services in palliative care to a new level, particularly in the area of mental health. As is often the case, care delivery is seen as something patients, families, and communities 'gravitate to'. Because of stigma, discrimination, and the mental health symptoms that accompany these experiences, it may be the case that palliation needs to 'go to' patients and families even in communities where it may be unsafe or difficult to access [10]. It may also be the case that palliative care in communities could benefit from case managers or healthcare navigators who represent those living with HIV infections because they are living with HIV infection themselves. The need to demystify the notion that palliative care is not hospice or end of life care through caring conversations, especially in communities where 'giving up the fight' against a disease is seen less than the optimal healthcare they deserve is significant and needs to be addressed [11].

Lack of access to palliative care because of lack of knowledge to the benefits of this approach, to make important decisions about what one needs or wants or the inability or unwillingness for healthcare centers to offer expertise in palliative care for a variety of reasons, leaves individuals, families, and communities without coordinated services. These services include the provision of stability, support, and strength at the individual and aggregate level to recognize the point at which curative care in no longer appropriate by considering the quality of life as defined by patients, families, and communities as a way to manage symptoms. Those living with HIV infection can and should benefit from multi-disciplinary expertise.

Despite increasing awareness that palliative care is not only a valuable but necessary tool in the trajectory of illness, it is neither well recognized nor utilized to its fullest capacity in the HIV community of care. As educated clinicians, academicians, or researchers, we are taught the rigors of science, and become believers in the healing power that comes from our disciplinary training. Advancements in healthcare and health science have given us treatment options, more now than ever. This has allowed us to successfully treat and study many life-limiting conditions and often prolong life for decades. The onset of disease can come at any point – we often think of the elderly as a group with complex comorbidities, though many people are diagnosed with serious, life-limiting medical conditions throughout their lifespan such as those living with HIV infection. Palliative care is becoming a more recognized option for those diagnosed with serious medical conditions, who face longer lives across a trajectory of the chronic 'ups and downs' of aging in treatment approaches, quality of life, and advancement of symptoms and damage from the disease and comorbidities.

## Aging and Illness: Living with HIV Infection

Aging is part of the natural order of life and with it comes the general breakdown of body systems. However, living with HIV infection, as we have come to understand, is a gradual process. Serious, life-threatening illness such as HIV infection can affect any one at any point in their life, from the pediatric to geriatric population. Whenever illness occurs, early or later in life, there are numerous treatment options, which can often be complex and convoluted. The evolution of infectious disease health science has made amazing advances in how to prevent and treat HIV infection; however, our medical model in general has some significant disparities in the approach to treatment. Often clinicians and researchers focus on medical options that increase the quantity rather than the quality of life years – multiple medications, procedures, and treatments to be given or studied for their effects. We utilize every battery of testing, diagnostic exam, and specialist to help diagnose and treat conditions aligned with immunological challenges brought with HIV. In doing so, clinicians are taught to fight to the very end. As a result, we have difficulty admitting to ourselves and our patients, in the context of how and where they live, that the diseases we try so hard to fight and manage are no longer 'fightable', especially when we metaphorically state that we are 'fighting' a disease or problem and nobody wants to lose the fight. We forge ahead with treatments that may cause pain and suffering to patients and devastation to families as they watch loved ones exhaust every last effort in hopes for improvement. Palliative care, which was introduced in conjunction with the hospice movement in the 1970s, became an option for those suffering from a serious, chronic illness or illnesses that were given a poor long-term outcome though not given a prognosis of 6 months or less as in hospice care. It has become a more accepted and used option in the medical world, though not consistently utilized [8, 11]. There are a variety of reasons why it is being underutilized. One significant reason for underutilization is the challenge to train and nurture expertise in an area that is perceived as less prestigious and less profitable.

### Palliation, Health Providers, and Healthcare Disparities

The discussion of palliative care is necessary and difficult. It is often avoided until the very last option and the person has been exhausted – this is exemplified by the many patients who have transitioned to hospice care shortly before death, limiting the benefits obtained by hospice services as noted by chronic short length of stays in an area of care [11]. Most healthcare professionals spend the majority of training in understanding the disease processes and treating the disease itself through medications, surgeries, and various techniques, often in conjunction with each other. The study is often at the individual level, and rarely are interactions and effects of family and environments considered as contributing factors to health or wellness. There are specialists for every body system, and newer research is developing every day with the goal to eradicate many of the more deadly diseases including cancer and HIV/AIDS. Where we fall short is in the recognition of disease advancement and when to ask the question: is this enough or what would the patient, family, or community want, rather than what I as a professional caregiver would want? When diagnosed with a serious illness, a healthcare provider should be presenting all options objectively to the patient, including those that improve the quality of life and those that could cause significant discomfort. Attitudes about serious illness, hospice and palliative care, and the role of the clinician as a 'healer' often prevent basic palliative care knowledge from being applied. Fear of provoking emotion by initiating a difficult conversation, fear of peer pressure by discussing a comfort care approach, fear of a lawsuit for not doing 'everything' are attitudinal barriers, which prevent timely and compassionate care for our most vulnerable patients [12].

From an allied health standpoint (physical, occupational, and speech therapy), there are deficits in training to recognize those who could benefit from palliative care. Physical therapists, for example, have been trained to work with patients in achieving all goals and returning a patient to their 'premorbid function', maximizing functional potential and setting goals that include phrases such as 'return to independent mobility'. Unless supplemental courses of study or continuing education are offered, there are no curriculum courses that teach any type of rehabilitation therapy student how to treat those patients who are declining from serious illness. As a result, when a referral for a medically complex patient is received such as someone living with HIV infection, often the therapist does not know what to do when the patient does not achieve a stated reimbursable outcome. There is a perception that this patient population is inappropriate for allied health services, they are not motivated to meet the set goals, and they are often discharged due to noncompliance [5].

Palliative care is not profitable at the provider side of the reimbursement equation [13], which may be the reason why many health professionals do not enter it as a specialty but envision it as a sub-specialty in the context of a larger scope of their work. Currently, the continued development of bundled reimbursement rather than fee for services under the category of advanced disease management allows for seamless care to be given to any patient seeking palliative care under the direction of a licensed care provider or palliative care team [14, 15]. Whatever the patient, family, or community centered motivation for goal setting or advancing the quality of life with their provider, choosing palliation over curative care can experience counter-cultural issues unless providers and insurers support the approach from a pragmatic perspective. A Black woman living with HIV may not choose a therapeutic intervention such as hospitalization, as it may appear to add homecare costs including multidisciplinary home visits, delivery of medications, transportation costs to outpatient services. On the contrary, if the same woman was in the hospital and received palliation, there are significant reductions in per diem costs and total costs, and it can also generate savings [16]. Palliative care alongside usual care in recent randomized outpatient trials has maintained or improved the quality of care in patients while generating substantial cost savings. The data are mixed about the impact of palliative care consultation on inpatient length of stay because these hospitalizations are related to local patterns of care, consultation, and assumption of control of the course of care [16]. We are yet to study this area thoroughly in evolving populations where location or cultural beliefs have created barriers to the conversations that lead to a less invasive approach to care. Such is the case of those disproportionately living with HIV infection [16].

## HIV Treatment Outcomes Using Palliative Care

In the time before ART were available in combination to address HIV infection in adults and children, there is evidence that palliative care was effective in improving symptoms of anxiety and pain in particular and giving patients insights into the uncertainty of facing an illness without a cure [17]. There is continued need to measure palliative care treatment outcomes in the age of ART across a variety of individuals with characteristics that may vary across access to health insurance, national and global resources, age, gender, sexual orientation, family constellation, social support, drug use history, and mental health issues among many other key variables that may help in understanding the health behavior when one is living with HIV infections. Study considerations need to include the differences between outcomes of aging adults and children, and the unique needs of women who often are tested very late in the infection trajectory. In addition, new CD4 thresholds for treatment may bring individuals into ART where palliation gets postponed more readily.

In undertaking research, choosing the right research questions to be studied in HIV palliation is very important because as is the case with other life-threatening illness such as certain types of cancer, getting treatment does not necessarily decrease suffering, that is, the side effects of medications or other therapeutic approaches, opportunistic infections and comorbidities we see with HIV and early aging (diabetes, cardiovascular disease, hypertension, renal compromise, peripheral vascular disease, congestive heart failure).

The presence of HIV/palliative care clinics can be a place where not only direct care can be given but also where unintended findings are observed through symptoms or symptom clusters that are observed and subsequently studied. For example, low back pain is a frequent complaint in HIV/palliative care clinics [18]. HIV seropositive patients do not receive diagnostic imaging routinely for low back pain even though they are at risk for cancer or fractures. In a retrospective study of low back pain complaints and MRI use, one study found that 76 of 137 patients complained of back pain ranging in age from 40 to 51 years of age. Although their HIV status was considered well controlled, 29% of this group had an MRI and 11% had degenerative disc disease and 4 had concerning results indicative of possible malignancies [18]. In this case, an opportunity presented itself to learn more about how palliative care can identify symptom or symptom clusters that may need routine follow-up to support intervention care earlier than later in an age trajectory.

### Why a Multidisciplinary Team Approach to HIV Palliative Care

Palliative care utilizes a multidisciplinary approach that encompasses a myriad of specialties that, as a group are better able to minister to the various aspects of physical, spiritual, psychosocial, and cultural elements that constitute a holistic approach to patient and family care (Krishna). This multifaceted, multi-talented, and multi-trained complementary and interdependent approach has been validated in a number of settings and found to be effective in meeting the goals and complex needs of patients and their families. A multidisciplinary approach is well supported and necessary in any palliative care approach, allowing for the involvement of all members of the team, including physician, nurse, allied heath (physical, occupational, and speech therapists), social workers, chaplain, and ancillary staff throughout all areas of the healthcare spectrum working toward the same patient- and family-centered goals. 'Each discipline has a clear knowledge of its roles, and through appropriate consideration of clinical and psychosocial issues and cultural and spiritual issues relevant to the patient and family unit, decision making and care provision will move beyond a purely clinical approach into one that is keeping with the central tenets espoused by palliative care [5], knowledge of the roles of different members of a multi-professional team and the part they can play in contributing to quality care is key in promoting communication between practitioners; a team approach utilizes all disciplines in a multifaceted arena to promote a joint effort in care for providing symptom management, communication, coordination, and building a relationship that promotes discussion of concerns with honesty. A multidisciplinary team utilizes all members in 3 main areas.

*Communication*

Perhaps the largest issue between clinicians and patients in HIV specialty care or in primary care is the lack of communication. Physicians who often do not have open discussion of medical care with their seriously ill patients are specifically targeted. Medical schools place far more importance on the capacity of students to show expertise in scientific reasoning, mathematical skills, and memorization at the expense of the ability to communicate [19]. As a result, physicians will order batteries of tests, prescribe treatments and medications, and recommend procedures, which may be beneficial for those who have a treatable illness with a reasonable prognosis. But when dealing with a terminal prognosis; however, it may not be favorable, where the burden and risk of suffering are high and the benefits minimal. Americans receive some of the best healthcare but they also experience some of the worst deaths in the developed world because of the failure of physicians to openly discuss medical care with their seriously ill patients [19]. Communication is an art and a science that takes practice and skill to be effective. Communicating with the patient effectively will aid in decreasing anxiety regarding his/her concerns and will clarify patients' goals of care. Asking the right questions, an essential piece to understanding, where the patient and family are in the process, will help determine what needs to be done [20]. Asking the following questions can lead to a value-driven approach to HIV care that is patient, family, and community centered:

'What do you understand about your diagnosis?';
'What are your concerns for what lies ahead?';
'What kind of trade-offs are options for you?';
'How do you want to spend your time?';
'Who will make decisions for you when you cannot?';
'What kinds of things are important to you?';
'What makes you happy?';

'What fears do you have about getting sick or needing medical care?';

'If you were very sick, are there any specific medical treatments that might be too much for you?', and;

'Do you have any beliefs that guide you?'.

Two thirds of terminal cancer patients had no discussion with their doctors about their goals [15]. Communication can lay the framework that guides patient care and will allow the patient and family to keep an open and honest communication between team members. Communication can be through many forms, including family conferences in person, in the hospital, office or home setting, or via phone or video-conferencing. Team members often discuss individual cases in person at weekly or monthly meetings.

*Education and Resources*

Through individual disciplines and team collaboration, we provide education to the patient and family throughout their journey. Information is given from each discipline and tailored to the patient's need, including disease process and progression and what to expect medically, functionally, emotionally, and spiritually; for example, a therapist would focus on functional and safety during periods of latency and transition, a social worker would focus on spiritual concerns and life review, also advanced care planning including initiating or updating advance directives. Many resources are provided to our patients throughout the course of their illness, from the hospital setting to the home.

*Counseling*

Whether it be a new diagnosis of cancer or an illness that has been present for years and is now progressing, palliative care offers the open space for patients and families to discuss their feelings and concerns with honesty. Patients may be concerned about issues including further debilitation and dependency, pain and suffering, consequences for dependents, arranging affairs, an uncertain future, dying alone, loss of control, changing relationships, and existential concerns [21]. All palliative care professional team members should be trained in the skill to provide active and reflective listening. Active and reflective listening is a communication technique in which listeners focus on what the patient says and provide reassurance that they understand. Active listening refers to being present and in the moment, and reflective listening refers to expressing oneself with clarity and sensitivity which allows the patient and family to express feelings of grief, sadness, and frustration in a non-judgmental environment. It also allows the patient to feel comfortable enough to discuss spirituality if they wish – expressing their beliefs, motivations, allowing them to explore what may be unfinished, and to make decisions based on their beliefs and motivations [22]. All team members should be trained on active/reflective listening, as the patient or family may have many questions to any and all clinicians working with them in the right moment.

## A Model for HIV Palliative Care Now and in the Future

In conclusion, we would like to emphasize the relevance of palliative care for those living with HIV nationally and internationally in the direction of not just conversation and reflection but ACTION. In other words, how do we make palliative care relevant to others and available to them? How do we advance use of palliation sooner than later? How do we get professionals equipped to do this work well and with positive results/outcomes for patients, families, and communities living with disproportionate burden of HIV infection? The Robert Wood Johnson Foundation (RWJF) mission is to improve the health of all Americans through a current initiative that focuses on creating a 'culture of health', that is, recognizing health's central importance in our lives [23]. Although a national mission and model for the United States, the idea and aspiration of this position is a worldwide goal for the WHO as it relates to all types of illness including HIV infection [23]. RWJF has championed a recent action model, with a set of tangible measurements, to help our nation and others to broaden the discussion about health, set goals, and integrate efforts to move forward. This framework is meant intentionally to translate to many actors, and the many facets of a culture of Health and is divided into 4 interconnected areas of ACTION. We share these 4 areas with the focus on HIV palliative care.

*Making Health a Shared Value*
We need to increase the number of people in communities who understand what palliative care offers in general, and in particular in the chronic care of those aging with HIV infection through sharing of best practices. HIV consumers/peers who have had successful experiences can be key. We also need to address the value of palliation through recognized leaders by educating others in the context of HIV care organizations or in health organizations in general and more specifically in primary care about what palliation 'is' and what 'it is not' with accuracy. We need to help communities and families value decisions about quality of life, and understand how adequate social support for families and friends can increase community strength [24]. We need to do this by understanding that culture and beliefs of certain groups may continue to define best practices. Lastly, we need to create more opportunities for interdisciplinary education related to palliative care, and palliative care specifically in areas of key chronic conditions. In public health terms, this would be a significant contribution to 'assurance' of competency which is a key public health principle and goal aligned with accurate assessment of community needs and establishing data-based policy that makes sense in all communities [25].

*Fostering Cross-Sector Collaboration to Improve Well-Being*
We need to create formal collaborative relationships between city, town, state health departments and community organizations, faith-based organizations, and employers to promote health through palliation by offering information and campaigns that

help increase collaborative referrals to help individuals, families, and communities care for those living longer with HIV infection [26]. Increasing assistance in how to navigate complex collaborating systems is also needed [27]. Developing stage-specific models of care that can allow collaborations to be more specific and address needs in a timely manner is also important in advancing well-being [28].

*Creating Healthier, More Equitable Communities*

We can advance community and neighborhood infrastructures that allow for aging and palliative care to intersect in a healthy way such as increasing grocery store access, farmers' market access, and safe sidewalks, and disability access in communities and affordable housing [29].

*Strengthening Integration of Health Services and Systems*

We continue to advance comprehensive follow-up and care of individuals aging with HIV infection in particular through advancing electronic data that can be shared across all the intersections of care that often do not connect such as pharmacies, in a context of polypharmacy in aging adults, primary care, specialty care, and out of state systems [30]. The need for clinicians, health systems, and individual patients to connect accurately without barriers is critical to a smooth and seamless approach to having palliative care honored and supported in a complex health delivery system [31]. We also need more collaborative community-based practices where home visits are a significant part of their care delivery while integrating comprehensive care that should include palliation that is, the notion of Gero-Palliation or Gero palliative care [30].

## References


1 World Health Organization: Definition of palliative care. http://www.who.int/cancer/palliative/definition/en/ (retrieved October 15, 2015).

2 World Health Organization: Palliative care: for all ages and all diseases. http://www.who.int/features/2015/south-africa-palliative-care/en/ (retrieved October 15, 2015).

3 Simms V, Higginson IJ, Harding R: Integration of palliative care throughout HIV disease. Lancet Infect Dis 2012;12:571–575.

4 American Association of Critical Care Nurses: End-of-Life Nursing Education Consortium (ELNEC) Core Curriculum Participant Outline 2010. Module 1: Palliative Nursing Care M1–M60.

5 Krishna L: Palliative care imperative: a framework for holistic and inclusive palliative care. Ethics Med Int J Bioethics 2013;29:41–61.

6 Dahlin Y, Heiwe S: Patients' experiences of physical therapy within palliative cancer care. J Palliat Care 2009;25:12–20.

7 Baldwin M, Woodhouse J: SAGE Key concepts series: key concepts in palliative care. Hospice movement and the evolution of palliative care. 2011. http://search.credoreference.com/content/entry/sageukjlcz/hospice_movement_and_evolution_of_palliative_care/0 (retrieved July 15, 2015).

8 Weissman DE: Next gen palliative care. J Palliat Med 2012;15:2–4.

9 Huang YT: Challenges and responses in providing palliative care for people living with HIV/AIDS. Int J Palliat Nurs 2013;19:218, 220–225.

10 Kayser K, DeMarco RF, Stokes C, DeSanto-Madeya S, Higgins PC: Delivering palliative care to patients and caregivers in inner-city communities: challenges and opportunities. Palliat Support Care 2014;12: 369–378.

11 Weissman DE, Meier DE: Identifying patients in need of a palliative care assessment in the hospital setting: a consensus report from the center to advance palliative care. J Palliat Med 2011;14:17–23.

12 Mack JW, Paulk ME, Viswanath K, Prigerson HG: Racial disparities in the outcomes of communication on medical care received near death. Arch Intern Med 2010;170:1533–1540.
13 O'Neill SM, Ettner SL Lorenz KA: Paying the price at the end of life: a consideration of factors that affect the profitability of hospice. J Palliat Med 2008;11: 1002–1008.
14 Centers for Medicare and Medicaid Services: Bundled Payments for Care Improvement (BPCI) Initiative: General Information. https://innovation.cms.gov/initiatives/bundled-payments/ (retrieved October 25, 2015).
15 Spettell CM, Rawlins WS, Krakauer R, Fernandes J, Breton ME, Gowdy W, Brodeur S, MacCoy M, Brennan TA: A comprehensive case management program to improve palliative care. J Palliat Med 2009; 12:827–832.
16 Smith TJ, Cassel JB: Cost and non-clinical outcomes of palliative care. J Pain Symptom Manage 2009;38: 32–44.
17 Lowther K, Simms V, Selman L, Sherr L, Gwyther L, Kariuki H, Ahmed A, Ali Z, Jenkins R, Higginson IJ, Harding R: Treatment outcomes in palliative care: the TOPCare study. A mixed methods phase III randomised controlled trial to assess the effectiveness of a nurse-led palliative care intervention for HIV positive patients on antiretroviral therapy. BMC Infect Dis 2012;12:288.
18 Molony E, Westfall AO, Perry B, Tucker R, Ritchie C, Saag M, Mugavero M, Sullivan JC 3rd, Merlin JS: Low back pain and associated imaging findings among HIV-infected patients referred to an HIV/palliative care clinic. Pain Med 2014;15:418–424.
19 Volandes AE: The Conversation: A Revolutionary Plan for End-of-Life Care. New York, Bloomsbury USA Publishing, 2015.
20 Gawande A: Being Mortal, Medicine and What Matters in the End. New York, Metropolitan Books, Henry Holt and Company LLC, 2014.
21 Hedlund S: Hope and communication in cancer care: what patients tell us. Cancer Treat Res 2008;1: 65–77.
22 Davis J. Asuncion M, Rabello J, Silangcruz C, van Dyk E: A qualitative review of occupational therapist's listening behaviors and experiences when caring for patients in palliative or hospice care. OTJR 2013;33:12–20.
23 Robert Wood Johnson Foundation: Weaving the threads of health. http://www.rwjf.org/en/library/annual-reports/presidents-message-2015.html (retrieved October 10, 2015).
24 Kovacs PJ, Bellin MH, Fauri DP: Family-centered care: a resource for social work in end-of-life and palliative care. J Soc Work in End of Life Palliat Care 2006;2:13–27.
25 Harkness GA, DeMarco R: Community and Public Health Nursing: Evidence for Practice. Philadelphia, Lippincott, Williams, and Wilkins, 2016.
26 Selman LE, Higginson IJ, Agupio G, Dinat N, Downing J, Gwyther L, Mashao T, Mmoledi K, Moll T, Sebuyira LM, Ikin B, Harding R: Quality of life among patients receiving palliative care in South Africa and Uganda: a multi-centred study. Health Qual Life Outcomes 2011;9:21.
27 DeMarco RF: Palliative care and African American women living with HIV. J Nurs Educ 2010;49:462–465.
28 Merlins JS, Tucker RO, Saag MS, Selwyn PA: The role of palliative care in the current HIV treatment era in developed countries. Top Antivir Med 2013; 21:20–26.
29 Harding R, Easterbrook P, Higginson IJ, Karus D, Raveis VH, Marconi K: Access and equity in HIV/AIDS palliative care: a review of the evidence and responses. Palliat Med 2005;19:251–258.
30 Greene M, Covinsky KE, Valcour V, Miao Y, Madamba J, Lampiris H, Cenzer IS, Martin J, Deeks SG: Geriatric syndromes in older HIV-infected adults. J Acquir Immune Defic Syndr 2015;69:161–167.
31 Daub S, Goldhar J, Purbhoo D: One client, one team. Health system integration of leaders. Healthcare Management Forum 2016;29:153–157.

Rosanna F. DeMarco, PhD, RN, PHCNS-BC, APHN-BC, FAAN
Department of Nursing, College of Nursing and Health Sciences
University Massachusetts Boston
100 Morrissey Boulevard, Boston, MA 02125-3393 (USA)
E-Mail rosanna.demarco@umb.edu

Brennan-Ing M, DeMarco RF (eds): HIV and Aging. Interdiscipl Top Gerontol Geriatr.
Basel, Karger, 2017, vol 42, pp 234–239 (DOI: 10.1159/000448567)

# Ageism, Aging and HIV: Community Responses to Prevention, Treatment, Care and Support

Rosanna F. DeMarco[a] · Mark Brennan-Ing[b] · Shelly M. Brown[c, d] · Courtenay Sprague[a, c]

[a]Department of Nursing, College of Nursing and Health Sciences, University of Massachusetts Boston, Boston, Mass., [b]ACRIA, Center on HIV and Aging, New York University College of Nursing, New York, N.Y., [c]University of Massachusetts Boston, Department of Conflict Resolution, Human Security, and Global Governance, John W. McCormack Graduate School of Policy and Graduate Studies, and [d]Boston University, Department of Health Sciences, College of Health and Rehabilitation Sciences: Sargent College, Boston, Mass., USA

**Abstract**

Ageism, in the form of prejudice, stereotyping, and discrimination targeting older adults, represents a barrier to addressing the graying of the HIV epidemic. There is widespread misperception on the part of older adults themselves, as well as service providers and society in general that HIV risk is low as one ages. In addition, internalized ageism may play a role in poorer physical and mental health outcomes, as the negative stereotypes associated with aging become a self-fulfilling prophecy. A number of steps can be taken to address HIV and aging in the context of ageism with regard to: prevention, education, and outreach; treatment guidelines for older adults with HIV; funding to address the aging of the epidemic; engagement of communities, health and social service organizations, and other providers around mental health and social support, and addressing the needs of special populations. Caring for an aging population with HIV represents a challenge, which is exacerbated in low and/or middle-income countries that typically lack the infrastructure of high resource settings. How we address the aging-related issues of the HIV epidemic across regions and settings could serve as a model in dealing with aging in our society in general regardless of HIV status.



The preceding chapters in this volume have presented the state of our current scientific knowledge around aging with HIV. However, ageism is a significant barrier in addressing HIV among older people, from prevention programs to medical care that includes messaging in all sectors of the treatment cascade. Ageism has been defined differently depending on one's worldview. But in general, ageism is a phenomenon that involves prejudice on the part of one age group towards another age group [1], or more specifically, prejudice and discrimination against older people [2, 3]. The lack of perceived HIV risk in late adulthood among older people themselves, as well as providers and society in general, inhibits investment in education, testing, and programmatic responses to address HIV and aging. Ageism perpetuates the invisibility of older adults, which renders current medical and social service systems unprepared to respond to the needs of aging people with HIV infection. While ageism may result in positive treatment, such as discounts for services, rent reductions, pharmacologic cost reductions, for example [1], it is the negative aspects of ageism that must be addressed in determining the appropriate response to aging in the HIV epidemic at the community level.

Ageism is perceived by many of those aging with HIV. The title of Charley Emlet's seminal paper on this topic, 'You're Awfully Old to Have this Disease', was derived from a comment by one of his research participants. It encapsulates the enduring misperception that HIV is a disease of the young, and in particular, young gay and bisexual men [4]. In Emlet's study, more than two-thirds of participants affirmed that they had experienced stigma due to both HIV and aging. This phenomenon of age-related stigma may be even more pronounced among gay and bisexual men who account for approximately 60% of the older adult HIV-infected population [5]. Wight et al. [3] note that some middle-aged and older gay men feel stigmatized on the basis of both age and sexual orientation, and can experience a psychological accelerated aging. In their study, Wight et al. [3] found that internalized ageism was related to depression in this population, and this depression could be buffered by perceptions of mattering, or in other words, being resilient because these gay and bisexual men perceived that they are still important, and hence not irrelevant or invisible, to the world around them.

In addition to depression among sexual minority men, there is also evidence that ageism can more broadly affect physical and behavioral health in older adults, regardless of gender or sexual identities. Thus, ageism represents a particularly relevant threat to those growing older with HIV, who already face multiple challenges in the health domain. Levy [6] has proposed that internalized negative age stereotypes impact health through psychological, behavioral, and physiological pathways. The psychological pathway represents expectations around aging, with evidence that those holding more negative age stereotypes perform more poorly on cognitive tests. The behavioral pathway involves healthy practices that may be curtailed due to beliefs that aging leads to inevitable health problems and physical decline. The physiological pathway involves the autonomic nervous system and environmental stress; those with internalized negative age stereotypes demonstrate a heightened response to stress that can result in health issues such as cardiac disease. These mechanisms may be responsible for empirical findings that internalized ageism is related to both chronic disease and longevity [7, 8].

While it may not be possible to reduce ageism at macro-levels of culture and society, in developing a community response to the aging of the HIV epidemic, there are opportunities at the meso-level of providers of health and human services to buffer or reduce the impact of ageism for those who are infected or at-risk for HIV. We present a number of recommendations to mitigate the effects of ageism as our society responds to the graying of this epidemic.

### Training of Health Providers in HIV Screening, Early Diagnosis, and Initiation of Combination Anti-Retroviral Therapy in Older Populations and Integration of Key Services

Across regions and settings, healthcare providers have been less likely to recognize signs and symptoms of HIV in older patients. This means that an important entry point for HIV diagnosis is being missed for older adults with delayed HIV diagnosis across regions, including high resource settings. This is illustrated by findings that over 40% of those 50 and older in the US receive a concurrent AIDS diagnosis (stage 3) at the time of HIV diagnosis, indicative of late testing in this age group [5]. Late entry into HIV care, especially for women generates additional risks of morbidity, mortality, and reduces prospects for achieving optimal health outcomes including viral suppression [9, 10]. This underscores the need to increase vigilance on HIV case detection, ensure early diagnosis, and rapid initiation of combination anti-retroviral therapy (cART) in older populations. To do so requires training of health personnel in screening, detection, case finding and in rapid linkage to care for older men and women. This includes education to address misperceptions or assumptions around aging, such as considering older persons to be at low to no risk for HIV acquisition. The call for integration of HIV services with other health services has been a trend in the high HIV prevalence countries, and should continue, given the increasing burden of non-communicable diseases and multiple morbidities. Finding ways to include HIV screening in other routine service delivery for mature individuals is recommended as a venue for reaching older cohorts, through annual physical examinations or routine screening for particular conditions in older individuals.

### Prevention, Education, and Outreach

The absence of public health prevention and messaging by health authorities to sensitize older individuals about HIV risk and inform them about testing and treatment options is critical. This approach often falls to departments of health to reach older populations, through 'test and treat' strategies. Messages need to be tailored to communicate risk of HIV infection to older adults and encourage behavioral change. Education, social, and behavioral interventions could target individuals in their 40s who are at risk. While efforts have been underway in some locations with large populations of older adults with HIV [11], these initiatives need to be expanded globally.

### Treatment Guidelines for Older Individuals with HIV

Though debates have emerged in the US about whether HIV treatment guidelines for those aged 50 and over, currently absent, should be developed, or whether care should be individualized [9]. Many countries rely on guideline-driven approaches and cannot afford individualized approaches to care, particularly the low- and/or middle-income countries (LMICs). As such, World Health Organization guidelines for older individuals should be developed.

### Funding in Line with Aging of the HIV Population

Support for research, training of health and social service providers, guideline development, public health messaging, and cART administration in older populations will be needed from governments, foundations, and private sources. Funding needs and priorities should be developed with an eye toward sustainability, and with attention to reporting, accountability, and transparency [12]. In some LMICs, up to 80% of health budgets are externally funded, including HIV services [12]. Different financing mechanisms exist by country and these should be reviewed to ensure older people with HIV can access screening and diagnostic tests and treatment, not only for HIV but also for comorbid conditions, including mental health. In the US, for example, the AIDS Drug Assistance Program could be expanded to ensure coverage of aging populations who qualify [9]. There are funding implications for ensuring health and well-being in this sub-population, including social support grants and pensions for older individuals in countries where programs exist, such as in sub-Saharan Africa and other regions.

### Engagement of Communities, Community-Based Organizations, and Social Service Providers in Outreach, Mental Health, and Social Support

The HIV research community has learned that engaging key actors at the local and community levels is often most effective in addressing the needs of individuals and communities with HIV. Stigma and social isolation in older populations is a consistent theme in the published studies and in this volume. Individuals may be less likely to have sufficient social support. They may suffer from depression or loneliness, with fewer resources or less robust social networks than younger people. Older individuals may anticipate HIV stigma or practice self-stigmatization. Ensuring early entry into long-term continuous HIV care is essential and will likely require innovative methods to reach older populations who may be anxious, depressed, feel socially excluded, or face other health concerns. Thus, involvement of community-based organizations (CBOs) is essential. Linkage to support services through local non-government organizations or CBOs may be essential in offering psychosocial support, care, and a sense of community [13]. Such services often generate creative problem-solving that recognizes the dignity of each person in ways that are important for individuals living with HIV. Organizations that engage older persons may include different types of service providers, including AIDS Service Organizations, community-based social service organizations that encompass mental health professionals and social workers, as well as religious congregations and faith-based organizations that attract and retain older populations.

## Addressing the Needs of Special Populations

Many of the groups that have been and continue to be most affected by HIV are part of socially marginalized communities [14]. Aging populations with HIV or at-risk are also likely to be affiliated with these same key affected populations, including gay and bisexual men, transgender and gender non-conforming individuals, sex workers, people who inject drugs other users of non-injecting substances, justice-involved individuals, and women and girls in many countries who lack the power or voice to insist on condom use or experience physical or sexual violence from partners or non-partners [9, 12, 14]. In addition to gender inequality and other adverse sociocultural gender norms and factors, older women are at elevated risk of HIV acquisition, biologically, due to the thinning of the vaginal wall after menopause. Sex workers, gay and bisexual men, and transgender and gender non-conforming individuals experience criminalization policies by their governments, which drives epidemics underground [12]. Structural, behavioral, and biomedical interventions should be tailored accordingly, with an emphasis on national epidemic factors, and the needs of such key affected populations in countries and sub-regions. Enabling policy, legal and human rights laws and frameworks are essential to ensure that the health and well-being of older populations with HIV are protected and enabled.

## Conclusion

At the advent of the HIV epidemic, with near certain mortality and unimaginable suffering, few would have believed that in the 21st century we have arrived at the point of talking about people growing old with HIV. With this demographic shift in the HIV population and the elusiveness of a cure, addressing the care needs of this aging population are paramount. These challenges are exacerbated in LMICs who often lack vital resources to provide clinical and social services for this population. Thus, the aging of the HIV population is very challenging, but it provides an opportunity to mount a global response to address the needs of this population across regions and settings, and serve as a model for addressing aging regardless of HIV status.

## References


1 Levy SR, Macdonald JL: Progress on understanding ageism. J Soc Issues 2016;72:5–25.

2 Jönson H: We will be different! Ageism and the temporal construction of old age. Gerontologist 2013;53: 198–204.

3 Wight RG, LeBlanc AJ, Meyer IH, Harig FA: Internalized gay ageism, mattering, and depressive symptoms among midlife and older gay-identified men. Soc Sci Med 2015;147:200–208.

4 Emlet CA: 'You're awfully old to have this disease': experiences of stigma and ageism in adults 50 years and older living with HIV/AIDS. Gerontologist 2006;46:781–790.

5 Centers for Disease Control and Prevention: Diagnoses of HIV infection among adults aged 50 years and older in the United States and dependent areas, 2007–2010. HIV Surveillance Supplemental Report, 2013, vol 18. http://www.cdc.gov/hiv/topics/surveillance/resources/reports/#supplemental (accessed May 17, 2016).

6 Levy B: Stereotype embodiment: a psychosocial approach to aging. Curr Dir Psychol Sci 2009;18:332–336.

7 Allen JO: Ageism as a risk factor for chronic disease. Gerontologist 2016;56:610–614.

8 Levy BR, Slade MD, Kunkel SR, Kasl SV: Longevity increased by positive self-perceptions of aging. J Pers Soc Psychol 2002;83:261–270.

9 High KP, Brennan-Ing M, Clifford DB, Cohen MH, Currier J, Deeks SG, Deren S, Effros RB, Gebo K, Goronzy JJ, Justice AC: HIV and aging: state of knowledge and areas of critical need for research. A report to the NIH Office of AIDS research by the HIV and aging working group. J Acquir Immune Defic Syndr 2012;60(suppl 1):S1–S18.

10 Negin J, Cumming RG: HIV infection in older adults in sub-Saharan Africa: extrapolating prevalence from existing data. Bull World Health Organ 2010; 88:847–853.

11 Seidel L, Karpiak SE, Brennan-Ing M: Training senior service providers about HIV and aging: evaluation of a multiyear, multicity initiative. Gerontol Geriatr Educ 2015:1–21.

12 Piot P, Abdool Karim SS, Hecht R, Legido-Quigley H, Buse K, Stover J, Resch S, et al; UNAIDS-Lancet Commission: Defeating AIDS – advancing global health. Lancet 2015;386:171–218.

13 Brennan-Ing M, Seidel L, London AS, Cahill S, Karpiak SE: Service utilization among older adults with HIV: the joint association of sexual identity and gender. J Homosex 2014;61:166–196.

14 UNAIDS: The Gap Report. Geneva, UNAIDS, 2014. http://www.unaids.org/sites/default/files/media_asset/UNAIDS_Gap_report_en.pdf.



Rosanna F. DeMarco, PhD, RN, PHCNS-BC, APHN-BC, FAAN
Department of Nursing, College of Nursing and Health Sciences
University Massachusetts Boston
100 Morrissey Boulevard, Boston, MA 02125-3393 (USA)
E-Mail rosanna.demarco@umb.edu

# Author Index


Alberts, L.H. 74
Appelbaum, J.S. 119
Aronowitz, T. 134
Avihingsanon, A. 119

Brennan-Ing, M. 159, 204, 234
Brown, S.M. 1, 234
Brown, T.T. 59

Cody, S.L. 173
Cossarizza, A. 28
Cox, L.E. 204
Czajkowski, S.E. 85

DeMarco, R.F. 222, 234
Dupuis, G. 28

Emlet, C.A. 144

Feldpausch, M.N. 47
Fitch, K.V. 47
Frost, E. 28
Fülöp, T. 28

Guaraldi, G. 59

Halkitis, P.N. 187
Havlik, R. 11
Herbein, G. 28

Karpiak, S.E. 11, 159
Krause, K.D. 187

Larbi, A. 28
Leveille, S.G. 101
Looby, S.E.D. 47

Moneyham, L. 173

Pantalone, D.W. 85
Pawelec, G. 28

Sangarlangkarn, A. 119
Seidel, L. 159
Shorthill, J. 222
Sprague, C. VII, 1, 234

Taylor, S.W. 85
Thapa, S. 101

Vance, D.E. 173
Vieira, D.L. 187

Witkowski, J.M. 28

# Subject Index


Accelerated aging, see Aging
ACTIVE, see Advanced Cognitive Training for Independent and Vital Elderly
ADAP, see AIDS Drug Assistance Program
Advanced Cognitive Training for Independent and Vital Elderly (ACTIVE) 178–180, 182
Africa, demographics of aging and HIV 2, 3, 7
Ageism
 health impact 235
 mitigation in HIV patients
  community engagement in social support 237, 238
  funding 237
  prevention, education, and outreach 236
  screening, early diagnosis, and antiretroviral therapy initiation 236
  special population needs 238
  treatment guidelines 237
 overview 234, 235
Aging
 accelerated aging process in HIV
  clinical reports 21, 22
  HIV effect isolation 15, 17, 18
  origin of hypothesis 12–14
  prospects for study 23–25
  testing of hypothesis 14–16, 22, 23
  typical aging versus aging with HIV 18
 biological processes in HIV infection 20
 epidemiology in HIV 59, 60, 137, 138, 204
 frailty and HIV 19, 20
 HIV infection as premature state of immunosenescence 38–40
 immune system effects 29–32
 inflammation in HIV infection
  aging effect on inflammation 33, 34
  HIV effect on inflammation 35–37
  overview 18
 markers, see specific markers
 service utilization, see Service utilization
AIDS Drug Assistance Program (ADAP) 214, 215
Antiretroviral therapy
 adherence challenges 75, 79–81
 multimorbidity role in HIV infection 64, 65
 prospects for study 81, 82
 reformulation of drugs 79, 80
 treatment guidelines 77, 78
Antiretroviral therapy
 initiation 236
 T cell effects in HIV 37
Antiretroviral therapy, disability in HIV and aging 104, 105
ATHENA cohort 61, 62, 173
Atripla 79

Balance impairment, disability in HIV and aging 111
Behavioral health
 factors affecting in HIV and aging 86–89
 prospects for study 96, 97
 treatment approach in HIV and aging 95, 96

C-reactive protein (CRP), inflammation marker in HIV infection 51
Cabotegravir 81
Cardiovascular disease (CVD), disability in HIV and aging 105, 106
China, demographics of aging and HIV 6, 7
Chronic pain, disability in HIV and aging 110, 111
CMV, see Cytomegalovirus
Cognitive impairment

cognitive training
combination approaches 183, 184
everyday function outcomes 182, 183
global cognitive training 181, 182
memory training 180, 181
overview 178
reasoning/executive training 180
speed of processing training 178–180
disability in HIV and aging 106, 109
HIV-associated neurocognitive disorder
classification 176, 177
mechanisms 175, 176
testing 176, 177, 182
neurocognitive reserve 174, 175
Comorbidity, see Multimorbidity
Complera 79
Condoms, use in older adults 136
CRP, see C-reactive protein
CVD, see Cardiovascular disease
Cytomegalovirus (CMV), immune system effects in aging 32

D-dimer, coagulopathy marker in HIV infection 52
Depression
disability in HIV and aging 110
epidemiology in older adults with HIV 190, 191
Diabetes, disability in HIV and aging 105
Disability, HIV and aging
balance and gait impairment 111
chronic pain 110, 111
contextual factors
extra-individual factors 114
intra-individual factors 114
predisposing factors 113
depression 110
fatigue 109, 110
hearing impairment 109
measures 112, 113
overview 101, 102
pathology
antiretroviral therapy 104, 105
cardiovascular disease 105, 106
cognitive impairment 106, 109
diabetes 105
HIV infection and comorbidity 103, 104
neuropathy 106, 107
renal disease 105
sarcopenia 107
skeletal disease 107
pathway modeling 102, 103
performance limitations 111, 112
prevention and management 114, 115
vision impairment 109

Europe, demographics of aging and HIV 4

Fatigue, disability in HIV and aging 109, 110
Frailty
HIV and aging 19, 20, 48, 66–68
multimorbidity in HIV infection 66

Gait impairment, disability in HIV and aging 111
Genvoya 79
Geriatric Resources for Assessment and Care of Elders (GRACE)
case example
baseline in-home comprehensive assessment 123, 124
data 123, 124
health status summary 124–126
interventions
initial 127, 128
long-term 128, 129
mid-range 128
multimorbidity management 127
overview 121–123
system-level application
comprehensive health services 129, 130
coordination and monitoring across care settings 131
integration of geriatric and HIV networks of services 130, 131
multidisciplinary team 129
patient-centered outcomes 130
GRACE, see Geriatric Resources for Assessment and Care of Elders

Hearing impairment, disability in HIV and aging 109
Hepatitis, rates in HIV infection 17, 63

IL-6, see Interleukin-6
Immune risk phenotype (IRP), aging 30
Inflammation, HIV infection and aging
aging effect on inflammation 33, 34
HIV effect on inflammation 35–37, 48, 49
markers 49–51
overview 18

Interleukin-6 (IL-6), inflammation marker in HIV infection 50, 51
IRP, see Immune risk phenotype

Macrophage, aging effects 30, 31
Memory training, see Cognitive impairment
Mental health, see also Depression; Stigma
comorbidity in older adults with HIV 191, 192
prospects for study 199, 200
psychosocial challenges in older adults with HIV 189, 190
resilience in older adults with HIV
conceptualization 194–196
contextualization 193, 194
modeling 197–199
overview 192, 193
service utilization, see Service utilization
status in HIV and aging 89–91
Middle East, demographics of aging and HIV 4, 5
Mortality, predictors in HIV infection 53–56
Multimorbidity
burden in HIV infection 60–62
consequences 66
disability, see Disability, HIV and aging
geriatric care 120, 121, 126, 127
pathways in HIV infection
antiretroviral therapy 64, 65
behavioral factors 65, 66
immune activation 63, 64
polypharmacy 68, 69, 76
recommendations for reduction 69

Natural killer (NK) cell, aging effects 31
Neurocognitive impairment, see Cognitive impairment
Neuropathy, disability in HIV and aging 106, 107
Neutrophil, aging effects 30
NK cell, see Natural killer cell

Opiates, adherence effects in HIV patients 81

PACE, see Programs for All Inclusive Care of the Elderly
Palliative care
communication with patients 229, 230
counseling 230
disparities 224–227
education and resources 230
goals
cross-sector collaboration 231, 232
equitable communities 232
health as shared value 231
integration of health services and systems 232
HIV treatment outcomes 227, 228
living with HIV 225, 226
multidisciplinary team approach 228, 229
overview 222–224
providers 226, 227
Polypharmacy
adherence challenges 75, 79–81
drug-drug interactions 78, 79
multimorbidity in HIV infection 68, 69, 76
overview 74, 75
prospects for study 81, 82
reformulation of drugs 79, 80
treatment guidelines 77, 78
PRISMA, see Program of Research to Integrate Services for the Maintenance of Autonomy
Program of Research to Integrate Services for the Maintenance of Autonomy (PRISMA) 122, 129–131
Programs for All Inclusive Care of the Elderly (PACE) 122, 129–131

Renal disease, disability in HIV and aging 105
Research on Older Adults with HIV (ROAH) 162, 163, 170
ROAH, see Research on Older Adults with HIV

Sarcopenia, disability in HIV and aging 107
SASP, see Senescence-associated secretory phenotype
sCD14, see Soluble CD14
sCD163, see Soluble CD163
SEAR, see South-East Asia Region
Senescence-associated secretory phenotype (SASP), aging effects 32
Service utilization
Andersen model 205, 206
Enabling factors in older adults with HIV 208–210
medical services 212–215
need factors in older adults with HIV 210, 211
overview 204, 205, 211, 212
predisposing factors in older adults with HIV 206–208

prospects for study 217, 218
social supportive services 215–217
Sexual activity
healthcare-related clinical issues 136, 137
HIV interventions
positive adults 139, 140
prevention 138, 139
HIV risks in older adults 140, 141
prospects for study 141
research methodology concerns in older adults 135, 136
Short physical performance battery (SPPB), HIV and aging studies 111
SIPA, see System of Integrated Care for Older Persons
Skeletal disease, disability in HIV and aging 107
SMART, see Strategies for Management of ART
Smoking, rates in HIV infection 17, 94
Social support
community engagement 237, 238
HIV in older adults
clinical implications 170, 171
psychosocial factors 161
Research on Older Adults with HIV study 162, 163, 170
social networks
characterization 161, 162
informal assistance 165–167
measures and data analysis 162–164, 170
psychosocial factors and stigma 168, 169
sufficiency perceptions 167, 168
types 161, 169, 170
older adults 160
overview 159, 160
service utilization, see Service utilization
Soluble CD14 (sCD14), immune activation marker in HIV infection 52, 53
Soluble CD163 (sCD163), immune activation marker in HIV infection 53
South-East Asia Region (SEAR), demographics of aging and HIV 5, 6
SPPB, see Short physical performance battery
Stigma
components 145, 146
conceptualization 145–147
HIV stigma
overview 144, 145
definition 147
historical perspective 147, 148
types and components 148, 149
impact on older adults
health outcomes 151
prevention and testing 149
management 151, 152
risk factors 152, 153
protective factors 153
interventions 154
clinical implications 155
service utilization impact 209
Strategies for Management of ART (SMART) 48–50
Stribild 79
Substance abuse, HIV and aging 91–95
Supportive services, see Social support; Service utilization
System of Integrated Care for Older Persons (SIPA) 122, 129, 131

T cell
aging effects 31, 32
antiretroviral treatment effects in HIV 37
HIV effects 34, 35
HIV infection as premature state of immunosenescence 38–40
T helper cell, aging effects 31
Telomere shortening, HIV infection and aging 20
TFV 79
TLRs, see Toll-like receptors
Toll-like receptors (TLRs), aging effects 33

VACS index, mortality prediction in HIV infection 54–56, 127, 128
Veterans Aging Cohort Study, see VACS index
Vision impairment, disability in HIV and aging 109